P9-CDL-598

Teen Health Series

Death and Dying
SOURCEBOOK

Second Edition

Health Reference Series

Second Edition

Death and Dying
SOURCEBOOK

Basic Consumer Health Information about
End-of-Life Care and Related Perspectives and Ethical
Issues, Including End-of-Life Symptoms and Treatments,
Pain Management, Quality-of-Life Concerns, the Use of
Life Support, Patients' Rights and Privacy Issues,
Advance Directives, Physician-Assisted Suicide,
Caregiving, Organ and Tissue Donation, Autopsies,
Funeral Arrangements, and Grief

Along with Statistical Data, Information about the
Leading Causes of Death, a Glossary, and Directories
of Support Groups and Other Resources

Edited by
Joyce Brennfleck Shannon

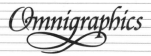

615 Griswold Street • Detroit, MI 48226

Bibliographic Note

Because this page cannot legibly accommodate all the copyright notices, the Bibliographic Note portion of the Preface constitutes an extension of the copyright notice.

Edited by Joyce Brennfleck Shannon

Health Reference Series

Karen Bellenir, *Managing Editor*
David A. Cooke, M.D., *Medical Consultant*
Elizabeth Barbour, *Research and Permissions Coordinator*
Cherry Stockdale, *Permissions Assistant*
Laura Pleva Nielsen, *Index Editor*
EdIndex, Services for Publishers, *Indexers*

* * *

Omnigraphics, Inc.

Matthew P. Barbour, *Senior Vice President*
Kay Gill, *Vice President—Directories*
Kevin Hayes, *Operations Manager*
David P. Bianco, *Marketing Director*

* * *

Peter E. Ruffner, *Publisher*
Frederick G. Ruffner, Jr., *Chairman*

Copyright © 2006 Omnigraphics, Inc.
ISBN 0-7808-0871-1

Library of Congress Cataloging-in-Publication Data

Death and dying sourcebook : basic consumer health information about end-of-life care and related perspectives and ethical issues, including end-of-life symptoms and treatments, pain management, quality-of-life concerns, the use of life support, patients' rights and privacy issues, advance directives, physician-assisted suicide, caregiving, organ, and tissue donation, autopsies, funeral arrangements, and grief; along with statistical data, information about the leading causes of death, a glossary, and directories of support groups and other resources / edited by Joyce Brennfleck Shannon. -- 2nd ed.
  p. cm. -- (Health reference series)
  Summary: "Provides basic consumer health information about end-of-life and related issues. Includes index, glossary of related terms, and other resources"-- Provided by publisher.
  Includes bibliographical references and index.
  ISBN 0-7808-0871-1 (hardcover : alk. paper)
  1. Death. 2. Terminal care.   I. Shannon, Joyce Brennfleck.
II. Series: Health reference series (Unnumbered)
  R726.8.D3785 2006
  362.1'75--dc22
2006015325

The information in this publication was compiled from the sources cited and from other sources considered reliable. While every possible effort has been made to ensure reliability, the publisher will not assume liability for damages caused by inaccuracies in the data, and makes no warranty, express or implied, on the accuracy of the information contained herein.

This book is printed on acid-free paper meeting the ANSI Z39.48 Standard. The infinity symbol that appears above indicates that the paper in this book meets that standard.

Printed in the United States

Table of Contents

Visit www.healthreferenceseries.com to view *A Contents Guide to the Health Reference Series*, a listing of more than 12,000 topics and the volumes in which they are covered.

Part III: Medical Decisions Surrounding the End of Life

Part IV: End-of-Life Care Facilities

Part V: End-of-Life Caregiving

Part VI: Death and Children: Information for Parents

Part VII: Legal and Economic Issues at the End of Life

Part VIII: Final Arrangements

Part IX: Mortality Statistics

Part X: Additional Help and Information

Preface

About This Book

Although people are living healthier and longer lives, more than two million Americans die annually. Some die suddenly; others pass away after long-term struggles with chronic disabilities or disease. Considering the dying process in advance allows people to talk about their choices concerning end-of-life medical preferences. Discussing these topics can be difficult, but appropriate planning allows people to remain in charge of their health care even after they are no longer able to make decisions. Additionally, knowledge about loved ones' wishes can help friends and families cope with the shock and grief of death.

Death and Dying Sourcebook, Second Edition provides information about end-of-life perspectives and the medical management of symptoms that can occur as death draws near. It discusses palliative care and describes issues surrounding life support choices, the termination of life-sustaining treatment, and the donation process for organs and tissues. A special section addresses caregiver concerns and another provides information about children and death. Facts about legal and economic issues at the end of life, funerals and other final arrangements, and grief are also included, along with statistical data, a glossary, and directories of support groups and other resources.

How to Use This Book

This book is divided into parts and chapters. Parts focus on broad areas of interest. Chapters are devoted to single topics within a part.

Part I: End-of-Life Perspectives begins with a dying person's advice concerning health care and the decision-making process. Cultural and spiritual concerns that impact end-of-life decisions are also discussed, and research findings about end-of-life care are described.

Part II: Medical Management of End-of-Life Symptoms explains treatments for pain, fatigue, and other symptoms during palliative care. It describes artificial hydration and nutrition, wound care, and cognitive disorders common at the end of life. Specific information for cancer and dementia patients is also included.

Part III: Medical Decisions Surrounding the End of Life presents facts about life support choices, termination of treatments, organ and tissue donation, physician-assisted suicide, and autopsies. It also provides specific information for commonly experienced end-of-life issues related to Alzheimer disease, advanced cancer, and HIV/AIDS.

Part IV: End-of-Life Care Facilities offers guidelines for evaluating care facilities and selecting options based on the needs of patients and caregivers. Hospice care, long-term care, home care, and other alternatives are described.

Part V: End-of-Life Caregiving has practical information for caregivers about coordinating communications among patients, families, and healthcare and support service providers. Topics include how to help at the end of life, the dying process, what to do when death occurs, and self-care tips for caregivers.

Part VI: Death and Children: Information for Parents provides advice about caring for terminally ill children and grieving the death of a child. Guidance for helping children cope with death, funerals, and grief is also presented.

Part VII: Legal and Economic Issues at End of Life presents guidelines for advance directives, powers of attorney for healthcare, living wills, financial assistance, taxes, and social security issues. It also describes patients' legal rights, the Family and Medical Leave Act (FMLA), and the duties of an executor.

Part VIII: Final Arrangements offers practical information about types of burials and expenses, planning funerals or memorial services, certification of death, and how to facilitate arrangements if death occurs while traveling. Chapters on grief which address bereavement, how to help grieving people, and tips for working through grief are also included.

Part IX: Mortality Statistics includes global and national mortality trends along with information about the leading causes of death in the United States, life expectancy at birth, and common causes of fatalities. Disparities in deaths from stroke and use of health care resources at the end of life are also discussed.

Part X: Additional Help and Information includes a glossary of end-of-life terms, a directory of support groups for end-of-life concerns, and a directory of organizations able to provide more information about death and dying.

Bibliographic Note

This volume contains documents and excerpts from publications issued by the following U.S. government agencies: Administration on Aging (AoA); Agency for Healthcare Research and Quality (AHRQ); Centers for Disease Control and Prevention (CDC); Centers for Medicare and Medicaid Services; Federal Trade Commission (FTC); National Cancer Institute (NCI); National Heart, Lung, and Blood Institute (NHLBI); National Institute on Aging (NIA); National Institute of Child Health and Human Development (NICHD); National Institutes of Health (NIH); National Women's Health Information Center (NWHIC); NIH Clinical Center; Office of Minority Health (OMH); Social Security Administration (SSA); Substance Abuse and Mental Health Services Administration (SAMHSA); U.S. Department of Health and Human Services (HHS); U.S. Department of Labor (DOL); and the U.S. Department of State (DOS).

In addition, this volume contains copyrighted documents from the following organizations: American Academy of Family Physicians (AAFP); American Association for Respiratory Care; American College of Physicians (ACP); American Geriatrics Society Foundation for Health in Aging; American Health Care Association; American Hospice Foundation; American Public Health Association; American Society of Clinical Oncology; Bereaved Parents of the USA; Beth Israel Medical Center; Children's Hospice International; First Candle/SIDS Alliance; Family Caregiver Alliance; Funeral Consumers Alliance; Hospice Association of America; Indiana Association for Home and Hospice Care; Joint Commission on Accreditation of Healthcare Organizations (JCAHO); Mountain Valley Hospice; National Family Caregivers Association; National

Hospice and Palliative Care Organization; National SHARE Office; RAND Corporation; Safe Kids USA; Sage Publications, Inc.; Society of Critical Care Medicine; United Services Automobile Association Educational Foundation; University of Hawaii at Manoa; University of Washington School of Medicine; and the World Health Organization (WHO).

Full citation information is provided on the first page of each chapter. Every effort has been made to secure all necessary rights to reprint the copyrighted material. If any omissions have been made, please contact Omnigraphics to make corrections for future editions.

Acknowledgements

In addition to the listed organizations, agencies, and individuals who have contributed to this *Sourcebook*, special thanks go to managing editor Karen Bellenir, research and permissions coordinator Liz Barbour, and document engineer Bruce Bellenir for their help and support.

About the Health Reference Series

The *Health Reference Series* is designed to provide basic medical information for patients, families, caregivers, and the general public. Each volume takes a particular topic and provides comprehensive coverage. This is especially important for people who may be dealing with a newly diagnosed disease or a chronic disorder in themselves or in a family member. People looking for preventive guidance, information about disease warning signs, medical statistics, and risk factors for health problems will also find answers to their questions in the *Health Reference Series*. The *Series*, however, is not intended to serve as a tool for diagnosing illness, in prescribing treatments, or as a substitute for the physician/patient relationship. All people concerned about medical symptoms or the possibility of disease are encouraged to seek professional care from an appropriate health care provider.

Locating Information within the Health Reference Series

The *Health Reference Series* contains a wealth of information about a wide variety of medical topics. Ensuring easy access to all the fact sheets, research reports, in-depth discussions, and other material contained within the individual books of the *Series* remains one of our highest priorities. As the *Series* continues to grow in size and scope, however, locating the precise information needed by a reader may become more challenging.

A Contents Guide to the Health Reference Series was developed to direct readers to the specific volumes that address their concerns. It presents an extensive list of diseases, treatments, and other topics of general interest compiled from the Tables of Contents and major index headings. To access *A Contents Guide to the Health Reference Series*, visit www.healthreferenceseries.com.

Medical Consultant

Medical consultation services are provided to the *Health Reference Series* editors by David A. Cooke, M.D. Dr. Cooke is a graduate of Brandeis University, and he received his M.D. degree from the University of Michigan. He completed residency training at the University of Wisconsin Hospital and Clinics. He is board-certified in Internal Medicine. Dr. Cooke currently works as part of the University of Michigan Health System and practices in Brighton, MI. In his free time, he enjoys writing, science fiction, and spending time with his family.

Our Advisory Board

We would like to thank the following board members for providing guidance to the development of this *Series*:

- Dr. Lynda Baker,
  Associate Professor of Library and Information Science,
  Wayne State University, Detroit, MI

- Nancy Bulgarelli,
  William Beaumont Hospital Library, Royal Oak, MI

- Karen Imarisio,
  Bloomfield Township Public Library, Bloomfield Township, MI

- Karen Morgan,
  Mardigian Library, University of Michigan-Dearborn,
  Dearborn, MI

- Rosemary Orlando,
  St. Clair Shores Public Library, St. Clair Shores, MI

Health Reference Series *Update Policy*

The inaugural book in the *Health Reference Series* was the first edition of *Cancer Sourcebook* published in 1989. Since then, the *Series* has been enthusiastically received by librarians and in the medical community. In order to maintain the standard of providing high-quality health information for the layperson the editorial staff at Omnigraphics felt it was necessary to implement a policy of updating volumes when warranted.

Medical researchers have been making tremendous strides, and it is the purpose of the *Health Reference Series* to stay current with the most recent advances. Each decision to update a volume is made on an individual basis. Some of the considerations include how much new information is available and the feedback we receive from people who use the books. If there is a topic you would like to see added to the update list, or an area of medical concern you feel has not been adequately addressed, please write to:

Editor
Health Reference Series
Omnigraphics, Inc.
615 Griswold Street
Detroit, MI 48226
E-mail: editorial@omnigraphics.com

Part One

End-of-Life Perspectives

Chapter 1

A Dying Person's Guide to Dying

Guidelines from Roger C. Bone, M.D., A Dying Person

Planning near the end of life is helpful. By thinking ahead about what could happen, and about how you will deal with problems if they do happen, you can create a better life and a better quality of life for yourself and for the people who love and care about you. What I have to say is for the person who, like me, is dying. We, too, need to plan, to think ahead, in order to fashion out of the time remaining, the best of what is possible.

As I am dying from cancer, I have learned some things that I think are important for a dying person to know in order to plan. I am a physician, but what I have learned has little to do with my medical training. I have learned this as a person; perhaps my medical experience was helpful because I have paid close attention to the actions and reactions of people around me.

First, it is likely that you will be surrounded by persons who mean well, but in the end you must die your own death. Dying can be considered a journey one takes alone with a crowd. Family and friends are the first to gather around you, and they offer the most comfort.

Here are some pieces of advice to remember in those first few days after you learn the bad news.

Reprinted with permission from *ACP Home Care Guide to Advanced Cancer*, © 1997 American College of Physicians. All rights reserved. Reviewed in December 2005 by Dr. David A. Cooke, M.D., Diplomate, American Board of Internal Medicine.

1. One or two people—probably family members—will make enormous personal sacrifices to help you. If you are married, your spouse is likely to do this, but don't be surprised if others—a daughter, a brother-in-law, or even a friend, step forward to offer extraordinary help. Be grateful and graciously accept help from whatever source.

2. Some family members, but especially friends, will treat you differently. Even before you show signs of serious illness, people will have a different look in their eyes as they talk with you. You might consider this patronizing or overbearing. It may be difficult, but it is best to ignore their attitudes and treat them as you always have. They will come around to their normal selves when they get over the shock.

3. Happily accept all gifts from family and friends. It makes them feel better and you might receive something you really like and appreciate.

4. Don't be afraid to ask to be alone. We need time to be by ourselves. Some family and friends may feel driven to fill your every waking moment with activities; perhaps they are trying to take your mind off your impending death, but they may also be doing the same thing for themselves.

5. Be your own counsel. No one, including your physician, religious counselor, spouse, or friends can understand 100% what you want and need. It surprised me that some people seemed to bully me with advice when they learned that I was terminally ill. Remember Immanuel Kant's advice to avoid accepting someone else's authority in place of our own powers of reason. We are the ones who should be considering alternatives and making choices. We can and should ask for advice, make telephone calls, and read books, but ultimately we should make our own decisions.

6. Slow down and ask your family and friends to slow down. There may not be a lot of time, but there is sufficient time in all but the most extreme cases to think, plan, and prepare.

There are things you need to know from your doctors and other health care staff. You need not ask all of the following questions or ask them in this order. Still, these questions deal with crucial issues that need to be addressed and, hopefully, resolved.

Questions to Ask

What is my disease?

You should find out as much as possible about your disease. What it is it? How will it affect you? And very importantly, how will it cause your death? First, ask your physician. Additionally, many popular books are available in bookstores and libraries which can give you a basic sense of your disease process and disease terminology. National organizations, such as the American Cancer Society, and, often, local hospitals can provide brochures, video tapes, or even lay experts to help you and your family understand your particular disease. Ignorance is not bliss; the more you and your family know, the better able everyone will be able to cope with what is happening.

Should I seek a second opinion about my disease and my condition?

Seek a second opinion. A second opinion will relieve your mind and resolve doubts one way or another that a major mistake has not been made. More importantly, a second opinion will offer a slightly different perspective that may help everyone to understand it. Don't be embarrassed about asking for a second opinion or think that you will make your physician angry. Second opinions are perfectly acceptable, and many physicians are happy when their patients seek second opinions. The original diagnosis is usually confirmed, and you are then more prepared to follow prescribed treatments.

What health professional do I especially trust?

Search for and then put your trust in a single individual. This does not mean you should not listen to all health professionals and follow reasonable directions and advice. But focus on one individual as the final helper. This normally will be the specialist physician in charge of your case. However, you may know your family doctor better than you know your specialist. If this is the case, your family doctor may be the one to choose. But, if you do, make certain that your family doctor knows that he or she is serving that role.

Why am I going into the hospital?

There are four basic reasons why a terminally ill person would be hospitalized, but not all four necessarily apply to every patient. They are:

- to confirm the diagnosis and analyze how far the disease has progressed;

- to provide treatment that can only be given in the hospital;

- to treat a severe worsening of the disease; and

- to treat the final phases of the disease, if this cannot be done at home or with hospice.

You should know which applies to you so that you can understand why things are done to you and what benefits you might expect.

What are the hospital rules about terminally ill patients?

Hospitals and medical centers have written rules and procedures that outline in detail how the hospital will deal with terminally ill patients. These are not treatment rules. These protocols, or guidelines, deal with how to handle end-of-life issues, such as whether the patient (or the patient's family speaking for the patient) wishes extraordinary, heroic measures to be used to keep the patient alive. Hospitals are obligated, and very willing, to share these protocols or guidelines with patients and families. Consider getting a durable power of attorney in which you name one or two people to make decisions or choices on your behalf if you should be incompetent or incapable of making decisions yourself. Read the "Do Not Resuscitate" policies of the hospital. Death should be peaceful, and you should not ask for anything that gives you prolonged agony.

You should be aware that nurses and other hospital staff may not know that you are terminally ill. This fact may not be written in your chart, which can lead to conflicts between families and hospital staff. The family may assume that everyone in the hospital shares their grief, and will not understand the work-a-day attitude of nurses, dietitians, or others. It is okay for the family to tell the hospital staff that you are dying since they may not know.

What resources are available from the health care community?

Most hospitals have many services available to patients and families to help with nonmedical aspects of your care. These include social services and psychological, financial, and religious counseling. For example, a visit before hospitalization to the hospital financial counselor by a family member to check on insurance and payment plans is a wise move. In the rush to admit a patient, important information may not get recorded. A fifteen minute meeting with counselors can avoid stress and anger over incorrect bills. Similarly, meeting with the hospital social worker may be very helpful in arranging home care. Use these services.

What can I do if it seems that nothing is being done or if I don't understand why certain things are done to me?

Hospitals, clinics, and doctors' offices can be confusing places. You can begin to feel you have no control over what is being done to you, and you may wonder if anyone really understands your case. This is the time to call the health professional that is your primary contact—the one you decided you fully trust—your physician specialist or family physician. Ask this person to explain what is going on. Have him or her paged or even called at home if your situation is very upsetting. It is the physician's responsibility to help you, and he or she will not be angry that you called.

How will I and my family pay for my treatment?

Financial professionals employed by hospitals understand billing and what may or may not be covered by Medicare, Medicaid, or private insurance. Consult them and be sure to ask every question to which you and your family need an answer. It is important that you and your family do not panic over billing. Ask for advice and help. Sometimes the hardest part about dying is the effect it has on your family and friends. Helping them deal with your death helps you find peace and comfort. If you are not at peace with your death, ask the health professional you especially trust to help you find peace. That person will help or will get whatever help is needed. After all, it is the goal of all health professionals, to give you comfort and health during life and peace to you and your family at death.

Chapter 2

Culture and the Dying Process

What Is Culture?

Culture refers to learned patterns of behaviors, beliefs, and values shared by individuals in a particular social group. It provides human beings with both their identity and a framework for understanding experience. When culture is referred to, it usually brings to mind a group of people with similar ethnic background, language, religion, family values, and life views.

Culture and nationality, however, are not synonymous. The United States (U.S.), for example, is a country made up of individuals from many countries and traditions, each with a unique culture. For many years, this country was viewed as the great melting pot of the world; however, this vision is being rejected. The truth is that the U.S. is a multicultural, or pluralistic society, including members of different ethnic, racial, religious, or social groups living side by side and sharing aspects of the dominant U.S. culture, but maintaining their own values and traditions.

Since culture provides individuals with a framework for understanding experience, it is of great importance to consider culture in the medical setting. Each cultural group has its own views about health, illness, and health care practices. Cultural views affect how individuals respond to illnesses and their symptoms including pain; identify and select medical care; and comply with prescribed care.

Excerpts from *A Clinical Guide to Supportive and Palliative Care for HIV/AIDS, 2003 Edition*, U.S. Department of Health and Human Services (HHS).

9

Hispanic Cultural Values and Disease

The first point that must be considered when referring to Hispanics is that the term is a label of convenience for a cultural group with a common cultural heritage stemming from Spain's colonization of the Americas. Hispanics can be of any racial group (for example, indigenous American, Negroid, Asian, Caucasian, or of multiple racial ancestry). Hispanics include several subgroups, each with important social and cultural differences. The major Hispanic subgroups in the United States traditionally have been Mexican Americans, Puerto Ricans, and Cubans. However, the dramatic increase in Hispanics observed in the 2000 census was fueled primarily by immigration from Central and South America.

There are some differences among Hispanic subgroups, related to country of origin, that country's racial/ethnic makeup, different histories of immigration to this country, or as in the case of Puerto Rico, the population's experience with colonization. However, these subgroups share a common language, religion, traditional family structure, and several common Hispanic values.

In addition to differences in subgroups, Hispanics in the U.S. also differ in terms of their level of acculturation or assimilation into mainstream culture. Language use is one very good example of these differences. For instance, while many Hispanics in the United States are bilingual, the degree to which they speak either Spanish or English varies considerably.

One value shared by most Hispanics is their religion. Although individuals' degree of practice and church participation varies, the majority of Hispanics are Christian, predominantly Roman Catholic. However, many Hispanics practice other religious beliefs that they have incorporated into their Christianity, such as forms of ancestor worship with rituals dating back to pre-Columbian times in Central American Indians. Many Caribbean Hispanics practice Santería, a syncretism of Catholicism and the Yoruba religion brought to Cuba by African slaves. Hispanic religious/spiritual beliefs include views on dying and death. For example, it is common to hold a continued vigil over an older family member with a terminal illness. After death, it is common practice to offer daily masses or light candles in honor of the deceased. These and other practices honor the loved one and form part of the bereavement ritual.

Family plays a very strong role for most Hispanics, with ties that exist within an extended network of uncles, aunts, cousins, grandparents, and family friends. Included in the important role the family plays is the concept of *familismo*, emphasis of the family welfare over that of the individual.

In addition to language, religion, and family, there are five more cultural themes that influence Hispanic culture.

- *Personalismo*: Trust building over time based on the display of mutual respect.

- *Jerarquismo*: Respect for hierarchy.

- *Presentismo*: Emphasis on the present, not the past or the future.

- *Espiritismo*: Belief in good and evil spirits that can affect health and well-being.

- *Fatalismo*: The belief that fate determines life outcomes, including health, and that fate is basically unbeatable.

Hispanic Values, Beliefs, and Practices Influence End-of-Life Care Preferences

Patient Autonomy

In a study in Los Angeles comparing Mexican, Korean, African, and European Americans on several issues relating to patient autonomy, researchers found that Mexican and Korean Americans were less likely to believe that a patient should be told about a terminal diagnosis or make decisions about using life support. Instead, the researchers found that Mexican and Korean American elders were more likely than African and European American elders to want family members to make these decisions. This study also found differences among Mexican Americans by income, degree of acculturation, and age; that is, younger and more acculturated respondents and those with higher incomes were more likely to favor truth-telling about the diagnosis.[1]

Advance Directives

The Los Angeles study on patient autonomy among Mexican, Korean, African, and European Americans also compared knowledge on completion of advance directives. They found that while Mexican and European Americans were significantly more knowledgeable than Korean and African Americans on advance directives, only 22% of the Mexican Americans actually possessed advance directives, in comparison to 40% of the European Americans. They also found that the Mexican Americans who had advance directives were more highly acculturated than the ones who did not. Three years earlier, at the University of Miami in Florida, Caralis, Davis, Wright, and Marcial had conducted a multicultural study examining the influence of ethnicity on attitudes toward advance directives, life-prolonging treatments, and euthanasia. Regarding advance directives, the researchers found that Hispanic Americans, the majority being of Cuban heritage, were less knowledgeable than African and non-Hispanic white Americans regarding living wills.[2]

Life-Prolonging Treatments

When it came to the issue of life-prolonging treatments at the end of life, Caralis and others found that Hispanic and African Americans were more likely than non-Hispanic whites to report wanting their doctors to keep them alive regardless of how ill they were (42% and 37% vs. 14%, respectively). Furthermore, only 59% of Hispanics and 63% of African Americans agreed to stop life-prolonging treatment, compared to 89% of non-Hispanic whites. This disparity may have been due partly to the Bible commandment, "Thou shalt not kill." A religious Christian might interpret withdrawing or withholding treatment as an infraction of this commandment.

Hospice

A few studies have suggested that Hispanics are low users of hospice services. This may be due to unfamiliarity with hospice, insurance coverage issues, language barriers, unpleasant experiences with or distrust of the health care system. In addition, Wallace and Lew-Ting proposed that the low utilization of hospice among Hispanics may be due to physician referral patterns—a physician might not refer Hispanic patients to hospice because they observe families providing care themselves and believe that hospice might be unnecessary or culturally inappropriate.[3]

African American Culture

In 2000, the population of the U.S. was approximately 281 million, of which 35 million were African Americans. They are the largest minority group in the U.S. While the term African American refers to a racial group, like Hispanics, they are heterogeneous and are comprised of several subgroups. Most African Americans are the descendants of slaves and were part of the U.S. population even before this country's independence from England. Some are immigrants from other places in the Americas, particularly the West Indies. More recently, there has been an influx of immigrants from the African continent. To one degree or another, African Americans share a legacy of slavery, segregation, and discrimination, and like most minorities, they experience a high degree of unemployment and overall poverty.

These challenges are reflected in a lower life expectancy and higher death rate for African Americans. In a 1996 CDC report, the 1993 age-adjusted death rates for African Americans were higher than those for the Caucasian population for all causes of death combined and for eight of the ten leading causes of death. Life expectancy for African American males was 8.5 years less than that for Caucasian males; this difference is attributed to higher death rates for homicide, heart disease, cancer, human immunodeficiency virus/acquired immune deficiency syndrome (HIV/AIDS), and perinatal conditions. The life expectancy for African American females was 5.8 years less than that for Caucasian females for similar conditions.

African American Core Values

Despite a long history of adversity, African Americans have remained strongly bound together by the importance they place on family, which they view as an extended network of kin and community, and a series of core values described by Sudarkasa as the *Seven Rs*:[4]

- Respect: The respect of others from parents and relatives to elders or leaders in the community.

- Responsibility: Being accountable for self and for those less fortunate in one's own extended family and even one's community.

- Reciprocity: Giving back to family and community in return for what has been given to one (mutual assistance).

- Restraint: Giving due consideration to the family or community/group when making decisions.

- Reverence: Deep awe and respect firstly toward God, toward ancestors, and toward many things in nature.

- Reason: Taking a reasoned approach to settling disputes within the family or the community.

- Reconciliation: The art of settling differences; that is, putting a matter to rest between two parties.

The Role of Religion

Religion is another core value among African Americans, just as it is among Hispanics. Historically, the church has been the center of the African American community serving as the single most important institution advocating improvements in health, education, and financial welfare.

While the majority of African Americans are Protestant Christians, a large proportion being Baptist, some are Roman Catholic. Certain African American subgroups, however, such as those from Haiti, have beliefs in voodoo, hexes, and curses which will also have a direct effect on health care views and practices. The history of deportation from the African continent, slavery, and oppression in the new world coupled with their Christian heritage has determined how African Americans view end-of-life decisions. Many believe in the God of the Old Testament, an all-powerful and fighting God, who liberated the Hebrews from the oppression of the Egyptians, and who liberated African Americans from slavery. From this comes the notion of divine rescue and thus the belief that God's power can conquer all, and that miraculous interventions can occur when all hope seems lost. The notion of divine intervention and rescue might influence patients to oppose continuing aggressive medical treatment, in order to allow "God's will" to be done.

African American Experiences Influence End-of-Life Care Preferences

Research findings indicate that African Americans are less likely than other groups to trust health care providers, communicate treatment preferences, complete advance directives, and withhold or withdraw life-prolonging treatments in the face of futility.

Issues of Trust

The long history of past and even current discrimination has led African Americans to display distrust in the institutions established by the dominant Caucasian society, including those institutions that provide health care. This institutional distrust is not without foundation, as there are several studies which document minorities' lack of access to available health care. Studies have suggested that certain procedures such as coronary bypass operations and organ transplants have been performed less frequently on African Americans than on Caucasian Americans. A study documented lower survival rates in African Americans with Stage I lung cancer, the second most common cause of death among African Americans, and suggested that this was in part due to lower referral rates for African Americans for potentially curative surgical procedures as compared to Caucasian Americans.[5, 6]

Some authors have suggested that these differences are due to discriminatory practices that have led African Americans not to trust Caucasians or their social institutions. The 40-year-old Tuskegee Syphilis Study, in which the U.S. Public Health Service lied to and denied standard treatment to 400 poor African American sharecroppers, is a reminder of why African Americans feel they cannot trust the health care system. In fact, one recent study of 520 African American males sampled door-to-door showed that 27% believed that HIV/AIDS was a government conspiracy against black people.

Discriminatory practices also extend to pain management. In studies in various medical settings, such as emergency rooms[8, 9] and cancer centers,[10, 11] pain severity was more likely to be underestimated and effective analgesia less likely to be prescribed for African Americans and Hispanics than for Caucasian Americans. These and other studies clearly document a racial bias on the part of medical care providers. Thus the distrust demonstrated by African Americans is warranted, as subtle discrimination continues. In addition, the studies document that the medical care received by minorities is less than optimal, which has led to African American distrust of health care institutions and has affected how African Americans view end-of-life care.

Communication of Treatment Preferences

The same distrust appears to have inhibited many African Americans from effectively communicating end-of-life decisions. In a study of communication of treatment preferences among 1,031 AIDS patients, researchers found that Caucasian patients were twice as likely as African American patients to have discussed their treatment preferences with their physicians. Perhaps not coincidentally, the study also found that African Americans were half as likely as Caucasians to prefer a treatment approach that focused on pain relief as opposed to extending life.[12] Suspicion about proposed palliative treatments may deter African American patients from honest, open communication with health care providers. Without adequate communication, the patient and family inadvertently give the decision-making power to the health care provider, which becomes a form of paternalism by permission and decreases patient autonomy.

Advance Directives

A retrospective chart review of 1,193 frail elderly in South Carolina found that African Americans were less likely than Caucasians or Hispanics to have completed advance directives, while in another study African Americans were less likely than Caucasians or Asians to complete durable power of attorney for health care.[13] While reasons for this are several, lack of access to medical care in general is of primary importance. If an advance directive to withhold life-prolonging therapies is seen by African Americans as yet another way of limiting their access to adequate health care, then they might be more inclined not to complete one.

Along with the decreased use of advance directives among African Americans is a low use of hospice services when compared to Caucasians. This is partially due to lack of access to and lack of education regarding hospice care.

Life-Prolonging Treatment

In an article concerning the implementation of the Patient Self-Determination Act of 1991, Young and Jex pointed out that African Americans tend to equate life-support with life, and view the withholding of any life-sustaining therapies as another attempt at genocide by the system. Therefore, African Americans might be reluctant to consider palliative care as a treatment option for fear that it might result in neglect or being allowed to die prematurely.

In a study comparing attitudes toward life-prolonging treatments among 139 patients at a general medicine clinic, only 63% of African Americans approved of stopping life-prolonging treatments, compared to 89% of Caucasians. Furthermore, 35% of Caucasians approved of physician-assisted suicide, compared with only 16% of African Americans.[2] Finally, Caralis and others, in their 1993 study found that African Americans were more likely than the general population to choose life-prolonging treatments, even in the face of a poor outcome.[2]

Conclusion

While health care providers cannot become familiar with every cultural issue related to medicine, they can become more sensitive to the role that culture plays in how people access and experience palliative care services. Recognizing the role of culture and being familiar with the core values of a cultural group will not only aid in eliminating barriers to treatment, but also optimize patient care, particularly end-of-life care.

References

1. Blackhall LJ, Murphy DT, Frank G, Michel V, Azen S. Ethnicity and attitudes toward patient autonomy. *JAMA* 10:820–5, 1995.

2. Caralis PV, Davis B, Wright K, Marcial E. The influence of ethnicity and race on attitudes toward advance directives, life-prolonging treatments, and euthanasia. *J Clinl Ethics* 4:155–65, 1993.

3. Wallace SP, Lew-Ting C. Getting by at home: community-based long-term care of Latino elders. *West J Med* 157:337–44, 1992

4. Sudarkasa N. African and Afro-American family structure. In Colle JB, ed. *Anthropology for the Nineties*. New York: Collier Macmillan, 1988.

5. Bach PB, Cramer LD, Warren JL, Begg CB. Racial differences in the treatment of early-stage lung cancer. *N Engl J Med* 341:1198–205, 1999.

6. Greenwald HP, Polissar NL, Borgatta EF, McCorkle R, Goodman G. Social factors, treatment, and survival in early-stage non-small cell lung cancer. *Am J Pub Health* 88:1681–4, 1998.

7. Klonoff EC, Landrine H. Do blacks believe that HIV/AIDS is a government conspiracy against them? *Prev Med* 28:451–7, 1999.

8. Todd KH. Pain assessment and ethnicity. *Ann Emerg Med* 27:421–3, 1996.

9. Todd KH, Samaroo N, Hoffman JR. Ethnicity as a risk factor for inadequate emergency department analgesia. *JAMA* 269:1537–9, 1993.

10. Anderson KO, Mendoza TR, Valero V, et al. Minority cancer patients and their providers: pain management attitudes and practice. *Cancer* 88:1929–38, 2000.

11. Cleeland CS, Gonin R, Baez L, Loehrer P, Pandya KJ. Pain and treatment of pain in minority patients with cancer. The

Eastern Cooperative Oncology Group Minority Outpatient Pain Study. *Ann Intern Med* 127:813–6, 1997.

12. Mouton CP, Teno J, Mor V, Pette J. Communication of preferences for care among human immunodeficiency virus-infected patients: barriers to informed decisions? *Arch Fam Med* 6:342–7, 1997.

13. Rubin SM, Strull WM, Fialkow MF, Weiss SJ, Lo B. Increasing the completion of the durable power of attorney for health care: a randomized controlled trial. *JAMA* 271:209–11, 1973.

Chapter 3

Spirituality in End-of-Life Care

Spiritual Care

Illness is a major life event that can cause people to question themselves, their purpose, and their meaning in life. It disrupts their careers, their family life, and their ability to enjoy themselves—three aspects of life that Freud said were essential to a healthy mind.

Palliative care has long recognized that in addition to physical and psychological symptoms patients with advanced illness will suffer existential distress as well. Existential distress is probably the least understood source of suffering in patients with advanced disease for it deals with questions regarding the meaning of life, the fear of death, and the realization that they will be separated from their loved ones.

A number of surveys and studies demonstrate the importance of considering spirituality in the health care of patients and document the relationship between patients' religious and spiritual lives and their experiences of illness and disease. These findings are particularly relevant in the delivery of palliative care. From the very early years of the modern hospice movement, spiritual aspects of health, illness, and suffering have been emphasized as core aspects of care.

This chapter includes excerpts from "Spiritual Care," Chapter 13 in *A Clinical Guide to Supportive and Palliative Care for HIV/AIDS, 2003 Edition,* Health Resources and Services Administration, U. S. Department of Health and Human Services (HHS); and excerpts from PDQ® Cancer Information Summary: "Spirituality in Cancer Care (PDQ®): Supportive Care–Patient," National Cancer Institute; Bethesda, MD, updated January 2006, available at http://cancer.gov. Accessed March 1, 2006.

A 1997 Gallup survey showed that people overwhelmingly want their spiritual needs addressed when they are close to death. Other studies have found spirituality to be an important factor in coping with pain, in dying, and in bereavement. For example, patients with advanced cancer who found comfort from their spiritual beliefs were more satisfied with their lives, were happier, and had diminished pain compared with those without spiritual beliefs. An American Pain Society survey found that prayer was the second most common method of pain management after oral pain medications, and the most common non-drug method of pain management.

Quality-of-life instruments used in end-of-life care measures often include an existential domain which measures purpose, meaning in life, and capacity for self-transcendence. Three items were found to correlate with good quality of life for patients with advanced disease:

- if the patient's personal existence is meaningful
- if the patient finds fulfillment in achieving life goals
- if life to this point has been meaningful

Spiritual Care

It is important to include a spiritual assessment or history as part of the overall clinical assessment of a patient. Doing so enables the provider to assess spiritual needs and resources, mobilize appropriate spiritual care, and enhance overall caregiving. Spiritual assessment has been included in coursework on spirituality and medicine and is performed by many practicing clinicians in the U.S.

A compassionate spiritual assessment helps to integrate spiritual concerns into therapeutic plans. Clinicians should strive to discuss these concerns in a respectful manner and as directed by the patient. Providers should always respect patients' privacy regarding matters of spirituality and religion and must be vigilant to avoid imposing their own beliefs. Providers can encourage religious and spiritual practices with their patients if these practices are already part of the patient's belief system. However, a nonreligious patient should not be told to engage in worship any more than a highly religious patient should be criticized for frequent church attendance.

Patients may ask health care providers to pray with them. It is appropriate to allow a moment of silence or a prayer. Not respecting such a request may leave the patient with a sense of abandonment. If the provider feels conflicted about praying with patients, he or she need only stand by quietly as the patient prays in his or her own tradition.

Once a spiritual assessment has been made, appropriate spiritual intervention should be offered. While spiritual and religious interventions can be provided by any clinician, integrating a pastoral care provider in the health care team will ensure that the team becomes familiar with religious and spiritual issues and that patient's spiritual needs are met. Some examples of spiritual practices are meditation, guided imagery, art, journaling, spiritual direction, pastoral counseling, yoga, religious ritual, and prayer.

Appropriate referrals to chaplains and other pastoral care providers are as important to good health care practice as are referrals to other specialists. It has been argued that discussions with patients about spiritual matters should be initiated solely by chaplains. Others recognize that health care providers can use spiritual histories as a screening tool to understand the role that a patient's beliefs play in his or her health and illness. Some patients may have complicated ethical and spiritual issues. Providers need not feel that they must solve these dilemmas; most physicians are not trained to deal with complex spiritual crises and conflicts. Chaplains and other spiritual caregivers are trained and often work with physicians in the care of patients.

It is important that health care providers be aware of their own values, beliefs, and attitudes particularly toward their own mortality. A spiritual perspective on care recognizes that the clinician and patient relationship is ultimately a relationship between two human beings. Confronting personal mortality enables a provider to better understand and empathize with what the patient is facing, to better handle the stress of working with seriously ill and dying people, and to form deeper and more meaningful connections with the patient.

The Role of the Chaplain

In recent years, the chaplain has become an increasingly important member of the health care team. Traditionally, the role of the chaplain has been to minister to the patient with certain prayers and rites particular to the patient's religion. Today, the role of a chaplain is often much broader. The chaplain can act as an extension of the patient's personal and community support system as well as be a source of spiritual support for the patient. When the chaplain has a regular presence in a health care setting, the opportunity exists to provide support to the staff as well.

It is the spiritual aspect of human nature that raises questions about ultimate meaning and purpose, questions for which medicine and science do not have answers. These issues require a unique language in which symbolism, story, and ritual are often involved. Chaplains have expertise in this form of communication and are often best able to answer such questions.

Chaplains are not necessarily clergy, although they can be, but all clinical pastoral education (CPE) certified chaplains know how to work with patients with different religious or spiritual beliefs. These chaplains can also work with atheists and agnostics.

Religious and Cultural Rituals

Every faith or cultural tradition is rich with practices and rituals that are of great support to the believer, particularly in moments of crisis. The most common religious ritual is prayer. Many patients have set times in the day when they pray and are helped by having this practice included in their care plans so that the ritual is facilitated.

Along with prayer, the reading of texts sacred of the patient's spiritual tradition can be of great support. This too should be included in the care plans so that the patient has time set aside for this reading. When a patient is too infirm to read the texts, a caregiver can offer to read to the patient.

Both prayer and reading serve as effective methods of relaxation. There are also many rituals that patients may find comfort in from their own cultures, and some families and patients have rituals they have created themselves.

Other rituals can be provided either by the chaplain or by the patient's spiritual or cultural leader. It is important that there be good communication between chaplaincy services and the patient's community in order to help the patient remain connected with his or her community.

Religious and cultural beliefs may impact practical decisions as well. For example, diet may be an important aspect of a patient's religious observances. Many hospitals make provisions to meet these special dietary needs as long as the patient's health is not compromised. Some religions recommend that articles of clothing be worn in the hospital or offer ways to prepare the bodies of the deceased once death occurs. Chaplains are good resources to find out this information. Whatever form it takes, the active practice of spirituality can bring resolution to existential concerns, particularly the fear of death.

Care Providers and Spiritual Care

All care providers (doctors, nurses, chaplains, social workers, therapists, family, and faith communities) can participate in the spiritual dimension of a patient's life. Each professional is trained to deal with

22

spiritual issues in a different way. The interdisciplinary model of palliative care that includes spiritual support is intended to ensure that patients receive the best care and opportunity for healing possible in a compassionate, caring, health care system.

Relation of Spirituality to Quality of Life

Spiritual and religious well-being may be associated with improved quality of life. It is not known for sure how spirituality is related to health. Some research shows that spiritual or religious beliefs and practices promote a positive mental attitude that may help a patient feel better. Spiritual and religious well-being may be associated with improved quality of life in the following ways:

- reduced anxiety, depression, and discomfort
- reduced sense of isolation (feeling alone)
- better adjustment to the effects of illness and its treatment
- increased ability to enjoy life during treatment
- a feeling of personal growth as a result of living with illness or disease
- improved health outcomes

Spiritual distress may contribute to poorer health outcomes. High levels of spiritual distress may interfere with the patient's ability to cope with illness and treatment and may contribute to poorer health outcomes. Health care providers may encourage patients to seek advice from appropriate spiritual or religious leaders to help resolve their conflicts which may improve their health and ability to cope.

Screening and Assessment

A spiritual assessment may help the doctor understand if a patient will use religious or spiritual beliefs to cope with the diagnosis and treatment. Knowing the role that religion and spirituality play in the patient's life may help the doctor understand how religious and spiritual beliefs affect the patient's response to the diagnosis and decisions about treatment. Some doctors or caregivers may wait for the patient to bring up spiritual concerns. Others will ask for some initial information in an interview or on a form called a spiritual assessment.

A spiritual assessment will include asking about religious preference, beliefs, and spiritual practices. A spiritual assessment may include questions relating to the following issues:

- religious denomination
- beliefs or philosophy of life
- important spiritual practices or rituals
- use of spirituality or religion as a source of strength
- participation in a religious community
- use of prayer or meditation
- loss of faith
- conflicts between spiritual or religious beliefs and treatments
- ways the caregivers may address the patient's spiritual needs
- concerns about death and the afterlife
- end-of-life planning

Additional Information

George Washington Institute for Spirituality and Health (GWish)
2131 K Street, N.W., Suite #510
Washington, DC 20037-1898
Phone: 202-496-6409
Fax: 202-496-6413
Website: http://www.gwish.org

National Association of Catholic Chaplains
3501 S. Lake Dr.
P.O. Box 070473
Milwaukee, WI 53207-0473
Phone: 414-483-4898
Fax: 414-483-6712
Website: http://www.nacc.org
E-mail: info@nacc.org

Association of Professional Chaplains
1701 E. Woodfield Rd., Suite 760
Schaumburg, IL 60173
Phone: 847-240-1014
Fax: 847-240-1015
Website: http://www.professionalchaplains.org
E-mail: info@professionalchaplains.org

Chapter 4

Chronic Illness in Old Age

Most older Americans now face chronic illness and disability in the final years of life. These final years can prove painful and difficult for sick and/or disabled elderly people who may have difficulty finding care to meet their needs. This period is often stressful and expensive for families. As currently configured, health care and community services simply are not organized to meet the needs of the large and growing number of people facing a long period of progressive illness and disability before death.

The New Demographic: Aging and Dying in 21ˢᵗ Century America

How Americans live and die has changed dramatically in the past century. In 1900, an American's life expectancy was much shorter, averaging 47 years. Illness and disability were more common at every age. Death, when it arrived, came abruptly. The most frequent causes of death in 1900 tended to be acute: pneumonia, tuberculosis, diarrhea, enteritis, and injuries. Few people lingered for many years with worsening disabilities arising from an eventually fatal chronic illness. The time from onset of a serious disability to death was measured in days or weeks, not years. Families bore the bulk of the medical expenses, and the main caregivers were family members, especially women—mothers, wives, and daughters. People generally lived their final days at home among family members.

Now, most Americans are healthier in every phase of life and live in good health into old age. In 2000, the average life expectancy for Americans was about 75 years (77 for women and 73 for men). Improved public health and medical treatments have translated into far fewer deaths from acute causes such as childbirth or infections. Currently, the most common causes of death are heart disease, cancer, stroke, chronic respiratory disease, injury, and diabetes. Dementia and multi-factorial frailty shape the last years of life for a large part of the population. Medicare pays for most physician and hospital expenses at the end of life, not families. Most Americans live out the end of their lives in hospitals rather than at home, and paid professionals provide most of the visible and costly health care. Americans will usually spend two or more of their final years disabled enough to need someone else to help with routine activities of daily living because of chronic illness.

These improvements in life expectancy and relative freedom from disease and injury in part pay tribute to America's health care system. Indeed, the fatal conditions of 1900 are precisely those that healthier living conditions and better health care have been most effective at averting. As a result, many more Americans survive into old age. However, the health care system has been slow to adapt to the chronic illness and disability that elderly Americans are likely to face at the end of their longer lives.

Changes in the way Americans die are mirrored in health care cost patterns. The overwhelming preponderance of U.S. health care costs now arise in the final years of life. Indeed, if one were to estimate costs across a lifespan, the shape of the expenditures reflects the new health and demographic circumstances. The final phase of life, when living with eventually fatal chronic illnesses, has the most intense costs and treatments. A similar curve for the U.S. population in 1900 would have been flatter, both because serious illness was more common throughout life and because death often occurred suddenly. Neither clinical services delivery nor Medicare has kept pace with the changes in the pattern of needs that underlie these costs.

So, although the overall health picture for Americans has improved dramatically, health problems have become clustered in the last years of life. In effect, the average American now lives a long, healthy life with only intermittent health problems or chronic conditions that are compatible with normal life. However, increasingly fragile health and complicated care needs ordinarily mark the years just before death.

Here Come the Boomers

In the next 30 years, the number of older Americans will continue to grow at an accelerating rate. In 2000, 4.2 million Americans were 85 or older. By 2030, the baby-boom cohort of the 1950s will begin to hit age 85 and faces the prospect of substantial disability. At that time, nearly 9 million Americans will be over 85.

While there has been some evidence that the prevalence of disability in old age and the number of years of disability in old age are both declining a little, a lengthy period of disability is still in store. The rising number of people who will be facing old age by 2030 makes it likely that supporting elderly persons with serious chronic illness will be a dominant challenge for health care in the next half-century.

The looming financial consequences of this aging tide are also worrisome. In fiscal year 2000, Medicaid paid for 45 percent of the $137 billion annual cost of formal, long-term care (paid care that does not include volunteer services by family members). The U.S. government forecasts that the cost of long-term care will reach $379 billion, in current dollar values, by 2050. Medicaid spending on health care and supportive services for the poor is now outpacing Medicare spending on health care for the elderly and disabled. Medicaid spending has become the second largest expenditure for states, behind education, and is projected to continue growing rapidly.

At the same time, caregivers for the elderly are becoming scarce. Para-professional workers provide more than three-quarters of care in nursing homes and more than 90 percent of care at home. By 2010, when the baby boomers start to retire, the pool of middle-aged women who staff most of these positions will be substantially smaller than it is now. Likewise, family caregiving—long the backbone of long-term care will be heavily burdened. Smaller family sizes and changed family structures are leaving a smaller potential group of family caregivers. Longer durations of illness and greater numbers of women working outside the home also place greater burdens on the pool of potential caregivers. Meeting the need for caregivers may prove even more difficult than the financial strain imposed by the aging baby boomers.

Chronic Illness among the Elderly

Most elderly people experience some chronic conditions. In planning for health care, these conditions may be split into three categories:

nonfatal chronic illness, serious and eventually fatal chronic illness, and frailty.

Nonfatal Chronic Illness

Common, nonfatal, chronic conditions include arthritis and hearing or vision problems. Most elderly people live for many years with these conditions, which gradually worsen but seldom pose a threat to life. These chronic conditions can contribute substantially to disability and health care costs.

Serious, Eventually Fatal, Chronic Conditions

An important subset of chronic conditions, however, tends to worsen and eventually cause death. The common fatal chronic conditions are cancers, organ system failures (including those affecting the heart, liver, kidney, or respiratory system), dementia, and strokes. Nine out of ten elderly who die when covered by Medicare have one or more of these conditions in their final year of life. While most older people eventually have to live with one of these, probably only about one-quarter of the elderly are actually ill or disabled by their eventually fatal chronic conditions at any given time. While no research yet has directly estimated this rate, the fact that 40 percent of the years past age 65 include some disability provides an upper limit. Conversely, recent work on Medicare claims shows that most elderly decedents were already sick with their eventually fatal conditions three years before death. With a life expectancy of about 15 years past age 65, the lower bound of the estimate would be 20 percent. Thus, two apparently contradictory statements are true: Most elderly people are relatively healthy; however, nearly all can expect to be chronically ill for an extended period at the end of their lives.

Frailty

Frailty is the fragility of multiple body systems as their customary reserves diminish with age and disease. Frailty may already be a major path through the end of life, but the standard classifications of illness often fail to recognize it. Therefore, persons in a general state of decline are often misleadingly labeled with heart failure or some other specific manifestation of their more general decline. In a sense, fatal chronic conditions are those that occur when the rest of the body's systems have substantial reserves. In contrast, frailty is a fatal chronic condition in which all of the body's systems have little reserve and small upsets bring about cascading health problems.

Shortcomings in the Current System

America is still learning how to think about and respond to these changes in living at the end of life. Shaped largely in the two decades after World War II, the U.S. health care system is designed mainly to prevent illness and to engineer dramatic rescues from injury or illness—mostly with surgery and medication. This concept works well for younger, basically healthy people. Indeed, its success has contributed to the dramatic improvements in American life expectancy.

However, the system has been slow to adapt to the new challenge of chronic illness in old age. Commonplace experience, buttressed by studies of current care arrangements for the chronically ill elderly, suggests that these patients must navigate a fragmented care system, offering them a patchwork of uncoordinated services that do not meet their needs. Indeed, the experience of an increasing number of families confirms the point that health care arrangements for persons with chronic illness often do not work smoothly, reliably, or well.

Our current health care delivery system is organized by setting: nursing home, hospital, home, and doctor's office. This setup determines how insurance pays bills, providers meet patients, and regulations are applied. Each care provider generally works in only one setting. Patients needing chronic care change settings often and may do so for several years; however, they have an overriding need for continuity of care, both across settings and across the changing challenges of worsening illness.

Likewise, much of how doctors and nurses think is organized around diagnosis, and this drives the course of care and treatment. However, chronically ill people coming to the end of life ordinarily have multiple diagnoses, none of which may be particularly revealing about aggregate severity of illness. Furthermore, a specific diagnosis may not shed light on their needs. For example, a person may have greater need for help in daily functioning—grocery shopping or in-home supervision—than for a particular course of medical treatment.

For elderly people, living with chronic conditions can resemble walking at the edge of a cliff. The slightest blow—such as a cold or the flu—will stress their already fragile systems and might push them over the edge. Very often, the health care system will label this final blow the cause of death, when the cause was more accurately the cumulative effect of illnesses or frailty. However, predicting the timing of the "big fall" is often difficult. Those with serious chronic illness may live reasonably well for many years or succumb quickly to early complications.

Envisioning Care for Chronic Illness in Old Age

One of the fundamental challenges that chronic illness poses for the current system is the way in which it blurs traditionally distinct concepts of health care. Diagnosis and cause of death in the chronically ill elderly have become ambiguous because most people have overall decline and multiple conditions. The value of preventing or curing any one illness diminishes greatly when patients have multiple conditions or face the onset of new symptoms as part of a broad deterioration.

Likewise, the concept of dying itself has become less clear. At one time, a person was healthy, then sick and either recovered or died quickly. Only mental illness and tuberculosis regularly violated this pattern. The recognition in the late 1960s that some patients were dying and thus not appropriately treated with aggressive interventions was a radical one in American health care and spawned the hospice movement in the 1970s. However, this model does not apply well to most chronically ill elderly. It presumes a sharp transition in which patients come to be dying by becoming terminally ill, and thus needing a different type of care from patients who might recover or remain stable. Many chronically ill elderly people have ambiguous medical prognoses: They may be sick enough to die, but could also live for many years. A more useful way to think about this near death condition is to focus on fragility rather than time to death. From this point of view, people living with serious illness at the end of life can be identified not from certainty of timing of death, but from living on thin ice—suffering long periods of illness or disability, diminished functioning, and potential exacerbation of symptoms, any of which could prove fatal. They could keep living on thin ice for some years, or die in a week.

Policy makers and the general public also lack terms to capture the types of care that individuals facing eventually chronic illness may need most. Many in the health care arena talk of end-of-life care as palliative or comfort-oriented care, but there is still no widely accepted definition of the term. The language typically associated with palliative care often assumes that it means a turning away from conventional care. However, chronically ill elderly patients routinely blur this distinction by needing a mix of both kinds of care. Early in the course of their illness, many need both curative treatment as well as palliative care aimed at treating symptoms; and late in life, some treatments may still stall the progression of illness, even while most needs are for relieving symptoms and providing support.

Trajectories of Chronic Illness: Service Needs across Time

One useful way of envisioning care for elderly people who are sick enough to die follows from classifying them into three groups, using the trajectory of decline over time that is characteristic of each major type of disease or disability. Each trajectory corresponds to a different rhythm and set of priorities in care.

- **Short period of evident decline**—typical of cancer. Most patients with malignancies maintain comfort and functioning for a substantial period. However, once the illness becomes overwhelming, the patient's status usually declines quite rapidly in the final weeks and days preceding death. Hospice is an important part of the care for this trajectory.

- **Long-term limitations with intermittent exacerbations and sudden dying**—typical of organ system failure. Patients in this category often live for a relatively long time and may have only minor limitations in everyday life. From time to time, some physiological stress overwhelms the body's reserves and leads to a worsening of serious symptoms. Patients survive a few such episodes but then die from a complication or exacerbation, often rather suddenly. Ongoing disease management, advance-care planning, and mobilizing services to the home are key to optimal care.

- **Prolonged dwindling**—typical of dementia, disabling stroke, and frailty. Those who escape cancer and organ system failure are likely to die at older ages of either neurological failure (such as Alzheimer disease or other dementia) or generalized frailty of multiple body systems. Supportive services at home such as Meals on Wheels and home health aides, followed by institutional long-term care facilities are central to good care for this trajectory.

Analyses of Medicare claims show that about one-fifth of those who die have a course consistent with the first group (mostly cancer patients); another fifth share the course of the second group (mostly organ system failure patients); and two-fifths follow the third course (frailty/dementia). The last one-fifth of decedents is split between those who die suddenly and others we have not yet learned to classify.

Chapter 5

Research Findings about End-of-Life Care and Outcomes

Improvements in medical science and health care have gradually changed the nature of dying. Death is no longer predominately likely to be the sudden result of infection or injury, but is now more likely to occur slowly, in old age, and at the end of a period of life-limiting or chronic illness. As a result, a demographic shift is beginning to occur that will include an increase in the number of seriously ill and dying people at the same time that the relative number of caregivers decreases. To meet this challenge, the best evidence that science can offer must be applied to guarantee the quality of care provided to the dying individual and their surviving loved ones.

Defining the Transition to End of Life

The evidence does not support a precise definition of the interval referred to as end of life or its transitions. End of life is usually defined and limited by the regulatory environment rather than by the scientific data. A regulatory definition is a barrier to improving care and research relating to end of life. End of life should not be defined by a specific time-frame unless evidence can support reliable prognostication.

There are individuals for whom identification of end of life is relatively clear; however, data support that this is relatively uncommon. The data demonstrate that it is not possible to accurately predict an individual's time of death.

Excerpted from "State-of-the-Science Conference Statement on Improving End-of-Life Care," National Institutes of Health (NIH), December 6–8, 2004.

There has been a lack of definitional clarity related to several concepts and terms, such as palliative care, end-of-life care, and hospice care. Too often these terms are used interchangeably and the distinctions for each term must be clarified to patients and their families, providers, policy makers, and investigators.

Respect for choice (patient or proxy), especially at the end of life, is a central value. However, patient and provider expectations and/or the desire for resource-intensive therapies with a small chance of benefit may clash with societal priorities.

Components of End of Life

There is no exact definition of end of life; however, the evidence supports the following components: (1) the presence of a chronic disease(s), symptoms, or functional impairments that persist but may also fluctuate; and (2) the symptoms or impairments resulting from the underlying irreversible disease that require formal (paid, professional) or informal (unpaid) care and can lead to death. Older age and frailty may be surrogates for life-threatening illness and comorbidity; however, there is insufficient evidence for understanding these variables as components of end of life.

Transitions to End of Life

Life is a continuum and individuals traverse this continuum facing illnesses and limited functionality. Evidence does not support defining end of life as crossing an arbitrary threshold. Administrative thresholds may be justifiable but should be based on solid science. The end-of-life process includes numerous transitions: physical, emotional, spiritual, and financial. There are also transitions in health care systems exacerbated by the lack of continuity among caregivers, challenges to social support networks, lack of sharing of clinical information, and multiple physical locations for care. Family members experience role transitions, stress, and, ultimately, bereavement as their loved one traverses life's continuum. Family and professional caregivers face similar challenges as well.

Outcome Variables That Are Important Indicators of the Quality of the End-of-Life Experience

Examples of broad outcome domains related to end of life include physical or psychological symptoms, social relationships, spiritual or philosophical beliefs, hopes, expectations and meaning, satisfaction, economic considerations, and caregiver and family experiences. Quality of life is a domain commonly proposed as an end-of-life outcome. However, the association between quality of life and end-of-life care could be strengthened by clear definitions and consistent measurements of quality of life,

The outcome domains are influenced by structure and process variables. Examples of structural variables of care include settings, provider education, demographics, geography, information systems, political systems, policies, regulations, and finances. Examples of processes of care domains include disease, syndrome and symptom management, continuity, goals and plans, monitoring and quality management, decision-making, and communication.

Patient, Family, and Health Care System Factors Associated with Improved or Worsened Outcomes

In general, research on the patient, family, and system factors that improve or worsen outcomes is limited. The research that has been conducted has used small samples and studies of narrowly defined populations. Thus, the results may not be applicable to larger groups or patients with diverse racial and ethnic backgrounds. Among the most important factors to be considered are: race, culture and ethnicity, socioeconomic status, sexual orientation, disease states, age, settings of care, and level of disability. All require further study.

Although race, culture, and ethnicity are difficult to define, they are associated with disparities in access to health care, quality of health care delivery, and health care outcomes. The reasons for these disparities are multiple, including provider factors (stereotyping and provider bias), patient factors (different values, attitudes, beliefs, and preferences in end-of-life care), and other health care system factors (inadequate translation and interpreter services). Disparities have been shown in the treatment of pain and symptom management in end-of-life care. Some minority groups have shown a preference for more intense therapy rather than hospice at the end of life. Additionally, minorities are underrepresented in end-of-life research.

Disease state can also affect end-of-life care. Whether one has cancer, heart disease, or dementia affects the pattern of functional decline, ability to interact with health care providers, attitudes of health care providers and caregivers, and manifestation of symptoms. Most of the end-of-life research has been done in patients with specific single disease states, such as cancer, and to a lesser extent in dementia.

Moreover, the sickest patients and those with comorbidities are often excluded from research studies.

Assessment and management of symptoms have been most thoroughly studied in patients with cancer. However, other life-limiting illnesses, such as congestive heart failure, end-stage renal disease, chronic obstructive pulmonary disease, liver failure, and dementia, present their own unique challenges in end-of-life care. For example, in the case of dementia, providers often do not recognize dementia as a terminal illness. Communication is more complex, often due to cognitive deficits and the need for surrogate decision-makers. Tools for measuring end-of-life care and to evaluate outcomes have not been validated in patients with dementia.

Setting of care, level of disability, and age are other factors that influence outcomes in end-of-life care and bereavement. The level of training of staff varies across settings and types of care (for example, nursing homes, community hospitals, university hospitals, and hospice). The most functionally disabled patients require substantial support for basic activities of daily living.

Of special note, there is a dearth of evidence on end-of-life treatment of children. The evidence comes from small, single site studies. What evidence there is suggests that fear of being forgotten, fear of pain, and fear of causing family sorrow, while common across patients of all ages, may represent unique challenges for children and their families. Recent reviews show that there are no instruments available for measuring the end-of-life experience in children. Due to this lack of data, it is difficult to draw broad conclusions. Researching the end-of-life experience in children and adults is complicated by the fact that institutional review boards are especially sensitive to the distress of the dying children and their families as well as to other vulnerable populations and, therefore, are reluctant to approve such studies.

General system factors can also affect outcomes. At the health care system level, one of the biggest problems noted is that care is fragmented, consisting of multiple providers, and requires the patients to make many transitions in their care. Other problems include lack of flow of information across providers and settings as well as different skill levels of providers and financial incentives that perpetuate discontinuity and discourage high-quality care.

The design of the current Medicare hospice benefit limits the availability of the full range of interventions needed by many persons at the end of life. These design limits include a six-month prognostication to death; a forced choice between skilled care and hospice care for Medicare patients entering nursing homes from hospitals; limitations on the availability of therapies, such as radiation for symptom management; and requirements for pass through payments between hospice and nursing home providers. Furthermore, although hospice has been a leader in the evolution of end-of-life care, the research on the hospice program is limited. The two randomized studies were conducted more than 20 years ago. More recent observational studies suffer from selection bias because they are limited to those who have chosen the hospice benefit.

Attention must also be paid to how State Medicaid policy affects end-of-life care for the significant number of patients who are dually eligible for Medicare and Medicaid. In theory, this creates the potential for integrated care (as demonstrated in PACE—the Program for All-Inclusive Care for the Elderly). However, there is evidence that state policy often creates barriers to care that need to be identified and addressed.

Processes and Interventions Associated with Improved or Worsened Outcomes

There is a growing body of research related to specific care interventions designed to improve outcomes for the end-of-life experience for patients and families. These include interventions in symptom management, spiritual aspects of dying, withdrawal of life-sustaining treatments, family caregiving, and bereavement. Effective communication is critical to the success of these interventions.

The following findings from these studies are of note.

- The quality of evidence on symptom management appears to be limited, with the exception of pain management. Although considerable research has been done regarding the use of medications in the management of pain, these protocols have not been widely incorporated into practice.

- Studies in the area of bereavement interventions indicate that, for some groups of adults, interventions are most effective when requested by the grieving party.

- Encouragement to initiate advance directives (for example, legal documents, such as living wills and health care powers of attorney) alone have not been shown to improve outcomes among individuals with diseases other than dementia; however, the reasons for this are not well-known.

- Communication among providers, patients, and families is believed to improve care. Communication is important as the common pathway to the relief of suffering; it generates gratitude and complaints and is an important component of palliative care.

- Effective multidisciplinary communication may be particularly important in the case of children where parents are the primary decision-makers. In particular, the absence of realistic hope with regard to pain and suffering has been shown to diminish the responsiveness of parents to initiating end-of-life discussions.

- Spirituality is consistently defined as a critical domain in end-of-life care; research on interventions to improve spiritual well-being is very limited. Preliminary evidence of a specific intervention—dignity therapy—shows positive outcomes for both the patient and family in terms of satisfaction and heightened sense of dignity, purpose, meaning, and grief management.

- Research on withholding and withdrawing life-sustaining treatment has been conducted most often in the intensive-care setting.

- Family caregivers are central to end-of-life care because they provide emotional support and essential help with activities of daily living, medications, and eating, as well as communicate with health care professionals. Although both educational and supportive interventions have been tested, only a limited number of randomized clinical trials have been conducted with caregivers of patients near end of life. There is limited information, aside from dementia, and little information about culturally diverse populations.

Future Research Directions for Improving End-of-Life Care

End-of-life care has emerged as a field of scientific inquiry in the past two decades. It is a vitally important area to public health in terms of resource considerations and to individuals. All people will die. Most deaths are not sudden. Most persons will also experience death as caregivers or family.

While there is a growing body of research covering a wide range of issues, the research is, in many ways, still in its infancy in terms of rigorous testing and evaluation of models of care, in terms of patients and family outcomes, and in terms of resource utilization. Research is needed to understand patient, caregiver, and health care system influences on these outcomes.

Conclusions

- Circumstances surrounding end of life are poorly understood, leaving many Americans to struggle through this life event.

- The dramatic increase in the number of older adults facing the need for end-of-life care warrants development of a research infrastructure and resources to enhance that care for patients and their families.

- Ambiguity surrounding the definition of end of life hinders the development of science, delivery of care, and communications between patients and providers.

- Current end-of-life care includes some untested interventions that need to be validated.

- Subgroups of race, ethnicity, culture, gender, age, and disease states experience end-of-life care differently, and these differences remain poorly understood.

- Valid measures exist for some aspects of end of life; however, measures have not been used consistently or validated in diverse settings or with diverse groups.

- End-of-life care is often fragmented among providers and provider settings, leading to a lack of continuity of care and impeding the ability to provide high-quality, interdisciplinary care.

- Enhanced communication among patients, families, and providers is crucial to high-quality end-of-life care.

- The design of the current Medicare hospice benefit limits the availability of the full range of interventions needed by many persons at the end of life.

Part Two

Medical Management of End-of-Life Symptoms

Chapter 6

What Is Palliative Care?

Palliative Care

Palliative care is an essential part of cancer control and can be provided relatively simply and inexpensively. Palliative care improves the quality of life of patients and families who face life-threatening illness by providing pain and symptom relief and spiritual and psychosocial support from diagnosis to the end of life and bereavement.

Palliative care:

- provides relief from pain and other distressing symptoms;

- affirms life and regards dying as a normal process;

- intends neither to hasten or postpone death;

- integrates the psychological and spiritual aspects of patient care;

- offers a support system to help patients live as actively as possible until death;

- offers a support system to help the family cope during the patient's illness and in their own bereavement;

- uses a team approach to address the needs of patients and their families, including bereavement counseling if indicated;

This chapter includes: Excerpts from "Palliative Care," © 2005 World Health Organization, reprinted with permission; and, excerpts from "Survivorship and the Changing Role of Palliative Care," by Dorie Hightower and Peggy Vaughn, *Benchmarks*, Vol. 3, Issue 4, National Cancer Institute (NCI), July 25, 2003.

- will enhance quality of life, and may also positively influence the course of illness;

- is applicable early in the course of illness, in conjunction with other therapies that are intended to prolong life, such as chemotherapy or radiation therapy, and includes those investigations needed to better understand and manage distressing clinical complications.

In most of the world, the majority of cancer patients are in advanced stages of cancer when first seen by a medical professional. For them, the only realistic treatment option is pain relief and palliative care. Effective approaches to palliative care are available to improve the quality of life for cancer patients.

Survivorship and the Changing Role of Palliative Care

The field of palliative care, once largely confined to providing comfort to the dying, has broadened to include the physical, social, psychological, and spiritual aspects of coping with cancer over the entire continuum of cancer care. This change in perspective is due in part to medical advances that have resulted in more people experiencing cancer as a chronic disease. Two key palliative care experts at the National Cancer Institute (NCI) were interviewed to learn more about this changing field and its role in controlling symptoms and eliminating suffering for people with cancer.

Andrea M. Denicoff, R.N., M.S., C.A.N.P., coordinates palliative care initiatives in the Office of the Deputy Director for Extramural Science. In order to integrate the institute's palliative care, symptom control and end-of-life initiatives, education and research, she chairs NCI's Palliative Care Working Group and serves as a locus for developing partnerships in palliative care.

Julia Rowland, Ph.D., is the director of NCI's Office of Cancer Survivorship. Her research focuses on both pediatric and adult cancer survivorship. She has published extensively on women's reactions to breast cancer, as well as the roles of coping, social support, and developmental stages in a patient's adaptation to cancer. She co-edited the groundbreaking text, *Handbook of Psycho-Oncology*.

Why is there a need for palliative care research?

Dr. Rowland: Very few of our current therapies are benign and without side effects. NCI and the oncology community have realized that it's not enough just to search for a cure; we have to look at the negative consequences of cancer treatment. In fact, as a two-time cancer survivor himself, NCI Director Dr. Andrew von Eschenbach is committed to NCI's role in eliminating suffering and finding ways to improve the quality of care and quality of life for cancer patients and their families.

Ms. Denicoff: Increasingly we're treating cancer as a chronic disease—one that a patient may live with for many years. We know that palliative care plays a critical role from the moment of diagnosis through treatment and survival.

How would you define palliative care?

Ms. Denicoff: I would certainly define it beyond the traditional definition of providing comfort to the dying. Several decades ago, the hospice movement in the United Kingdom sparked a new philosophy towards palliative care based on attitudes and skills that for the first time considered the psychological issues of patients and their families. In 2001, the Institute of Medicine (IOM) issued a report called "Improving Palliative Care for Cancer" that defined palliative care as beginning at the diagnosis of cancer or any other chronic or potentially life-threatening disease. The World Health Organization expanded its definition the following year as improving the quality of life of patients and their families during the entire course of an illness. So gradually, palliative care has evolved beyond end-of-life care to providing symptom management and other aspects of palliative care much earlier in the course of disease, along with tumor-directed therapies, and continues across the entire disease trajectory.

How did changing the definition change the field of palliative care research?

Dr. Rowland: In expanding the definition, the IOM recommended more attention be given to the emotional, spiritual, and practical needs of patients and their families. Nobody with cancer does it alone and does it well. It takes a medical team to treat you medically and a secondary team of family and friends to help you get through it. We're treating cancer as a chronic illness now, and that's a whole new philosophy. It ensures that palliation does not get orphaned at the end of life.

Can doctors palliate and treat an illness at the same time?

Ms. Denicoff: Yes, it should never be an either/or choice. The challenge is that doctors are trained to diagnose and cure illness and patients naturally focus on living and not dying. There's real avoidance of the "elephant in the room," because culturally, Americans don't like to discuss death. Things began to improve when the definition of palliative care took on a broader meaning and it was no longer an either/or choice. We began to appreciate palliative care as a way of improving the quality of life for a patient at all stages (of illness).

Dr. Rowland: It helps to put this in a historical perspective. Early in the 20th century, there was a lot of hope that all diseases could be cured in the way we cured tuberculosis and polio. But in reality, most common medical conditions such as cardiac disease, diabetes, flu, and viruses are palliated. We're treating the symptoms, not curing the illnesses. With cancer, we are—albeit reluctantly—beginning to accept that we may not necessarily be able to cure the disease, but we can definitely control it for the vast majority of people.

Isn't palliative care considered to be a sort of extra—not really part of treating the disease?

Ms. Denicoff: Palliative care is actually an integral part of cancer care. For example, when an oncologist is treating a woman with metastatic breast cancer that has spread through the bones, of course a major goal will be to try to stop the spread of disease. But, the doctor should also discuss symptom management, long-term prognosis, and what to expect during this course of illness with the patient and her family. None of this should ever be considered extra care, but a regular part of high-quality cancer care.

Dr. Rowland: Cancer can disrupt lives at so many levels. Dealing with the fatigue and pain, with continuing to work or attend school, and concerns over insurance and medical treatments can overwhelm the patients and their families. Palliative care addresses all the communication and decision-making aspects of coping with cancer, as well as the treatment of such medical problems as nausea and lymphedema.

Chapter 7

Common Problems of Critical Illness

There are many reasons a person may need care in an Intensive Care Unit (ICU). This chapter will attempt to explain some of the more common problems and conditions that either bring a patient to the ICU or develop while the patient is in the unit.

Shock

When in shock, the organs of the body do not get enough oxygen and blood pressure for them to function normally. There are many causes of shock. The four most common causes and their treatments are:

- **Hypovolemic Shock:** Severe dehydration or massive blood loss. Treatment is intravenous fluids (IV) and/or blood transfusions.

- **Cardiogenic Shock:** Cardiac or heart failure. Treatment is medications or devices to improve heart function.

- **Septic Shock:** Severe infection resulting in organ failure. Treatment is intravenous fluids (IV) and medications to increase blood pressure and treat the infection.

- **Systemic Inflammatory Response Syndrome (SIRS):** Can be caused by any massive trauma to the body such as a car accident, severe infection, or by some medical conditions such as pancreatitis. Treatment is intravenous fluids (IV) and medications to increase blood pressure.

If shock cannot be reversed in a matter of days, the body's organs will start to shut down. This may lead to death.

Acute Respiratory Failure

The lungs remove CO_2 (carbon dioxide) from the blood and resupply the blood with O_2 (oxygen). Acute respiratory failure occurs when the lungs do not work sufficiently. Acute respiratory failure may be the reason for admission to an ICU or a complication that occurs in the ICU from many different causes. Acute respiratory failure can range from mild to severe.

Causes of mild acute respiratory failure include a variety of conditions such as pneumonia or heart failure. These are usually treated with oxygen and respiratory treatments to help strengthen breathing and bring up phlegm.

Moderate respiratory failure may be caused by more severe pneumonia or chronic obstructive pulmonary disease (COPD). Usually, these patients need some type of mechanical support to help their breathing. Support may be provided by a tight-fitting mask that delivers oxygen under pressure or through the insertion of an endotracheal tube (breathing tube) into the trachea (windpipe). A variety of support can be provided through this tube.

The most severe form of acute respiratory failure is called acute respiratory distress syndrome (ARDS). In ARDS, the lungs cannot supply oxygen to the blood, and a ventilator (breathing machine) may be needed. ARDS is always caused by something, but that list is very long. Common examples of causes are: pneumonia, aspiration (foreign liquid gets into the lungs), trauma, severe infections, and pancreatitis. There is no single therapy for ARDS. The goal is to support the patient until the lungs heal.

Chronic Respiratory Failure

If patients remain critically ill for a long period, they become very weak. This weakness often prevents them from having the strength to breathe on their own. The respiratory muscles need to be exercised and slowly built up before the patient will be able to breathe on his or her own again. This may take as long as two to three months. When the use of a breathing machine is needed for more than a few weeks, it may be necessary to move the tube from the mouth or nose to the neck (tracheostomy). This is done to improve patient comfort and help the patient breathe well enough to be removed from the ventilator. A feeding tube may also need to be inserted.

Infections

Infections can also develop while a patient is in the ICU. Infections occur for many reasons. Usually, the illness that has brought the patient to the ICU has weakened him or her and lessened the ability to fight off infections. In addition, a patient often needs devices like a breathing tube and intravenous lines. These medical devices are necessary, but foreign to the body and can lead to infections. The most common infection in a patient on a ventilator is pneumonia or an infection of the lung. Sometimes the pneumonia can be mild and is treated with antibiotics. Sometimes the pneumonia can be severe and cause sepsis and ARDS.

Another severe infection that can occur is bacteremia or infection of the blood. This infection may be caused by the presence of intravenous lines that the patient needs to receive medications. This is called a line infection or line sepsis. If this occurs, the intravenous line needs to be removed and a new line placed in a different location. Most of the time, line sepsis can be successfully treated with antibiotics. Line sepsis can also lead to hypotension and ARDS.

Other infections that can occur include urinary tract infections (UTI) from a Foley catheter or tube inserted into the bladder to drain urine. There may be infections in the bowel that may cause diarrhea. Wound infections may occur from a recent surgery in which the surgical incision has not completely healed. These infections are usually treated fairly easily with antibiotics.

Sepsis and Severe Sepsis

Infections are a common cause of ICU admission and are also a frequent complication. The severity of infection, as well as the age and medical conditions affecting the patient, may put them at risk for an uncontrolled inflammation in response to their infection and/or injury. This inflammatory response is called sepsis. Severe sepsis occurs when this inflammation begins to affect the function of the body (for example, renal failure or acute respiratory failure), and the patient becomes very sick. Aggressive antibiotics, fluids, other medications, and sometimes surgery may be used to treat sepsis and severe sepsis, while other forms of support such as dialysis or ventilation may be needed to support the body's function. Septic shock is when blood pressure becomes low. Specific drugs (vasoconstrictors) are used to address septic shock.

Renal Failure

The kidneys remove water and toxins from the body. Kidney or renal failure is very common in the ICU and can be the reason the patient came to the ICU. It may also develop at any time while the patient is in the ICU. The kidneys are very sensitive to any severe illness, and many different illnesses can lead to renal failure.

Two major problems occur with renal failure. First, the body is unable to remove extra water from the body. The skin is a common place the water is stored and results in swelling of the arms, legs, and face. The patient will often look puffy. That extra water also builds up in the organs of the body and can cause trouble breathing and problems with the function of other organs.

The second function of the kidneys is to remove toxins from the body. When those toxins start to build up they affect the brain, and the patient gets sleepy and can become unresponsive (goes into a coma). These toxins are not damaging the brain, and the patient should wake up again if the toxins can be removed. If the toxins build up enough, the heart may stop and the patient will die from renal failure.

Renal failure can be mild to severe. Mild causes can be treated with intravenous fluids and sometimes medications to help the kidneys work better. Severe renal failure can lead to the need for dialysis (a machine to take over the function of the kidneys and remove the toxins and the extra water). Dialysis does not make the kidneys improve faster. The kidneys must heal by themselves. Dialysis only allows the body to stay alive while the kidneys are improving.

There are two major types of dialysis—intermittent or continuous. Intermittent dialysis is a treatment that uses a machine for three to four hours a day or every other day. Continuous dialysis is a machine that stays connected to the patient 24 hours a day. The sicker a patient is the more likely they will need continuous dialysis.

An important question about renal failure is: Will the kidneys ever recover? This is a hard question to answer because every patient and every situation is a little different. A general rule is that if the patient had normal kidney function before they got sick, they have a good chance of not having permanent renal failure. If their kidneys were not normal before they came to the ICU, then the chances of their kidneys' improving are much lower. If the kidneys are to improve, it may occur while they are in the ICU, but it may take weeks to months before the kidneys improve. Sometimes patients even go home on dialysis and improve several months later.

Neurological Conditions

A variety of neurologic (brain) disorders are seen in the ICU. These may include traumatic brain injuries, strokes, infections, or changes that occur when a patient is critically ill. The patient may be sleepy, disoriented, frightened, or agitated. The patient may become paranoid and scared requiring calming medications and/or restraints to prevent self-harm. The patient may not be awake at all while they remain critically ill. These changes are related to how sick the patient is, and usually resolve if the overall condition improves. Elderly patients are extremely susceptible to these changes due to the unfamiliar environment and the change in sleep patterns that occur in the critical care unit.

Bleeding and Clotting

Two other common problems deserve mention. The critically ill patient can develop bleeding from the stomach from a stress ulcer. Most critically ill patients are given medication to prevent this, but it can occur even if medication is given. Usually, the bleeding stops by itself, but it often requires blood transfusions. Occasionally, surgery or another procedure needs to be considered.

Critically ill patients also are at risk for developing blood clots in their legs and lungs. Most critically ill patients are given medications, or devices are placed on their legs to prevent this; however, it can occur even with these measures. The blood clot can be minor and only need anticoagulation to treat, or it can be life-threatening.

Multiple Organ Dysfunction Syndrome (MODS)

Any type of critical illness that brings a patient to the ICU has the potential to affect the other organs in the body. These organs may not have been affected at first, but slowly one organ after another starts to fail. This is called Multiple Organ Dysfunction Syndrome or MODS. There is no specific treatment for MODS, only supportive care. The first and most commonly affected organs are the lungs and the kidneys, followed by the brain and the immune system (fights off infection). Other organs then begin to be involved: the heart, liver, blood, intestines, and any other organs. Chances of surviving decrease if a patient develops MODS. The more organs that fail, the more likely it is that the patient will not survive.

Additional Information

Society of Critical Care Medicine
701 Lee St., Suite 200
Des Plaines, IL 60016
Phone: 847-827-6888
Fax: 847-827-6886
Website: http://www.sccm.org
E-mail: info@sccm.org

Chapter 8

Pain Management and Assessment

Chapter Contents

53

Section 8.1

Pain Management

Reprinted with permission from StopPain.org, Beth Israel Medical Center, New York, NY. © 2000–2005 Continuum Health Partners, Inc.

Pain

Many serious diseases, such as cancer and acquired immune deficiency syndrome (AIDS), cause pain. Pain can be intermittent or constant, and can vary in severity from mild to severe. It can have many different qualities, such as burning, shooting, aching, piercing, or pinching. Many factors influence the perception of pain including mood, activity level, stress, and the availability of pain-relieving therapies. Pain can be caused by:

- the activation of pain receptors by something that injures pain-sensitive tissues (nociceptive pain), for example, tissue damage from a mass (like a tumor) or from inflammation can cause this type of pain;

- nerve damage (neuropathic pain) from a virus, chemotherapy, trauma, or a disease such as multiple sclerosis.

Treating pain is important. Unrelieved pain can cause patients to:

- experience depression;
- experience disruptions in activity, appetite, and sleep;
- feel helpless and anxious;
- give up hope;
- reject treatment programs;
- stop participating in life to the fullest extent possible.

Pain usually can be controlled. There are many treatment options. To offer the best approaches for pain, doctors must recognize that pain is different in every person. All patients who experience pain deserve a detailed evaluation of the pain, the effect of the pain, and the diseases that may be causing the pain.

Pain in Cancer Patients

Many people with cancer experience pain. Thirty to 40 percent of patients in active cancer therapy and 70 to 90 percent of patients with advanced cancer report pain. Cancer pain can be caused by:

- tumors pressing on organs, nerves, or bone;

- treatment such as surgery, chemotherapy, or radiation;

- other conditions related to the cancer, such as stiffness from inactivity, muscle spasms, constipation, and bedsores;

- conditions unrelated to the cancer, such as arthritis or migraine.

In most cases, cancer pain can be controlled through relatively simple means. Doctors usually use medications, which are prescribed according to a plan that was first described by the World Health Organization and is called the Analgesic Ladder approach to cancer pain management. Other ways to alleviate cancer pain include:

- surgery, radiation, or chemotherapy to shrink tumors causing pain;

- antibiotic therapy or drainage for pain caused by infection;

- psychological therapies, and social and spiritual support, to influence the perception of pain;

- other pain treatments.

World Health Organization's Analgesic Ladder Approach for Relief of Cancer Pain

Step 1

Patients with mild to moderate pain should receive:

- a nonopioid analgesic, such as acetaminophen or a nonsteroidal anti-inflammatory drug (NSAID);

- adjuvant drugs if a specific indication exists.

Step 2

Patients with moderate to severe pain (or who have failed to achieve adequate relief with step 1) should receive:

- an opioid conventionally used for moderate pain (usually codeine, hydrocodone, dihydrocodeine, oxycodone, propoxyphene, or tramadol);
- a nonopioid analgesic, such as acetaminophen or a NSAID;
- an adjuvant drug in some cases.

Step 3

Patients with severe pain (or who have failed to achieve adequate relief with step 2) should receive:

- an opioid conventionally used for severe pain, such as morphine, oxycodone, hydromorphone, methadone, levorphanol, or fentanyl;
- a nonopioid analgesic in some cases;
- adjuvant drugs in some cases.

Pain in Acquired Immune Deficiency Syndrome (AIDS) Patients

Pain is just as common in AIDS as it is in cancer. Like cancer pain, AIDS-related pain can be caused by the disease itself and from therapies. AIDS patients commonly experience:

- pain due to nerve damage, such as peripheral neuropathy and postherpetic neuralgia;
- headaches from meningitis;
- abdominal pain from gastrointestinal disease;
- chest pain from pneumonia;
- muscle pains.

To find an appropriate treatment, a doctor should perform a detailed assessment.

Treatment of Pain

Treatments that can successfully control pain include:

Pharmacological Therapies (Medication)

- non-opioid pain relievers
- opioids
- adjuvant medications (drugs whose primary purpose is not for pain, but rather for other conditions)
- topical treatments (drugs are applied directly to the skin, as a patch, gel, or cream)

Because the effects of a medication can vary widely from person to person, treatment of pain needs to be tailored to fit each individual. Some patients may need to try many different kinds of treatments before they find the right balance between pain relief and side effects.

Patients should be sure their doctors are aware of all medications and over-the-counter drugs, such as aspirin, they are taking, even for conditions unrelated to their pain. Many medications should not be taken together because they increase or decrease each other's effects or produce new adverse reactions. Of course, the doctor should also be informed if the patient is pregnant or breastfeeding.

Non-Pharmacological Treatments

Non-pharmacological treatments (treatments that do not rely primarily on medication to achieve their effect) offer a variety of approaches to pain relief. Most are non-invasive. Simple, relatively safe non-pharmacological approaches include:

- physiatric approaches;
- non-invasive stimulatory approaches;
- psychological approaches;
- complementary/alternative approaches.

In most cases, these techniques should be used in addition to, not instead of, other approaches to pain relief. More invasive non-pharmacological treatments include:

- anesthesiologic approaches;
- invasive stimulatory approaches;
- surgical approaches.

Physiatric Approaches

Therapeutic Exercise

Exercising is important because it can:

- strengthen weak muscles;
- mobilize stiff joints;
- help restore coordination and balance;
- promote a sense of well-being;
- decrease anxiety and stress;
- keep the heart healthy;
- help maintain an appropriate weight.

A physical therapist, exercise physiologist, or certified athletic trainer can help patients get started safely and learn exercises designed specifically to target problem areas. Even bedridden patients can benefit from range-of-motion exercises.

Heat Therapy

Heat therapy can reduce pain, especially the pain of muscle tension or spasm. Sometimes patients with other types of pain benefit. Heat therapy acts to:

- increase the blood flow to the skin;
- dilate blood vessels, increasing oxygen and nutrient delivery to local tissues;
- decrease joint stiffness by increasing muscle elasticity.

Heat should be applied for 20 minutes. Patients can use hot packs, hot water bottles, hot and moist compresses, electric heating pads, or chemical and gel packs carefully wrapped to avoid burns. Patients can also submerge themselves or the painful part in warm water.

Heat therapy is not recommended on tissue that has received radiation treatment. Pregnant women should avoid using hot tubs or any method that subjects the developing baby to prolonged heat.

Deep heat delivered to underlying tissue by short wave diathermy, microwave diathermy, or ultrasound is also sometimes used to relieve pain. Deep heat should be used with caution by patients with active cancer and should not be applied directly over a cancer site.

Cold Therapy

Cold therapy, which constricts blood vessels near the skin, sometimes can relieve the pain of muscle tension or spasm. Other types of pain also benefit in some cases. It can also reduce swelling if applied soon after an injury.

Ice packs, towels soaked in ice water, or commercially-prepared chemical gel packs should be applied for 15 minutes. Cold sources should be sealed to prevent dripping, flexible to conform to the body, and adequately wrapped to prevent irritation or damage to the skin.

Non-Invasive Stimulatory Approaches

Transcutaneous Electrical Nerve Stimulation

Transcutaneous electrical nerve stimulation (TENS) is a method of applying a gentle electric current to the skin to relieve pain. Studies have shown that it can be effective in certain cases of chronic pain. A TENS unit is a small box-shaped device, which patients can put in their pocket or hang on their belt, transmits electrical impulses through wires to electrodes taped to the skin in the painful area. Patients describe the sensation of TENS as buzzing, tingling, or tapping.

The patient should experiment with the placement of the electrodes and the timing, intensity, amplitude, and frequency of the electrical current to find the most effective setting. Pain relief usually lasts beyond the period when current is applied. TENS can become less effective at relieving pain over time. TENS is usually safe and well tolerated. However, it is not recommended on inflamed, infected, or otherwise unhealthy skin, over a pregnant uterus (except for obstetric pain relief), or in the presence of a cardiac pacemaker.

Psychoeducational Approaches

Cognitive Behavioral Techniques

Cognitive behavioral techniques are used to reduce the body's unproductive responses to stress, helping to relieve pain or improve the ability to tolerate it.

Deep breathing: In this simple technique, the patient focuses his or her attention on breathing deeply. This may shift attention away from the source of pain.

Progressive muscle relaxation: In this technique, developed in the 1930s, patients contract and then relax muscles throughout the body, group by group. Progressive muscle relaxation can help patients learn about the tension in their body and the contrast between tense and relaxed muscles.

Imagery: In this technique, patients focus on pleasant thoughts, for example, waves gently hitting a sandy beach. One variation is to think of an image that represents the pain (such as a hot, blazing, concrete sidewalk), and then imagine it changing into an image representing a pain-free state (a pretty, snow-covered forest).

Meditation: In this technique, practiced routinely in Asia, the individual aims to empty his or her mind of thoughts, focusing instead on the sensation of breathing and the rhythms of his or her body.

Biofeedback therapy: Biofeedback is a method in which people learn to reduce their body's unproductive responses to stress, and thus decrease their sensitivity to pain. Children are particularly quick to learn from biofeedback. In biofeedback, electrodes are placed at various points on the patient's skin to measure:

- muscle tension—as a muscle contracts, electrical activity increases;
- temperature—the stress response is related to blood flow in the hands or feet, and blood flow determines temperature;
- heart beat;
- sweating.

Patients watch the monitor and listen to the tones measuring their stress indicators. They use these as a guide in learning to release tension throughout their body.

Distraction: Distraction is a pain management technique which has patients focusing their attention on something other than their pain and negative emotions. To distract themselves, patients can:

- sing;
- count;
- listen to music;
- watch television;

- listen to the radio;
- talk to friends or family;
- read;
- listen to stories being read.

Reframing: A pain and stress management technique that teaches patients to monitor negative thoughts and images and replace them with positive ones. Patients can learn to have a more positive outlook by recognizing some counterproductive thought patterns, such as:

- Blaming, in which the individual avoids taking responsibility. Thoughts such as, "It's my boss's fault I have this headache," can be replaced with, "I'm going to focus on what I can do to feel better."

- Should or must statements, which imply that someone has failed to live up to an arbitrary standard. Statements such as, "I should have been more careful," can be counteracted with, "I do not have to be perfect," or "I made the best decision I could have at the time."

- Polarized thinking, in which everything is black or white, with no shades of gray. Statements such as, "I'm still in pain, so this program is useless," can be counteracted with, "I wish I could be free of pain, but I have made some progress. Sometimes small improvements add up."

- Catastrophizing, in which the person imagines the worst possible scenario then acts as if it will surely come true. Statements such as, "This pain must mean I am going downhill," can be counteracted with, "I am jumping to conclusions," or "I'll find a way to cope with whatever happens."

- Control fallacy, in which the person sees himself or herself as completely controlled by others (or controlling everything). Thoughts such as, "My spouse doesn't think I need to see a counselor, so I can't go," can be counteracted with, "I am not a helpless victim," (or thoughts such as, "My family will fall apart without me," can be counteracted with, "Members of my family are not helpless").

- Emotional reasoning, in which the individual believes that what he or she feels must be true. Statements such as, "I'm so frightened the pain will never stop, I know it never will," can be counteracted with, "I'm scared, but that does not give me an accurate view of the situation," or "When I calm down, I will think about what this means."

61

- Filtering, in which people focus on one thing (such as pain) to the exclusion of any other experience or point of view. Statements such as, "I can't take it," can be replaced with, "I have coped before and can cope again."

- Entitlement fallacy, in which individuals believe they have the right to what they want. Statements such as, "Life is so unfair," or "I have been cheated," can be counteracted with, "No one promised me a rose garden. I will focus on finding ways to make things better."

Psychotherapy and Social Support

Psychotherapy and social support can help a patient cope with pain. Psychotherapy may be useful for anyone whose pain is difficult to manage, who has developed clinical depression or anxiety, or who has a history of psychiatric illness. Spiritual leaders are another potential source of support for patients. Among the goals of psychotherapy are the following:

- emphasize the patient's past strengths
- support the patient's use of previously successful coping strategies
- teach new coping skills
- establish a bond to decrease a patient's sense of isolation
- foster a sense of self-worth

Group approaches: Peer groups, in which a patient meets with others with the same condition, can help by:

- providing support;
- showing the patient how others have coped effectively;
- helping the patient maintain a social identity;
- providing access to information and material aid.

Complementary/Alternative Approaches

Acupuncture

Acupuncture, used in China for thousands of years, is an ancient method for relieving pain and controlling disease. It appears to be effective for some patients with chronic pain. During acupuncture, thin gold or metal needles, gently twirled for ten to twenty minutes can be used to stimulate acupuncture points which relieve pain in specific parts of the body (for example, a point on the leg targets stomach pain). Patients usually feel a tingling, warm sensation similar to that of transcutaneous electrical nerve stimulation. Acupuncture points can also be stimulated with deep massage (acupressure), electric currents (electroacupuncture), or lasers.

The risk of side effects is low. Side effects can include pain after the procedure, bleeding, bruising, dizziness, fainting, and local skin reactions. Rarely, organ damage can occur with deep needling techniques. Infection because of inadequately sterilized needles is a hazard; disposable needles are recommended. Acupuncture is not recommended for patients with serious blood clotting problems. Acupuncture should be used with caution by pregnant women.

Massage

Massage can be a useful addition to a pain management program, especially for patients who are bedridden. Massage can:

- stimulate blood flow;
- relax muscles that are tight or in spasm;
- promote a feeling of well-being.

Muscles can be stroked, kneaded, or rubbed in a circular motion. A lotion can reduce friction on the skin. Massage is not recommended in cases of swollen tissue. It should be used in addition to, and not instead of, exercise by patients who can walk.

Anesthesiologic Approaches

For patients with pain who fail conservative therapies, simple to complex interventional therapies such as nerve blocks, epidural steroid injections, intraspinal drug administration, or trigger point injections may be helpful. These therapies are typically provided by anesthesiologists with advanced training in pain management.

Nerve Blocks and Epidural Steroid Injections

Nerve blocks can relieve pain by inhibiting the impulses that travel along specific nerves in the body. To achieve a block, the doctor usually injects a local anesthetic along the course of a nerve or nerves. Al-though this is called a temporary block, in the best outcome, pain relief lasts for a long time. In very selected cases, the doctor can inject a solution that damages the nerve and produces a more permanent block.

Sympathetic nerve blocks inhibit the nerves of the sympathetic nervous system, which are responsible for increasing heart rate, con-stricting blood vessels, and raising blood pressure in response to stress. Sympathetic nerve blocks can be useful in treating some pains due to nerve damage, such as some types of complex regional pain syn-drome (also called reflex sympathetic dystrophy or causalgia).

Blocks of somatic nerves can be targeted to any area of the body. In some cases, nerve blocks fail to provide pain relief, or provide only a brief respite.

Epidural steroids, administered through injection, can help to in-terrupt the passage of painful impulses through nerves.

Spinal Infusion

Intraspinal drug administration involves the delivery of low doses of analgesic drugs, such as morphine or clonidine, through a catheter inserted directly into the spine. This approach is often used to man-age cancer pain.

Invasive Approaches

Invasive Nerve Stimulation

Invasive nerve stimulation can provide pain relief for some patients who have not responded to other therapies. In this technique, elec-trodes are implanted in the patient's body to send a gentle electrical current to nerves in the spinal column or the brain.

Spinal cord stimulation has been used for chronic back and/or leg pain following lumbar surgery, pain due to nerve damage (complex regional pain syndrome and postherpetic neuralgia), and intractable angina. Few controlled studies of this method exist.

Deep brain stimulation may help as many as half of patients with central pain, a challenging condition that can develop as a result of damage to the central nervous system from stroke. Disadvantages of this therapy include its high cost, risks of an invasive treatment (such as infection), and difficulty predicting before a trial which patients will benefit.

Surgical Approaches

Surgery to treat pain (rather than the underlying disease) is only appropriate in cases where more conservative approaches have failed and where trained neurosurgeons and follow-up care are available. A surgeon can cut a nerve close to the spinal cord (rhizotomy) or bundles of nerves in the spinal cord (cordotomy) to interrupt the pathways that send pain signals to the brain. In the best possible outcome, surgery relieves pain and the need for most or all pain medication. However, surgery carries the risk of:

- stopping the pain only briefly;

- creating new pain from nerve damage at the site of the operation;

- limiting the patient's ability to feel pressure and temperature in the region, putting him or her at risk for injury.

Section 8.2

Pain Assessment in Cancer Patients

Excerpts from PDQ® Cancer Information Summary. National Cancer Institute; Bethesda, MD. Pain (PDQ®): Supportive Care–Patient. Updated 12/2005. Available at: http://cancer.gov. Accessed March 1, 2006.

Cancer pain can be managed effectively in most patients with cancer or with a history of cancer. Although cancer pain cannot always be relieved completely, therapy can lessen pain in most patients. Pain management improves the patient's quality of life throughout all stages of the disease.

Flexibility is important in managing cancer pain. As patients vary in diagnosis, stage of disease, responses to pain and treatments, and personal likes and dislikes, management of cancer pain must be individualized. Patients, their families, and their health care providers must work together closely to manage a patient's pain effectively.

Assessment

To treat pain, it must be measured. The patient and the doctor should measure pain levels at regular intervals after starting cancer treatment, at each new report of pain, and after starting any type of treatment for pain. The cause of the pain must be identified and treated promptly.

Patient Self-Report

To help the health care provider determine the type and extent of the pain, cancer patients can describe the location and intensity of their pain, any aggravating or relieving factors, and their goals for pain control. The family and/or caregiver may be asked to report for a patient who has a communication problem involving speech, language, or a thinking impairment. The health care provider should help the patient describe the following:

- **Pain:** The patient describes the pain, when it started, how long it lasts, and whether it is worse during certain times of the day or night.

- **Location:** The patient shows exactly where the pain is on his or her body or on a drawing of a body, and where the pain goes if it travels.

- **Intensity or severity:** The patient keeps a diary of the degree or severity of pain.

- **Aggravating and relieving factors:** The patient identifies factors that increase or decrease the pain.

- **Personal response to pain:** Feelings of fear, confusion, or hopelessness about cancer, its prognosis, and the causes of pain can affect how a patient responds to and describes the pain. For example, a patient who thinks pain is caused by cancer spreading may report more severe pain or more disability from the pain.

- **Behavioral response to pain:** The health care provider and/or caregivers note behaviors that may suggest pain in patients who have communication problems.

- **Goals for pain control:** With the health care provider, the patient decides how much pain he or she can tolerate and how much improvement he or she may achieve. The patient uses a daily pain diary to increase awareness of pain, gain a sense of control of the pain, and receive guidance from health care providers on ways to manage the pain.

Assessment of the Outcomes of Pain Management

The results of pain management should be measured by monitoring for a decrease in the severity of pain and improvement in thinking ability, emotional well-being, and social functioning. The results of taking pain medication should also be monitored. Drug addiction is rare in cancer patients. Developing a higher tolerance for a drug and becoming physically dependent on the drug for pain relief does not mean that the patient is addicted. Patients should take pain medication as prescribed by the doctor. Patients who have a history of drug abuse may tolerate higher doses of medication to control pain.

Treating Older Patients

Older patients are at risk for under-treatment of pain because their sensitivity to pain may be underestimated, they may be expected to tolerate pain well, and misconceptions may exist about their ability to benefit from opioids. Issues in assessing and treating cancer pain in older patients include the following:

- Multiple chronic diseases and sources of pain: Age and complicated medication regimens put older patients at increased risk for interactions between drugs and between drugs and the chronic diseases.

- Visual, hearing, movement, and thinking impairments may require simpler tests and more frequent monitoring to determine the extent of pain in the older patient.

- Nonsteroidal anti-inflammatory drug (NSAID) side effects, such as stomach and kidney toxicity, thinking problems, constipation, and headaches are more likely to occur in older patients.

- Opioid effectiveness: Older patients may be more sensitive to the pain-relieving and central nervous system effects of opioids resulting in longer periods of pain relief.

- Patient-controlled analgesia must be used cautiously in older patients, since drugs are slower to leave the body, and older patients are more sensitive to the side effects.

- Other methods of administration, such as rectal administration, may not be useful in older patients since they may be physically unable to insert the medication.

- Pain control after surgery requires frequent direct contact with health care providers to monitor pain management.

- Reassessment of pain management and required changes should be made whenever the older patient moves (for example, from hospital to home or nursing home).

Section 8.3

Pain Assessment in Patients with Dementia

"Assessing Pain in Loved Ones with Dementia: A Guide for Family and Caregivers," used with permission from the American Geriatrics Society Foundation for Health in Aging, http://www.healthinaging.org, © 2005.

Dementia is a condition of declining mental abilities. A diagnosis of dementia means that the patient may have difficulty reasoning over time. The patient may have problems remembering things and even people they love. Your loved one may not be able to communicate his or her thoughts, feelings, needs, or physical problems. In fact, he or she may not even fully understand physical problems, such as pain.

Sadly, persistent pain is common among older persons, because they are more likely to suffer from problems such as arthritis and other chronic medical conditions. Many people think that pain is to be expected with aging and that nothing can be done. Older persons commonly have multiple medical problems which, when combined with dementia, can make diagnosis difficult. If your loved one has dementia, determining if he or she is experiencing pain may be up to you. Often, older persons deny that they have pain. Instead, asking your loved one whether he/she experiences discomfort, aching, or hurting may result in a more truthful answer. Even if dementia makes it impossible for your loved one to respond, your careful observation can reveal important clues to let you know that he or she is experiencing pain.

What are the clues?

- **Facial expressions:** Does your loved one frown, look frightened, grimace, wrinkle his or her brow, keep eyes closed tightly, blink rapidly, or exhibit any distorted expression?

- **Verbalizations/vocalizations:** Does he or she moan, groan, sigh, grunt, chant, call out, breathe noisily, ask for help, or become verbally abusive?

- **Body movements:** Is your loved one's body posture rigid and/ or tense? Does he or she fidget, pace, rock back and forth, have restricted movement, gait, or mobility changes?

- **Behavioral changes:** Does he or she refuse food or have an appetite change? Is there any change in sleep or rest periods? Has he or she suddenly stopped common routines or begun wandering?

- **Mental status changes:** Does he or she cry, become more confused, irritable, or distressed?

When does the pain occur?

- During movement: Does your loved one grimace or groan during personal care (such as bathing), walking, or transferring (from bed to chair, for example)?

- When no movement is involved: Does your loved one appear agitated or have other behavioral changes, such as trouble sleeping, loss of appetite, or reclusiveness?

The Pain Assessment

If you see any clues that indicate pain, talk to your health care provider right away. If your loved one has mild-to-moderate dementia and is able to communicate adequately, your health care provider will question him or her directly and should use pain evaluation tools and scales. The health care provider may ask the patient to give pain a number from one to ten, or use pictures of faces, or a pain thermometer to help measure the pain.

If your loved one is not able to communicate adequately, you must describe your loved one's signs of pain with as much detail as possible. Tell the health care provider what you have noticed and give examples. Focus on when the pain occurs. You can describe how it seems to be experienced (for example, burning, aching, stabbing, and whether the pain occurs with or without movement). Tell your health care provider what—if anything—relieves the pain. The health care provider will be able to make a diagnosis and offer a plan to help relieve the pain.

An important part of the pain assessment is a history of all prescription and over-the-counter medicines your loved one now takes and has taken in the past. Write down all medications and dosages the patient has taken and give it to the health care provider.

The health care provider should also perform a physical examination that will focus on the site(s) of pain, often the muscle, bone, and nervous systems. The health care provider will evaluate the patient's physical function (walking, range of motion of joints, etc.). Laboratory tests and/or x-rays may be performed, as well.

Treatments

Medication is the most common way of controlling pain in older persons. Around-the-clock doses of acetaminophen (Tylenol®) are effective for most patients with mild-to-moderate muscle and/or bone pain, like arthritis. Nonsteroidal anti-inflammatory drugs (NSAIDs), such as aspirin and ibuprofen, can be effective but may have more side effects in older persons. Because they have to be taken every day over a long period of time they may cause such problems as bleeding ulcers.

For more serious pain, there are the opioid drugs, such as Vicodin or Roxicet to name just a couple of the many different products that are now available for moderate to severe pain. These drugs can be very effective in some cases.

For pain that is due to damage to nerves, a wide variety of drugs used for control of depression and even epilepsy have been found to be helpful. If movement causes pain, the health care provider can prescribe medication to be taken before the movement. He or she may suggest ways to alter the movement or activity that causes pain. If the pain is caused by something other than movement, the health care provider will investigate other causes and ask questions like: Are the patient's basic needs being met? Is there an infection? Is the patient constipated? Treatment needs to be prescribed based on each patient's specific situation.

Pain is a serious problem for many older persons. Alleviating pain in patients with dementia often depends on the observations of the family and/or caregiver. You and your health care provider can work together to relieve the patient's pain and achieve a better quality of life for your loved one in his/her later years.

Additional Information

The AGS Foundation for Health in Aging
350 Fifth Avenue, Suite 801
New York, NY 10118
Toll-Free: 800-563-4916
Phone: 212-755-6810
Fax: 212-832-8646
Website: http://www.healthinaging.org
E-mail: staff@healthinaging.org

Chapter 9

Managing Fatigue and Other End-of-Life Symptoms

What Is Fatigue?

Fatigue is a feeling of weariness, tiredness, or lack of energy that varies in degree, frequency, and duration. Everyone has experienced normal fatigue, which improves with rest. Chronic fatigue associated with a disease or treatment of a disease does not improve with rest and can seriously affect a person's ability to function and quality of life. Fatigue can impact quality of life in many different ways—physically, emotionally, socially, and spiritually.

Acute Versus Chronic Fatigue

Acute fatigue has a recent onset and is temporary in duration. It is usually related to excessive physical activity, lack of exercise, insufficient rest or sleep, poor diet, dehydration, increase in activity, or other environmental factors. Acute fatigue can be a protective body function, alerting a person to rest. It is anticipated to end in the near future, with interventions such as rest or sleep, exercise, and a balanced diet.

Chronic fatigue persists, and recovery is not quickly anticipated. Chronic fatigue may be associated with numerous illnesses, such as

This chapter includes: "Pain Medicine and Palliative Care: Fatigue," and "Pain Medicine and Palliative Care: Symptom Management," from StopPain.org, Beth Israel Medical Center, New York, NY. © 2000–2005 Continuum Health Partners, Inc. Reprinted with permission.

cancer; acquired immune deficiency syndrome (AIDS); heart, lung or kidney problems; multiple sclerosis; and other medical conditions. Fatigue can also accompany psychological problems such as depression, or result from the use of medications.

Cancer-Related Fatigue

Fatigue symptoms are common, yet unrecognized in many cancer patients. Fatigue experienced by cancer patients can result from the course of the disease, preexisting physical or psychological conditions, effects of medication, or lack of exercise. Fatigue may also result from treatment such as surgery, chemotherapy, and radiation therapy.

Fatigue from cancer surgery can last for weeks or months, and may be caused by anxiety as patients prepare for surgery as well as the pre-admission testing for surgery. Pain after surgery, the effects of anesthesia, sedatives, or analgesics may also cause fatigue.

Fatigue from chemotherapy affects most patients, lasting for one to two weeks following treatment then decreasing gradually. Fatigue as a result of radiation therapy affects almost all patients and may worsen during the course of treatment, peaking at four to six weeks. Fatigue may lessen after radiation therapy is completed but still continue for weeks or even months. Many patients undergoing interferon or interleukin therapy also experience fatigue.

Patients may discuss adjusting therapeutic regimens with their doctors to relieve fatigue symptoms. Delaying chemotherapy treatments for one or two days to attend important life events, or changing the time of their treatment, may be considered.

Symptoms and Possible Causes

Fatigue is generally defined in terms of symptoms that occur over time, cause distress, or impair function, or are likely to result from disease or treatment of disease. The following symptoms, which vary from patient to patient, are associated with fatigue:

- diminished energy disproportionate to activity, causing distress

- diminished activity associated with lower physical or intellectual performance, for example, lack of focus, short attention span, memory problems

- diminished motivation, interest in activities

- exhaustion, apathy, lethargy

- generalized (whole body) weakness or tiredness

- sleep abnormalities

- irritability, impatience, sadness, changes in mood

Though little is known about fatigue prevention and treatment, fatigue may be related to a variety of medical and physical conditions and psychosocial factors. Fatigue can be caused by anemia or associated with major organ dysfunction, including severe heart or lung disease, kidney failure, or liver failure. Hypothyroidism (insufficient production of thyroid hormone) and adrenal problems, even if mild, can cause fatigue. Neuromuscular disorders, malnutrition, infection, dehydration, or electrolyte disturbances can also be associated with fatigue, as well as sleep disorders, immobility and lack of exercise, chronic pain, or the use of centrally-acting drugs such as opioids. Psychosocial factors associated with fatigue are anxiety and depression, stress, and those related to the reactions of others to the fatigue.

How Health Care Providers Assess Fatigue

Assessment of fatigue begins with a detailed description of its history, development, symptoms, and causes. This information is acquired from the patient's self-report, medical history, physical examination, and review of laboratory tests such as a complete blood count, thyroid function, and imaging studies (CT or MRI scan).

The onset of fatigue, course of the symptoms, severity or intensity, level of distress, and degree of interference with daily activities should be addressed. Factors that relieve fatigue or make it worse should also be examined. These factors may be emotional (moods, etc.), social (relationships with family and friends), and psychological (effect on thought process). These areas can be assessed using a verbal rating scale: none, mild, moderate, and severe; or a 0 to 10 scale (where 0 means no fatigue and 10 means the worst fatigue imaginable). One scale is usually adopted and consistently used.

Treatment

The treatment of fatigue includes identifying and managing the underlying cause and using a variety of interventions, including medication; education; exercise; sleep hygiene; stress management, and nutrition.

Treating Anemia

Anemia (below normal levels of red blood cells) can be a major factor in cancer-related fatigue. Lack of red blood cells and oxygen in the body creates an energy deficit, causing tiredness or fatigue. Blood transfusion therapy, as well as recombinant human erythropoietin (a hormone produced by DNA technology), is used to treat anemia. Erythropoietin stimulates bone marrow to produce red blood cells, thereby increasing the number of red blood cells in the body.

Adjusting Current Medications

Patients on medication who complain of fatigue may need their drug regimens reviewed or adjusted by their physicians. Centrally-acting drugs that are not essential may be eliminated or reduced (for example, antiemetics, hypnotics or anxiolytics, antihistamines, and analgesics). If opioids are taken for controlling pain, dosage reduction is done cautiously to see whether fatigue improves without making the pain worse.

Commonly Prescribed Medications

Drug therapy for treating fatigue associated with medical illness has not been evaluated through controlled studies. Some doctors consider the use of psychostimulants such as methylphenidate and pemoline. These drugs are often used to treat opioid-related cognitive impairment and depression in the elderly and medically ill.

Sometimes low-dose corticosteroids (such as dexamethasone or prednisone) are used in the treatment of cancer-related fatigue.

Amantadine has been used for many years in the treatment of fatigue due to multiple sclerosis.

An antidepressant drug may be used to treat fatigue due to clinical depression, preferably one of the serotonin-specific reuptake inhibitors, secondary amine tricyclics, or bupropion.

Patient / Caregiver Education

Patients and caregivers can be helped to understand the nature of fatigue symptoms, treatment choices, and expected outcomes through education and counseling. Patients can be prepared to anticipate fatigue as a normal part of the course of cancer and its treatment. Patients can be taught energy conservation and restoration strategies while undergoing these treatments.

Exercise

Exercise may be beneficial in relieving fatigue. The exercise program should be tailored to the individual according to age, gender, and physical and medical condition. Exercises should involve rhythmic and repetitive movement of large muscle groups (walking, cycling, or swimming). These exercises should begin gradually, several days a week, and not be performed to the point of exhaustion. Some contraindications to low-intensity exercise include cardiac abnormalities, recurrent or unexplained pain, and onset of nausea with exercise.

Change in Activity and Rest Patterns

Using a diary to assess fatigue may identify specific activities that increase fatigue. Patients can record changes in energy levels, and this information can help to modify, schedule, or pace these activities throughout the day.

Naps should be taken in the morning or early afternoon. Late afternoon or evening naps might interfere with sleep at night. Basic sleep hygiene principles, such as a specific bedtime and wake time, noise and light reduction, diversional activities (music, massage), avoidance of stimulants (caffeine, nicotine, steroids, methylphenidate) and central nervous system depressants (alcohol) prior to sleep should be employed. A specific wake time helps to maintain a normal sleep-wake rhythm. Consistent exercise tends to improve sleep and promote deeper sleep when done at least six hours before bedtime.

Stress Management and Cognitive Therapies

Using stress reduction techniques or cognitive therapies (relaxation, deep breathing, hypnosis, guided imagery, or distraction) can promote coping skills and relieve stress. Coping skills such as seeking more information about the illness and its interventions, planning and scheduling activities, delegating tasks, and developing solutions to daily problems associated with fatigue are helpful to patients. Mental fatigue may be relieved by activities that conserve and restore mental capacity, such as decreasing noise and distractions while trying to concentrate, walking outside, gardening, and other environmental activities.

Adequate Nutrition and Hydration

A balanced diet that combines adequate caloric intake including grains, green vegetables, legumes, and iron-rich foods can help maintain energy levels. Adequate fluid intake can prevent dehydration and hypotension which can intensify fatigue symptoms. Regular exercise may improve appetite and increase nutritional intake.

Other End-of-Life Symptoms

Shortness of Breath

The sensation of shortness of breath, or dyspnea, is common in patients with life-threatening conditions: between 20–80% of palliative care patients experience this symptom. Like pain, shortness of breath is subjective. It is partly independent of oxygen and carbon dioxide levels. There are many causes of shortness of breath, including:

- disease of the lung, such as emphysema, chronic bronchitis, cancer and many others
- fluid in the lungs
- infection
- anemia
- emotional factors, such as anxiety

Sometimes simple measures can relieve the sensation of shortness of breath, including:

- providing a familiar voice to reduce anxiety
- changing position
- using relaxation techniques
- improving air circulation by opening a window or turning on a fan

Medication can sometimes be useful, including:

- opioids, such as morphine
- sedatives, such as benzodiazepines
- oxygen through a face mask, in some cases
- corticosteroids, for patients with obstructive complications such as superior vena cava syndrome
- bronchodilators, if airway spasm is involved

Fatigue

Fatigue is common among those with life-threatening diseases. Fatigue can be caused by:

- the disease
- medical problems related to the disease or treatment, like anemia
- treatments for the disease (for cancer patients, as an example, fatigue may be caused by radiation or chemotherapy)
- other medication
- immobility
- sleep disturbance
- depression and anxiety

Management of fatigue can include having the patient:

- conserve energy whenever possible, and learn techniques of energy and time management
- learn to improve sleep
- learn to use exercise or physical therapy

Medications used to treat fatigue include:

- psychostimulants, such as methylphenidate or pemoline
- low-dose corticosteroids such as, dexamethasone or prednisone
- amantadine (for fatigue related to multiple sclerosis)
- antidepressants
- erythropoietin for fatigue caused by anemia

Friends and family can help by being responsive to the patient's pace. Activities and/or conversations can be saved for periods when the patient feels that he or she would enjoy them.

Dry Mouth

The sensation of a dry mouth, or xerostomia, is a common symptom in palliative care. A dry mouth can be caused by:

- dehydration

- erosion of the mucous membrane lining the mouth
- depression or anxioty
- chemotherapy or radiotherapy for cancer
- many medications, including some pain relievers, antidepressants, diuretics and tranquilizers

The sensation of a dry mouth can sometimes be relieved by simple measures, including:

- drinking lots of fluids
- good oral hygiene
- providing humidified air
- sucking on ice or vitamin C tablets
- chewing sugarless gum
- artificial saliva, provided in a spray form
- pilocarpine

Appetite Loss

Patients with life-threatening diseases often lose their appetite and may lose weight. When severe, this is called cachexia or wasting syndrome. Causes of weight loss (from the disease or treatments) include:

- inadequate intake of nutrients because the patient cannot or does not want to eat
- poor absorption of food that is consumed
- changes in the patient's metabolism

Management of weight loss depends on the patient's goals. It may include:

- eating small, frequent meals
- eating high-calorie, high-protein foods and nutritional supplements
- receiving nutritional counseling
- feeding through artificial means (such as a tube or IV)
- eating and drinking whatever the patient would like
- relieving thirst by sucking on ice chips or a moist cloth

Medication can include:

- corticosteroids, which stimulate appetite but do not usually increase weight

- megestrol acetate, which stimulates appetite and causes slight weight gain

- dronabinol, which prevents nausea and vomiting, and increases appetite, enhances a sense of well-being and causes weight gain

- cyproheptadine, which mildly enhances appetite, increases food intake and enhances weight gain

- pentoxifylline, which potentially acts to lower levels of a substance (tumor necrosis factor) that contributes to weight loss in cancer patients.

Gastrointestinal Symptoms

Gastrointestinal symptoms include such problems as nausea (feeling queasy or sick to one's stomach), vomiting (throwing up), constipation or diarrhea, anorexia (loss of appetite), and cachexia (severe weight loss). These difficulties can be caused by a number of illnesses, treatments, medications, and other factors, including:

- cancer, AIDS, and other diseases
- radiation therapy
- dehydration
- chemotherapy
- certain foods
- opioids, antibiotics, and other drugs
- lactose (milk) intolerance
- emotional distress and anxiety
- surgery
- taste changes

Help for Nausea/Vomiting

- Encourage the patient to take prescribed antinausea medication.
- Fix the patient frequent light meals throughout the day.
- Serve the patient's foods cool or at room temperature.

- Avoid fried foods, dairy products, and acidic foods such as citrus fruits, citrus juice, and vinegar.
- Stay away from spicy foods; stick to bland foods such as dry crackers.
- Make sure the patient's mouth is kept clean.
- Offer chewing gum or hard candy.
- Take the patient outside or open a window for fresh air.
- Encourage rest and relaxation.
- Make sure the patient drinks enough clear liquids, sipped slowly, to prevent dehydration.
- Avoid unpleasant or strong odors.
- Distract the patient with music, television, or other activities.

Call the doctor about nausea and vomiting:

- if there is blood or material that looks like coffee grounds in the vomit
- if vomit shoots out for a distance (projectile vomiting)
- if two doses of prescribed medications are not taken or kept down because of nausea or vomiting
- if the patient cannot keep liquids or food down
- if weakness or dizziness occur
- if severe stomach pains occur with vomiting

Help for Constipation

- Discuss the use of laxatives and stool softeners with the doctor and follow a regular schedule as directed.
- If the doctor agrees, give the patient foods high in fiber (whole grain cereal and bread, dried fruit, nuts, beans, and raw fruits and vegetables).
- Make sure the patient drinks enough liquids (up to 6–8 glasses per day).
- Offer the patient prune juice, hot lemon water, tea, or coffee which may stimulate the bowels.
- Encourage daily exercise, such as walking (in keeping with the doctor's advice).

Call the doctor about constipation:

- if the patient has not had a bowel movement in many days
- if constipation occurs with severe abdominal pain
- if constipation worsens and is followed by vomiting

Help for Diarrhea

- Give the patient medicine for diarrhea as directed by the doctor.
- Replace lost fluids and nutrients by offering clear liquids (clear juices, water, broth), often and between meals (2–3 quarts per day).
- Serve the patient foods low in fiber and high in potassium and protein (eggs, bananas, applesauce, mashed potatoes, rice, and dry toast).
- Serve many small meals throughout the day rather than three big meals.
- Avoid serving foods that may increase bloating (vegetables, beans, fruits).
- Avoid serving fatty or acidic foods (fatty meat, fried food, spicy food).
- Limit the patient's caffeine intake (coffee, tea, soda with caffeine, and chocolate).
- Avoid serving dairy or milk products.

Call the doctor about diarrhea:

- if the patient is losing a lot of fluid from severe diarrhea
- if there is blood in the diarrhea
- if diarrhea is oily in the toilet
- if there is a fever
- if the patient does not drink any liquids for more than two days

Helping Loss of Appetite/Weight Loss

- Do not force-feed the patient.
- Do not get angry if the patient does not want to eat.
- Prepare familiar, favorite foods.
- Try light exercise or walking before meals.

- Encourage eating meals at the table with others.
- Serve meals over a prolonged period of time in a relaxed environment.
- Serve meals on smaller plates with smaller servings more frequently.
- Cover up unpleasant odors.
- Serve a glass of wine before meals to stimulate appetite (as per the doctor's advice).
- Offer frequent high protein, high calorie snacks (pudding, ice cream, milk shakes).
- Try new spices or flavorings for foods.
- Prevent early feelings of fullness by: serving beverages between meals, not with meals; eating slowly; and avoiding too many vegetables and carbonated drinks.

Call the doctor about appetite/weight loss:

- if the patient reduces normal food intake for a long time
- if the patient loses five pounds or more in a short time
- if there is pain with chewing and/or swallowing
- if the patient experiences dizziness upon standing
- if the patient does not urinate for an entire day, or does not move the bowels for many days

Skin Problems

There are a number of skin symptoms that can accompany cancer, AIDS, sickle cell disease, and other illnesses. Such skin problems include dryness, rash, itching, sores, ulcers, and swelling. It is important for you to be aware of skin problems so that they can be treated as quickly as possible in order to reduce discomfort and the risk of infection.

Pressure Sores: Blisters or breaks in the skin caused when the body's weight stops the flow of blood to a certain area, causing a breakdown in the skin. Pressure sores are most likely to affect patients who are bedridden, underweight, malnourished, or dehydrated and usually occur in bony areas, such as the head, elbows, heels, hips, shoulders, and tailbone. Sores are made worse when the patient rubs against his/her sheets. Signs and symptoms of pressure sores include:

- red areas on the skin that do not go away when pressure is removed
- cracked, blistered, scaly, or broken skin
- an open sore on the skin's surface or invading deeper, underlying tissue
- yellowish stains on clothing or sheets
- pain at pressure points

Ulcers: Crater-like lesions on the skin which are usually caused by inflammation or infection of the area, or an underlying condition that may affect the skin's ability to heal.

Edema: Swelling of the skin that is caused by water and salt retention. Can occur from certain medications; heart, liver, or kidney failure; malnutrition; and obstruction of veins or lymph nodes. Signs and symptoms of edema include:

- swelling of feet and lower legs when sitting in a chair or walking
- tightness in the hands when making a fist
- swollen or distended abdomen

Itching: The desire to rub or scratch the skin that can be the result of dryness, allergies, and side effects of medications or treatments.

Rash: Bumpy, red, itchy skin commonly caused by an allergy, irritation, radiation therapy, or certain infections.

Dryness: Rough, flaky, red, sometimes painful skin due to a lack of water or oil in the skin layers that can be caused by dehydration, cold weather, heat, and side effects of treatments (such as chemotherapy and radiation).

To help pressure sores:

- keep skin dry and clean
- check skin daily for pressure sores and other skin irritations
- try to turn a bedridden person every few hours (or as often as possible), alternating positions
- encourage the patient to get out of bed as much as possible

- never leave the patient lying or sitting in wet clothes or bedding
- make sure the bedding is not wrinkled or irritating the patient's skin
- promote a balanced nutritious diet, high in protein (fish, poultry, and dairy products)
- do not open or break blisters
- put dry, clean gauze on any open areas

To help ulcers:

- Keep skin area clean and observe for signs of infection (pain, redness, drainage that looks like pus). Follow treatment instructions from the doctor, which may include wet dressings and topical antibiotics to control infection in open ulcers.

To help with edema:

- keep feet elevated when lying in bed or sitting
- take medication, and restrict fluids or salt intake, as prescribed by the doctor

To help with itching/rash:

- bath the patient with cool water
- add baking soda to bath water
- apply a cool, moist cloth to itchy areas
- wash sheets and towels in a mild laundry soap and change daily
- avoid harsh laundry detergents
- apply medications prescribed by the doctor for skin irritations

To help with dry skin:

- add mineral or baby oil to warm bath water
- apply moisturizers
- make sure the patient drinks 8–10 glasses of water per day
- do not scrub the patient's skin while bathing, and gently pat the skin dry

Call the doctor if:

- you see pressure sores (cracked, scaly, blistered, broken skin)
- a pressure sore is getting larger
- a cut becomes very red, sore, or swollen
- skin gets very rough, red, or painful
- a rash develops or hives appear
- pus comes out of a wound or cut
- severe itching lasts more than a few days
- a rash becomes worse after applying ointment or cream
- swelling spreads up legs or arms
- the patient's belly becomes swollen

Anxiety

Anxiety is a common symptom among patients with a life-threatening disease, sometimes occurring with depression. Characteristics of anxiety include:

- feelings of fear, worry, or apprehension
- additional symptoms, such as tension, restlessness, jitteriness, insomnia, fatigue, distractibility, shortness of breath, numbness, or muscle tension
- long duration (generalized anxiety) or short, intense bouts (panic attacks)

Causes of anxiety can include:

- difficulty adjusting to the illness
- common fears about death, including isolation and separation
- poorly-controlled pain
- side effects of medication
- withdrawal from benzodiazepines or opioids, if these are decreased abruptly
- medical conditions, such as dehydration, electrolyte imbalance, or withdrawal from drugs such as nicotine or alcohol.

Some anxiety is a normal response to the frightening situation facing patients with a life-threatening illness. However, if anxiety begins to cause the patient distress, there are several treatment options including:

- stress management techniques, such as progressive relaxation, guided imagery, and hypnosis
- counseling
- support from family, friends, spiritual leaders, and peers
- control of pain, side effects from medication and other medical conditions, where possible
- medication such as benzodiazepines and other tranquilizers, such as the phenothiazine and haloperidol; antihistamines, especially hydroxyzine; antidepressants; and opioids

Counseling can help patients with a life-threatening disease deal with anxiety by:

- establishing a bond to decrease the patient's sense of isolation
- fostering a sense of self-worth
- correcting misconceptions about the past and present
- integrating the present illness into a continuum of life experience
- emphasizing past strengths
- supporting ways of coping that the patient has used successfully in the past
- helping the patient meet interpersonal goals, such as reconciling differences with a family member or maintaining relationships with friends
- exploring issues of separation, loss, and the unknown that arise when facing death
- addressing practical concerns
- addressing needs of the family and other caregivers

Depression

Depression is common in patients with a life-threatening disease, and often affects members of the patient's family as well. Symptoms of depression can include:

- profound sadness, inability to experience joy

- withdrawal from friends, family, and associates
- dramatic changes in normal behavior patterns of eating, sleep ing, self-care, or interacting with others
- a feeling that everything is hopeless, nothing is enjoyable, and life is not worth living
- feelings of worthlessness and guilt
- thoughts of suicide
- alcohol or other drug use

Depression in patients can be related to:

- loss of the ability to function
- other losses, such as troubling change in body image or problems in intimate relationships
- medications and other medical problems
- pain and other symptoms, such as shortness of breath
- role changes in the family and concerns about being a burden
- limited social and financial support
- spiritual distress

Control of depression is important in alleviating a patient's distress. It can include:

- antidepressant medication
- management of pain and other distressing symptoms
- counseling
- support of spiritual leaders, family, friends, and peers found through support groups
- stress and pain management techniques, such as relaxation, guided imagery, and distraction

Confusion

Confusion is an aspect of delirium, which is common, especially in patients with advanced disease. Patients with a progressive medical disease often develop confusion or drowsiness before death. Delirium can be caused by:

- complications of the disease such as organ failure

- medications
- nutritional deficiencies
- other disorders that affect the brain

Some signs of delirium include:

- memory impairment or confusion
- change in mood
- illusions or hallucinations
- agitation
- disturbance in the sleep/wake cycle
- fluctuating level of consciousness
- disorientation to place, time, and/or person

Management of delirium can include:

- medications (for example, haloperidol, methotrimeprazine, thioridazine, chlorpromazine)
- general support for and communication with the patient and family
- encouraging the family's interaction with the patient
- any treatment that can help reverse the underlying cause

Chapter 10

Palliative Wound Care

Wound care, a form of palliative care, supports the health care needs of dying patients by focusing on alleviating symptoms. Although wound care can be both healing and palliative, it can impair the quality of the end of life for the dying if it is done without proper consideration of the patient's wishes and best interests. Wound care may be optional for dying patients.

The majority of people die from chronic degenerative diseases. As the population ages and the incidence and prevalence of chronic conditions are widespread, patients' needs are increasing in their complexity. Patients referred to palliative and hospice care are quickly becoming debilitated by the nature of their serious or life-threatening illness. Owing to advanced chronic conditions (for example, neurological, cardiac, or respiratory diseases) or malignancies, wound care can complicate care, increase the cost of care, and threaten the quality of life for patients.

In considering problems targeted by nurses in caring for dying patients, wound care is rarely discussed. Because dying patients may have surgical wounds, complicating wounds (for example, pressure ulcers), and malignant wounds, home health care nurses need to understand the critical issues facing patients nearing the end of their lives.

Planning Care: Palliative Care Versus Wound Healing

After patients' diseases are no longer responsive to curative treatment, patients can benefit from palliative or end-of-life care. The goal of palliative care is to promote the quality of life, being supportive by focusing on managing and controlling patients' symptoms to achieve the best possible quality of life for patients and their families, neither hastening nor postponing death. Pain is the most common symptom that is often undertreated, and the one that dying patients fear the most. Although certain aspects of palliative care, specifically comfort care, can be of benefit earlier in the course of illness, end-of-life palliative care enables patients to spend their last days with dignity by having elected care, not care that is forced upon them. Palliative care has a more holistic approach by focusing on the physical (including pain, nausea and vomiting, or dyspnea), psychosocial, and spiritual problems of the dying.

Providing wound care, although it is often curative, is also palliative. It may seem contradictory, but patients nearing the end of their lives may benefit from the curative aspects of wound care. Wound care may lead to wound healing, even among the dying. Physiologically, prior to a patient's death, body systems begin to shut down usually over a period of 10 to 14 days or within 24 hours and blood circulation slows down. In some instances, the wound will heal in the weeks or days preceding death. Although wound healing may be thwarted by the physiology of the terminally ill, poor wound care and management of symptoms can be responsible for patient discomfort and can have a devastating effect on patients' quality of dying.

When patients enter the last months, weeks, and days of their lives, the quality of their lives needs to be understood from the patient's subjective perspective in the context of the broader elements of their physical, functional, emotional, and social situations. Dying patients are generally weak and dependent on the care from others, often finding their ability to perform everyday functions impaired. Patients can often feel split between who they are and their illness. When possible, promoting self-care rather than having others perform all dressing changes or having others perform all essential activities of daily living can improve a patient's sense of dignity and wholeness and quality of life while dying.

Ethical Obligations and Patients' Rights

According to the principles of autonomy (or self-determination), providers and patients have an interdependent, shared decision-making relationship that is conducive to enabling patients' self-determination. Providers share their clinical knowledge and expertise, treatment recommendations, and values, and patients use their experience, perceptions, and values.

Legally, patients are considered competent to make decisions when they are informed and able to understand the facts; are able to make rational treatment decisions and understand their implications; and can communicate their choices. Clinicians must respect and not unduly pressure patients when they request withholding or withdrawal of treatment, even refusing some or all treatments. Yet when the patient is not competent, the best interest of the patient must then be considered by clinicians and the patient's loved ones; they are challenged to balance potential benefits with previously expressed wishes, if known.

Since the passage of the Patient Self-Determination Act, patients have legal rights to make health care decisions. Some patients have made advanced autonomous choices about their care at the end of life. These advanced directives or living wills, including do-not-resuscitate orders, are intended to reduce aggressive interventions. However, research has found that when patients have advanced directives, they are more likely to have more invasive and expensive care than patients without an advanced directive thus illustrating that their prior wishes are ignored, primarily after the patient becomes incompetent.

Care for dying patients with wounds consists of:

- Care that should be provided.
- Care that should not be provided.
- Care that can be considered optional.

Health care providers together with patients (and their families) should make decisions on the merits of a particular intervention or treatment. Determining whether a specific aspect of wound care is to be provided hinges on balancing benefits with burdens (including harms and risks). In all cases, patients' choices must be respected. However, if the patient is not competent and there are no advanced directives, then the intervention would be considered obligatory and should be provided. For example, treatment measures to relieve distressing symptoms, such as pain associated with a wound, should be provided.

Conversely, treatment should not be provided if:

- The competent patient refuses the treatment.

- The treatment is considered futile or clinically inappropriate if the treatment will not fulfill its purpose when the patient is imminently dying.

- The burden of treatment outweighs potential benefits.

If a clinician makes the decision to not treat on the basis of their knowledge and experience and considers the burdens to outweigh the benefits, then they may be justified in not offering the treatment.

In most instances, the balance of benefits to burdens is not clear in either direction, meaning that such interventions are considered optional. Part of the challenge in providing care is that predictions of life expectancies of the terminally ill are imprecise. As a result, palliative care for the dying may never be given, and patients may receive care that offers no benefit. Interventions such as antibiotics and wound irrigation would then be considered optional. Making the decision for or against optional interventions according to the merits of a particular intervention needs to be made jointly by health care providers and their patients (and their families). Although clinicians may feel obligated to continue life-sustaining treatments or reluctant to withdraw these interventions, nurses are obligated to represent and advocate for the best interests of the patient.

Nurses need to be effective advocates for dying patients to achieve what the Institute of Medicine (IOM) defines as a "decent and good death—one that is free from avoidable distress and suffering for patients, families, and caregivers; in general accord with patients' and families' wishes; and reasonably consistent with clinical, cultural, and ethical standards." As a patient's illness progresses and death nears, the goals of care, including wound care, may change by shifting from cure to comfort and from life extension to preserving dignity. Although there is no legal distinction between withdrawing or withholding treatment, not providing treatment to aid wound healing or ending wound treatment may be not only what the patient wants, but what can or should be done for the patient to be free from pain and other distressing symptoms before they die.

Transitioning from Home Health Care to Hospice and End-of-Life Care

Home health care nurses are challenged to care for patients that will be transitioning to hospice care or whose needs should have necessitated referral to hospice. Hospice and end-of-life care generally include palliative care at home, except for those who live alone or do not have a family member who can provide support and assistance. The philosophy behind hospice care is to assist patients and their families in achieving the best quality of life and to die peacefully and comfortably with dignity. One of the goals of hospice care is enhancing the quality of life through comfort care, not curative treatment. This includes management of pain and physical symptoms.

Efforts to improve end-of-life care through the timely referral to and use of hospice and palliative care are sometimes challenged by physicians' understanding what hospice care is and attitudes toward care of the dying. One of the most common reasons patients do not benefit from hospice care is that they die before they can make that transition. Even though decisions regarding when to transition to hospice may come only a few days before the patient dies, the patient's needs must be accurately assessed and conveyed.

Transitions from home health care to hospice are the time when patient safety issues are of more concern than when the person is in one setting or the other. It is the time when medication errors and patient treatment protocol errors are most likely to occur. Transferring patients requires expert communication between the nurses from each agency (or within an agency if the agency has both traditional home care and hospice care). For example, because many older adults take multiple medications (an average of five), they are at a higher risk for medication errors. If they slip (in patient safety language) and do not tell the hospice nurse about the medications, or if the home health nurse slips and does not tell the hospice nurse about the medications that the patient is taking, it is a medical error. Although the nurse intended to do the correct thing, the slip may have occurred because of system errors that have the nurse doing too many things at the same time.

In addition, communication between the hospice nurse and physician offers the potential for other communication errors. Careful consideration should be given to the mode of communication. Although the physician will eventually provide a written order form for hospice care, the transfer occurs between the nurses based on verbal communication with the physician. To decrease the chance of error from communication slips, communication should be written and verified by repeating back all verbal orders.

The goals of care in home care compared to hospice differ. Clinicians need to effectively communicate with the patient, family, and other caregivers as the transition to hospice and different care goals are made. In home health care, nurses focus on wound treatment, healing, and the use of medication therapies. In hospice care, nurses focus on the primary goal of symptom management, especially the relief from pain and less on what becomes the secondary need of wound treatment and healing. Pain management can be complicated by concerns of oversedation and untoward effects of medication which can result in the under treatment of pain. Since the goals of care change, hospice nurses should discuss the patient's care needs, including wound care, with physicians and specify how they differ from the former home health care needs.

Wound Care Treatment in Home Care Compared to Hospice

Issue of Comfort Verses Healing

Dying patients with existing wounds are at risk of wounds not healing, beginning, and/or becoming larger. The skin of dying patients can be fragile and sensitive and is subsequently at risk of being compromised from wound exudates, body fluids, pressure, and friction. Given the underlying life-threatening condition, wounds and the nature of pain associated with the wound should also be fully assessed and described. Patients should have an individualized, systematic approach to assessment, planning, treatment, and evaluation of their wounds in the context of their life-threatening illness.

Nurses are critical to assessing each patient's physiologic, psychosocial, and environmental factors with particular emphasis on impairments of the skin's integrity and potential for infection. A detailed assessment would include physical characteristics (size, location, and condition of surrounding tissue); risk factors (immobility, malnutrition, incontinence); and the effects of the wound on the patient's quality of life and on their family. The nurses' goals are to preserve and maintain the skin's integrity, prevent further deterioration of existing wounds, and to provide care that the patient would want to have. Some patients may not choose these goals.

Terminally ill patients often have compromised mobility, malnutrition and dehydration, functional incontinence, and in some instances, advanced age thereby making them particularly susceptible to developing pressure ulcers. The prevention and management of pressure ulcers for terminally ill patients is not only a clinical issue but an emotional and ethical issue as well. Pressure ulcers are painful causing suffering and complicating the care and quality of life for the dying. Contrary to the prevailing belief that pressure ulcers should be preventable even at the end of life, some research suggests that skin, the largest organ in the human body, begins to fail along with the other organ systems and such prevention is not possible.

Evidence suggests that even in the presence of aggressive preventive measures critically ill individuals will have alterations in tissue perfusion, immune functioning, and coagulation which compromise muscle cells and the overall healing response. In fact, pressure ulcer formation may be a visual biomarker that the critical illness has totally overwhelmed the body and that skin breakdown is neither preventable nor treatable.

As the current controversy regarding the contributing factors to pressure ulcer formation continues, wound care standards will depend on whether interventions should be focused on prevention, treatment, or palliation. Skin barriers, not adhesives, should be used for vulnerable skin to provide a protective film on or barrier for the unaffected skin. Yet, the exact treatment protocols and methods for treating wounds of the dying are not necessarily standardized. Part of the reason for the debate surrounding a recognized standard of wound care for dying patients is that there is little research on the factors that contribute to skin breakdown in this population.

Emotional concerns for family members of terminally ill patients surface because they can view pressure ulcer formation as a failure on the part of the health care staff caring for the patient, or even as their own failing if they are responsible for providing care. Hospice staff may feel that turning a patient frequently may contribute to an increase in pain, so standard preventive measures such as turning a patient every two hours may be suspended. Eisenberger and Zeleznik reported in 2003 that when patients experienced a single position of comfort—that is, when patients are more comfortable in a particular position due to advanced illness—overall comfort becomes of greater importance. In fact, some staff felt that prevention and treatment could potentially compromise the overall hospice philosophy of providing comfort care.

Often, clinicians have to strike a balance between the patient's quality of life and administering opioids. Although they relieve pain which often increases functional ability, they can decrease the patient's mental status thereby leading to a decrease in activity level which contributes to pressure ulcer formation. Additionally, when pressure ulcers are considered to be inevitable or have a small chance of healing, the goals of care can shift from prevention and treatment toward palliation and managing pressure ulcer pain and odor.

Wound and Skin Care in the Terminally Ill Cancer Patient

Terminally ill cancer patients are at risk for a number of dermatologic and mucous membrane alterations. The specific skin problems include ulcerating or fungating cutaneous metastasis, pressure ulcers, stomas and fistulas, peripheral edema, lymphedema, and pruritus. Among these problems, peripheral edema and lymphedema account for the largest proportion of skin problems in this population. Oral complications include xerostomia, oral mucositis, taste abnormalities, and halitosis.

For both skin and oral mucosal problems, pain is the major symptom afflicting terminally ill cancer patients. If not adequately managed, patients can develop severe emotional distress coupled with feelings of isolation and helplessness. In addition, patients are at risk for systemic infections, malnutrition, dehydration, and bleeding. Adequate support and teaching of family members to provide much of this care is critical to ensuring high quality care at the end of life.

The management of pressure ulcers in the terminally ill cancer patient is no different than for other terminally ill patients. A two-pronged approach, including pharmacotherapy and physical therapy, are keys to managing peripheral edema and lymphedema. Pharmacologic approaches include diuretics such as furosemide and spironolactone, and corticosteroids. A comprehensive nursing therapy program includes meticulous skin care, protecting the limb from trauma, use of compression bandages, lymphatic massage, and range-of-motion exercises. The nurse can teach these activities to family members.

Management of oral mucosa complications poses a number of challenges to family members and health care providers. With the onset of pain and xerostomia, patients often become anorexic and ultimately cachectic. Both topical and systemic analgesic treatment approaches are needed for adequate pain relief. Topical approaches include single agents such as lidocaine, benzydamine, and sucralfate, and combinations of agents such as milk of magnesia and diphenhydramine. Traditional general measures for the prevention and treatment of oral mucositis that have been employed for a number of decades remain the hallmark of care. These include serving bland, moist food at room temperature; performing regular mouth care; and using a soft toothbrush and mild solutions every four hours around the clock.

Managing skin alterations, both externally and orally, is important to relieving the pain and suffering that terminally ill cancer patients often experience. Evidence-based guidelines are very limited for these two problems, and more research is needed to discover the underlying mechanisms and novel therapies to alleviate the associated symptoms.

Chapter 11

Acute Respiratory Distress Syndrome

Acute respiratory distress syndrome (ARDS) is breathing failure that can occur in critically ill persons with underlying illnesses. It is not a specific disease. Instead, it is a life-threatening condition that occurs when there is severe fluid buildup in both lungs. The fluid buildup prevents the lungs from working properly—that is, allowing the transfer of oxygen from air into the body and carbon dioxide out of the body into the air.

In ARDS, the tiny blood vessels (capillaries) in the lungs or the air sacs (alveoli) are damaged because of an infection, injury, blood loss, or inhalation injury. Fluid leaks from the blood vessels into air sacs of the lungs. While some air sacs fill with fluid, others collapse. When the air sacs collapse or fill up with fluid, the lungs can no longer fill properly with air and the lungs become stiff. Without air entering the lungs properly, the amount of oxygen in the blood drops. When this happens, the person with ARDS must be given extra oxygen and may need the help of a breathing machine.

Breathing failure can occur very quickly after the condition begins. It may take only a day or two for fluid to build up. The process that causes ARDS may continue for weeks. If scarring occurs, this will make it harder for the lungs to take in oxygen and get rid of carbon dioxide.

In the past, only about four out of ten people who developed ARDS survived. But today, with good care in a hospital's intensive or critical

Excerpted from "ARDS (Acute Respiratory Distress Syndrome)," National Heart, Lung, and Blood Institute (NHLBI), August 2003.

care unit, many people (about seven out of ten) with ARDS survive. Although many people who survive ARDS make a full recovery, some survivors have lasting damage to their lungs.

Effects of ARDS

In ARDS, tiny blood vessels leak too much fluid into the lung. This results from toxins (poisons) that the body produces in response to the underlying illness or injury. The lungs become like a wet sponge, heavy and stiffer than normal. They no longer provide the effective surface for gas exchange, and the level of oxygen in the blood falls. If ARDS is severe and goes on for some time, scar tissue called fibrosis may form in the lungs. The scarring also makes it harder for gas exchange to occur.

People who develop ARDS need extra oxygen and may need a breathing machine to breathe for them while their lungs try to heal. If they survive, ARDS patients may have a full recovery. Recovery can take weeks or months. Some ARDS survivors take a year or longer to recover, and some never completely recover from having ARDS.

Other names for ARDS include:

- adult respiratory distress syndrome (ARDS)
- stiff lung
- shock lung
- wet lung

There is a similar condition in infants called infant respiratory distress syndrome (IRDS, RDS, and hyaline membrane disease). It mainly affects premature infants whose lungs are not well-developed when they are born.

What Causes ARDS?

The causes of ARDS are not well understood. It can occur in many situations and in persons with or without a lung disease. There are two ways that lung injury leading to ARDS can occur: through a direct injury to the lungs, or indirectly when a person is very sick or has a serious bodily injury. However, most sick or badly injured persons do not develop ARDS.

Direct lung injury. A direct injury to the lungs may result from breathing in harmful substances or an infection in the lungs. Some direct lung injuries that can lead to ARDS include:

- severe pneumonia (infection in the lungs)
- breathing in vomited stomach contents
- breathing in harmful fumes or smoke
- a severe blow to the chest or other accident that bruises the lungs

Indirect lung injury. Most cases of ARDS happen in people who are very ill or who have been in a major accident. This is sometimes called an indirect lung injury. Less is known about how indirect injuries lead to ARDS than about how direct injuries to the lungs cause ARDS. Indirect lung injury leading to ARDS sometimes occurs in cases of:

- severe and widespread bacterial infection in the body (sepsis)
- severe injury with shock
- severe bleeding requiring blood transfusions
- drug overdose
- inflamed pancreas

It is not clear why some very sick or seriously injured people develop ARDS, and others do not.

Who Gets ARDS?

ARDS usually affects people who are being treated for another serious illness or those who have had major injuries. It affects about 150,000 people each year in the United States. ARDS can occur in people with or without a previous lung disease. People who have a serious accident with a large blood loss are more likely to develop ARDS. However, only a small portion of people who have problems that can lead to ARDS actually develop it.

In most cases, a person who develops ARDS is already in the hospital, being treated for other medical problems. Some illnesses or injuries that can lead to ARDS include:

- serious, widespread infection in the body (sepsis)
- severe injury (trauma) and shock from a car crash, fire, or other cause
- severe bleeding that requires blood transfusions
- severe pneumonia (infection of the lungs)

- breathing in vomited stomach contents
- breathing in smoke or harmful gases and fumes
- injury to the chest from trauma (such as a car accident) that causes bruising of the lungs
- nearly drowning
- some drug overdoses

Signs and Symptoms of ARDS

The major signs and symptoms of ARDS are:

- shortness of breath
- fast, labored breathing
- a bluish skin color (due to a low level of oxygen in the blood)
- lower amount of oxygen in the blood

Doctors and other health care providers watch for these signs and symptoms in patients who have conditions that might lead to ARDS. People who develop ARDS may be too sick to complain about having trouble breathing or other related symptoms. If a patient shows signs of developing ARDS, doctors will do tests to confirm that ARDS is the problem.

ARDS is often associated with the failure of other organs and body systems. They include the liver, kidneys, and the immune system. Multiple organ failure often leads to death.

How Is ARDS Diagnosed?

Doctors diagnose ARDS when:

- A person suffering from severe infection or injury develops breathing problems.
- A chest x-ray shows fluid in the air sacs of both lungs.
- Blood tests show a low level of oxygen in the blood.
- Other conditions that could cause breathing problems have been ruled out.

ARDS can be confused with other illnesses that have similar symptoms. The most important is congestive heart failure. In congestive heart failure, fluid backs up into the lungs because the heart is weak and cannot pump well. However, there is no injury to the lungs in congestive heart failure. Since a chest x-ray is abnormal for both ARDS and congestive heart failure, it is sometimes very difficult to tell them apart.

How Is ARDS Treated?

Patients with ARDS are usually treated in the intensive or critical care unit of a hospital. The main concern in treating ARDS is getting enough oxygen into the blood until the lungs heal enough to work on their own again. Following are important ways that ARDS patients are treated.

Extra oxygen. The main treatment is giving a higher concentration of oxygen than that found in normal air, enough to raise blood levels of oxygen to safe levels. At first, this can sometimes be done with a face mask. A face mask can deliver oxygen at a concentration of 40–60 percent. As the ARDS progresses over hours or days, the patient may need a higher level of oxygen than a face mask can give.

As the patient becomes tired from breathing so hard, it may become necessary to connect the patient a breathing machine (ventilator). This can be done by placing a tube through the mouth or nose into the windpipe (trachea) in a procedure called endotracheal intubation (or just intubation) and connecting the tube to the ventilator. Sometimes the connecting tube is inserted through a surgical opening in the neck (tracheotomy). The breathing machine can be set to help or completely control breathing. It will deliver the minimum amount of air every minute. If the extra oxygen and help with breathing are not enough, the breathing machine can be set to positive end-expiratory pressure (PEEP) to maintain the surface for gas exchange.

PEEP keeps some air in the lungs at the end of each breath. It helps keep the air sacs open instead of collapsing. The setting can be adjusted to fit the needs of the patient. There are other settings on the ventilator that control the number of breaths per minute (rate control) and the amount of air the ventilator uses to inflate the lungs in each breath (tidal volume).

Medicines. Many different kinds of medicines are used to treat ARDS patients. Some kinds of medicines used include:

- antibiotics to fight infection
- pain relievers

- drugs to relieve anxiety and keep the patient calm and from fighting the breathing machine

- drugs to raise blood pressure or stimulate the heart

- muscle relaxers to prevent movement and reduce the body's demand for oxygen

Other treatment. With breathing tubes in place, ARDS patients cannot eat or drink as usual. They must be fed through a feeding tube placed through the nose and into the stomach. If this does not work, feeding is done through a vein. Sometimes a special bed or mattress, such as an air bed, is used to help prevent complications such as pneumonia or bedsores. If complications occur, the patient may require treatment for them.

Results (with treatment):

- Some patients recover quickly and can breathe on their own within a week or so. They have the best chance of a full recovery.

- Patients whose underlying illness is more severe may die within the first week of treatment.

- Those who survive the first week but cannot breathe on their own may face many weeks on the breathing machine. They may have complications and a slow recovery if they survive.

Recovering from ARDS

Some people who survive ARDS heal quickly and recover completely in a relatively short time. Some are able to have the breathing tube and breathing machine removed in a week or so. Survivors often recover much of their lung function in the first 3–6 months after leaving the hospital and continue to recover for up to a year or more.

Other people recover more slowly. Some ARDS survivors never recover completely and have continuing problems with their lungs. Every case is different. People who are younger and healthier when they develop ARDS are more likely to recover quickly than those who are older or who have more health problems.

ARDS patients who survive the first week but cannot breathe on their own may have to be on a breathing machine for several weeks or longer. These patients often develop complications such as infections or air leaks. While some of these patients will die, others will get better and be able to breathe on their own again. Their recovery is usually slow, and they may have continuing problems.

After leaving the hospital, ARDS survivors need to visit a doctor during recovery to check how well their lungs are doing. Doctors use lung function tests to check the lungs. Spirometry is the most commonly used lung function test. It involves taking a deep breath and blowing hard into a plastic tube. The doctor will also do an oxygen saturation (oximetry) test or a blood test to check the amount of oxygen in the blood.

After going home from the hospital, the ARDS survivor may need only a little or a lot of help. While recovering from ARDS at home, a person may:

- need to use oxygen at home or when going out of the home, at least for a while;

- need to have physical, occupational, or other therapy;

- have shortness of breath, cough, or phlegm (mucus);

- have hoarseness from the breathing tube in the hospital;

- feel tired and not have much energy;

- have muscle weakness.

Complications of ARDS

Anyone who stays in the hospital for a long time can get complications. Common complications in ARDS patients are infections with hospital-acquired bacteria and leaks of air out of the lungs into other body spaces.

- **Bacterial infections.** The lungs or other parts of the body may become infected. These infections are usually treated with antibiotics after a test to see what kind of bacteria is causing the infection.

- **Air leaks.** Leaks of air through holes in the lungs are caused by pressure from the breathing machine that is needed to be sure the patient gets enough air and from the very stiff lungs. Air from the injured lungs may enter the space between the lungs and the lining around the lungs (the pleura) and cause a pneumothorax (collapsed lung). Treatment involves using a chest tube and suction to remove the air and help the lungs reinflate. Air may also enter the space between the membranes that line the abdomen (pneumoperitoneum) or the soft tissue under the skin (subcutaneous emphysema). These are not usually treated.

Each complication is treated as it arises. Careful hand washing by hospital staff and visitors helps reduce infections, and new breathing machine methods help reduce air leaks.

Chapter 12

Artificial Hydration and Nutrition

When do people need artificial hydration and nutrition?

If a patient isn't able to swallow because of a medical problem, he or she can be given fluids and nutrition in ways other than by mouth. This is referred to as artificial hydration and nutrition. This is sometimes done when someone is recovering from a temporary problem. It may also be done when someone has an advanced, life-threatening illness and is dying.

What is involved in artificial nutrition and hydration?

An intravenous (IV) catheter (a thin plastic tube that slides in over a needle) may be placed in the vein under the patient's skin. Fluids and sometimes nutrition are given through the catheter.

Another method of artificial nutrition and hydration is through a plastic tube called a nasogastric tube (also called an NG tube). This tube is put through the nose, down the throat, and into the stomach. It can only be left in for a short time, usually one to four weeks. If the tube has to be in longer, a different kind of feeding tube may be used. It is placed into the wall of the stomach (also called a PEG tube or g-tube).

What happens if artificial hydration or nutrition are not given?

Persons who don't receive any food or fluids will eventually fall into a deep sleep (coma) and usually die in one to three weeks.

What are the benefits?

A person with a temporary illness who cannot swallow may be hungry and thirsty. A feeding tube may help. Sometimes a person may become confused because of dehydration. Dehydration is when the body does not get enough fluids. Giving a patient fluids through a tube helps dehydration and may lessen his or her confusion. Giving fluids and nutrition helps the patient as he or she is recovering. For a patient with an advanced, life-threatening illness who is dying, artificial hydration and nutrition may not provide many benefits. Artificial hydration and nutrition in these patients may make the patient live a little longer, but not always.

What are the risks?

There is always a risk when someone is fed through a tube. Liquid might enter the lungs. This can cause coughing and pneumonia. Feeding tubes may feel uncomfortable. They can become plugged up, causing pain, nausea, and vomiting. Feeding tubes may also cause infections. Sometimes, patients may need to be physically restrained or sedated to keep them from pulling out the feeding tube.

How do we decide whether to use artificial hydration and nutrition?

The patient and his or her family should talk with the doctor about the patient's medical condition and risks and benefits of giving artificial hydration and nutrition. Each situation is different. Your doctor can help you make the decision that is right for the patient and family.

Chapter 13

Nutrition Therapy in Cancer Care

Nutrition Screening and Assessment

Screening is used to identify patients who may be at nutritional risk. Assessment determines the complete nutritional status of the patient and identifies if nutrition therapy is needed. The patient or caregiver may be asked for the following information:

- Weight changes the patient has experienced over the past six months.

- Changes in the amount and type of food eaten compared to what is usual for the patient.

- Problems that have affected eating, such as nausea, vomiting, diarrhea, constipation, dry mouth, changes in taste and smell, mouth sores, pain, or loss of appetite.

- Ability patient has to walk and perform the activities of daily living.

A physical exam is part of the assessment. The physical exam will check the body for general health and signs of disease, such as lumps or growths. The physician will look for loss of weight, fat, muscle, and fluid buildup in the body. Ongoing assessment is completed by a

Excerpts from "Nutrition in Cancer Care PDQ®: Supportive Care–Patient," PDQ® Cancer Information Summary, National Cancer Institute, Bethesda, MD, updated December 2005, available at http://cancer.gov. Accessed March 1, 2006.

healthcare team with expertise in nutritional management. A nutrition support team will monitor the patient's nutritional status during cancer treatment and recovery. The team may include a physician, nurse, registered dietitian, social worker, and psychologist.

Goals of Nutrition Therapy

The goals of nutrition therapy for patients who have advanced cancer are designed to improve the quality of life. The goals of nutrition therapy for patients who have advanced cancer are to do the following:

- reduce side effects
- reduce risk of infection
- maintain strength and energy
- improve quality of life

Methods of Nutrition Care

Nutrition support provides nutrition to patients who cannot eat normally. Eating by mouth is the preferred method and should be used whenever possible, but some patients may not be able to take any or enough food by mouth due to complications from cancer or cancer treatment. A patient may be fed using enteral nutrition (through a tube inserted into the stomach or (intestine) or parenteral nutrition infused into the bloodstream directly). The nutrients are delivered in formulas—liquids that contain water, protein, fats, carbohydrates, vitamins, and/or minerals. The content of the formula depends on the needs of the patient and the method of feeding.

Nutritional support can improve a patient's quality of life during cancer, but there are risks and disadvantages that should be considered before making the decision to use it. The effect of nutritional support on tumor growth is not known. Also, each form of nutrition therapy has its own benefits and disadvantages. For example, enteral nutrition keeps the stomach and intestines working normally and has fewer complications than parenteral nutrition; nutrients are used more easily by the body in enteral feeding. These and other issues should be discussed with the patient's health care providers so that an informed decision can be made.

Patients with certain conditions are most appropriate for treatment with nutrition support. Nutrition support may be helpful for patients who have one or more of the following characteristics:

- low body weight
- inability to absorb nutrients
- holes or draining abscesses in the esophagus or stomach
- inability to eat or drink by mouth for more than five days
- moderate or high nutritional risk
- ability, along with the caregiver, to handle tube feedings at home

Advanced Cancer

Nutrition-related side effects may occur or become worse as cancer becomes more advanced. The most common nutrition-related symptoms in patients who have advanced cancer are:

- cachexia (a wasting syndrome that causes weakness and a loss of weight, fat, and muscle)
- weight loss of more than 10% of normal body weight
- feeling too full to eat enough food
- bloating
- anorexia (the loss of appetite or desire to eat)
- constipation
- dry mouth
- taste changes
- nausea
- vomiting
- inability to swallow

The usual treatment for these problems in patients with advanced cancer is palliative care to reduce the symptoms and improve the quality of life. Palliative care includes nutrition therapy and/or drug therapy.

Eating less solid food is common in advanced cancer. Patients usually prefer soft foods and clear liquids. Those who have problems swallowing may do better with thick liquids than with thin liquids. Terminally ill patients often do not feel much hunger at all and may be satisfied with very little food.

When cancer is advanced, food should be viewed as a source of enjoyment. Eating should not just be about calories, protein, and other nutrient needs.

Dietary restriction is not usually necessary, as intake of prohibited foods (such as sweets for a patient with diabetes) is not enough to be of concern. Some patients, however, may need certain diet restrictions. For example, patients who have pancreatic cancer, uterine cancer, ovarian cancer, or another cancer affecting the abdominal area may need a soft diet (no raw fruits and vegetables, no nuts, no skins, no seeds) to prevent a blockage in the bowel. Diet restrictions should be considered in terms of quality of life and the patient's wishes. The benefits and risks of nutrition support vary for each patient.

Decisions about using nutrition support should be made with the following considerations:

- Will quality of life be improved?

- Do the possible benefits outweigh the risks and costs?

- Is there an advanced directive? An advanced directive is a written instruction about the provision of health care or power of attorney in the event an individual can no longer make his or her wishes known.

- What are the wishes and needs of the family?

Cancer patients and their caregivers have the right to make informed decisions. The healthcare team, with guidance from a registered dietitian, should inform patients and their caregivers about the benefits and risks of using nutrition support in advanced disease. In most cases, the risks outweigh the benefits. However, for someone who still has good quality of life but also physical barriers to achieving adequate food and water by mouth, enteral feedings may be appropriate. Parenteral support is not usually appropriate.

Advantages of eternal nutrition are that it may:

- improve alertness

- provide comfort to the family

- decrease nausea

- decrease hopelessness and fears of abandonment

Disadvantages of enteral nutrition are that it:

- may cause diarrhea or constipation

- may increase nausea

- requires surgery for the placement of a tube through the abdomen

- increases risk of choking or pneumonia
- increases risk of infection
- creates a greater burden on the caregiver

Additional Information

National Cancer Institute (NCI)
6116 Executive Blvd.
Suite 3036A, MSC 8322
Bethesda, MD 20892-8322
Toll-Free: 800-4-CANCER (800-422-6237)
Toll-Free TTY: 800-332-8615
Website: http://www.cancer.gov
E-mail: cancergovstaff@mail.nih.gov

Chapter 14

Cognitive Disorders and Delirium

Cognitive disorders and delirium are conditions in which the patient experiences a confused mental state and changes in behavior. People who have cognitive disorders or delirium may fall in and out of consciousness and may have problems with the following:

- attention
- thinking
- awareness
- emotion
- memory
- muscle control
- sleeping and waking

Delirium occurs frequently in cancer patients, especially in patients with advanced cancer. Delirium usually occurs suddenly and the patient's symptoms may come and go during the day. This condition can be treated and is often temporary, even in people with advanced illness. In the last 24 to 48 hours of life, however, delirium may be permanent due to problems such as organ failure.

Excerpts from "Cognitive Disorders and Delirium PDQ®: Supportive Care–Patient," PDQ® Cancer Information Summary, National Cancer Institute, Bethesda, MD, updated November 2005, available at http://cancer.gov. Accessed March 1, 2006.

Causes of Cognitive Disorders and Delirium

Cognitive disorders and delirium may be complications of cancer and cancer treatment, especially in people with advanced cancer. In cancer patients, cognitive disorders and delirium may be due to the direct effects that cancer has on the brain, such as the pressure of a growing tumor. Cognitive disorders and delirium may also be caused by indirect effects of cancer or its treatment, including the following:

- Organ failure

- Electrolyte imbalances: Electrolytes are important minerals (including salt, potassium, calcium, and phosphorous) that are needed to keep the heart, kidneys, nerves, and muscles working correctly

- Infection

- Medication side effects: Patients with cancer usually take many medications. Some drugs have side effects that include delirium and confusion. The effects of these drugs usually go away after the drug is stopped

- Withdrawal from drugs that depress (slow down) the central nervous system (brain and spinal cord)

Risk factors for delirium include having a serious disease and having more than one disease. Other conditions besides having cancer may place a patient at risk for developing delirium. Risk factors include the following:

- advanced cancer or other serious illness

- having more than one disease

- older age

- previous mental disorder, such as dementia

- low levels of albumin (protein) in the blood

- infection

- taking medications that affect the mind or behavior

- taking high doses of pain medication

Early identification of risk factors may help prevent the onset of delirium or may reduce the length of time it takes to correct it.

Effects of Cognitive Disorders and Delirium on the Patient, Family, and Healthcare Providers

Cognitive disorders and delirium can be upsetting to the family and caregivers, and may be dangerous to the patient if judgment is affected. These conditions can cause the patient to act unpredictably and sometimes violently. Even a quiet or calm patient can suddenly experience a change in mood or become agitated, requiring increased care. The safety of the patient, family, and caregivers is most important.

Cognitive disorders and delirium may affect physical health and communication. Patients with cognitive disorders or delirium are more likely to fall, be incontinent (unable to control bladder and/or bowels), and become dehydrated (drink too little water to maintain health). They often require a longer hospital stay than patients without cognitive disorders or delirium.

The confused mental state of these patients may hinder their communication with family members and the healthcare providers. Assessment of the patient's symptoms becomes difficult and the patient may be unable to make decisions regarding care. Agitation in these patients may be mistaken as an expression of pain. Conflict can arise among the patient, family, and staff concerning the level of pain medication needed.

Diagnosis of Cognitive Disorders and Delirium

Possible signs of cognitive disorders and delirium include sudden personality changes, impaired thinking, unusual anxiety, or depression. A patient, who suddenly becomes agitated or uncooperative, experiences personality or behavior changes, has impaired thinking, decreased attention span, or intense, unusual anxiety or depression, may be experiencing cognitive disorders or delirium. Patients who develop these symptoms need to be assessed completely.

The symptoms of delirium are similar to symptoms of depression and dementia. Early symptoms of delirium are similar to symptoms of anxiety, anger, depression, and dementia. Delirium that causes the patient to be very inactive may appear to be depression. Delirium and dementia are difficult to tell apart, since both may cause disorientation and impair memory, thinking, and judgment. Dementia may be caused by a number of medical conditions, including Alzheimer disease. Some differences in the symptoms of delirium and dementia include the following:

- Patients with delirium often go in and out of consciousness.
- Patients who have dementia usually remain alert.
- Delirium may occur suddenly. Dementia appears gradually and gets worse over time.
- Sleeping and waking problems are more common with delirium than with dementia.

In elderly patients who have cancer, dementia is often present along with delirium, making diagnosis difficult. The diagnosis is more likely dementia if symptoms continue after treatment for delirium is given. Regular screening of the patient and monitoring of the patient's symptoms can help in the diagnosis of delirium.

Treatment of Delirium

Patient and family concerns are addressed when deciding the treatment of delirium. Deciding if, when, and how to treat a person with delirium depends on the setting, how advanced the cancer is, the wishes of the patient and family, and how the delirium symptoms are affecting the patient.

Monitoring alone may be all that is necessary for patients who are not dangerous to themselves. In other cases, symptoms may be treated or causes of the delirium may be identified and treated.

Controlling the patient's surroundings may help reduce mild symptoms of delirium. The following changes may be effective:

- putting the patient in a quiet, well-lit room with familiar objects
- placing a clock or calendar where the patient can see it
- reducing noise
- having family present
- limiting changes in caregivers

To prevent a patient from harming himself or herself or others, physical restraints also may be necessary.

Medical treatment of delirium may include the following:

- stopping or reducing medications that cause delirium
- giving fluids into the bloodstream to correct dehydration

- giving drugs to correct hypercalcemia (too much calcium in the blood)
- giving antibiotics for infections

Drugs called antipsychotics may be used to treat the symptoms of delirium. Drugs that sedate (calm) the patient may also be used, especially if the patient is near death. All of these drugs have side effects and the patient will be monitored closely by a doctor. The decision to use drugs that sedate the patient will be made in cooperation with family members after efforts have been made to reverse the delirium.

Delirium and Sedation

The decision to use drugs to sedate the patient who is near death and has symptoms of delirium, pain, and difficult breathing presents ethical and legal issues for both the doctor and the family. When the symptoms of delirium are not relieved with standard treatment approaches and the patient is experiencing severe distress and suffering, the doctor may discuss the option to give drugs that will sedate the patient. This decision is guided by the following principles:

- Healthcare professionals who have experience in palliative care make repeated assessments of the patient's response to treatments. The family is always included.
- The need to use drugs that sedate the patient is evaluated by a multidisciplinary team of healthcare professionals.
- Temporary sedation should be considered.
- A multidisciplinary team of healthcare professionals will work with the family to ensure that the family's views are assessed and understood.

Additional Information

National Cancer Institute
6116 Executive Blvd.
Suite 3036A, MSC 8322
Bethesda, MD 20892-8322
Toll-Free: 800-4-CANCER (800-422-6237)
Toll-Free TTY: 800-332-8615
Website: http://www.cancer.gov
E-mail: cancergovstaff@mail.nih.gov

Chapter 15

Clinical Trial Results That Impact End-of-Life Treatments

End-of-Life Care and Outcomes

More than 75 percent of Americans now live past age 65, and 83 percent of Americans now die while covered by Medicare. By 2050, life expectancy for women and men will likely increase to 84 and 80, respectively. A century ago, death came to most Americans suddenly. Today, many Americans live their last years with a chronic health condition, and about 40 million people—15 percent of the adult U.S. population—are limited in activities from such a condition. Population aging patterns suggest that in the coming decades, larger numbers of Americans will be coping with serious impairments late in life.

For the relatively healthy, a care system focused on curing acute intermittent illness is adequate. For persons living with advanced, chronic disease, neither prevention, nor cure is ordinarily possible. Instead, patients and families struggling with serious illness have other concerns including: managing pain and other symptoms; coordinating care among multiple providers and settings; ensuring that treatments reflect preferences and balance benefits and harms as well as medical appropriateness; achieving empathic communication and care; fostering well-being (including spiritual concerns); maintaining

This chapter includes an excerpt from "End-of-Life Care and Outcomes," Agency for Healthcare Research and Quality (AHRQ), December 2004; and excerpts from "Supportive Care Trial Results," National Cancer Institute (NCI), 2006.

121

function; and practically supporting family and caregivers through illness and bereavement.

Scientific evidence supports the association of satisfaction and quality of care with pain management, communication, practical support, and enhanced caregiving in end-of-life care. There are effective end-of-life interventions to improve satisfaction, ameliorate cancer pain, relieve depression in cancer, and non-pharmacologic interventions for behavioral problems in dementia.

Supportive Care Clinical Trial Results

Following are clinical trial results which may impact treatment for symptoms of terminal illnesses.

Surgery Helps Relieve Spinal Cord Compression Caused by Metastatic Cancer: Surgery followed by radiation is more effective than radiation alone in treating spinal cord compression caused by metastatic cancer (updated August 23, 2005).

Methylnaltrexone Relieves Constipation Caused by Pain Medication: Seriously ill patients in hospice or palliative care settings who were constipated from their pain medications got significant relief from the drug methylnaltrexone, according to findings presented at the 2005 meeting of the American Society of Clinical Oncology (June 1, 2005).

Palifermin Reduces Mouth Sores Caused by Cancer Treatment: An experimental drug called palifermin (Kepivance™) reduced both the severity and the duration of sores and ulcers in the mouth in patients who received intensive chemotherapy and radiation to treat lymphoma and other cancers of the blood, according to a report in the December 16, 2004 issue of the *New England Journal of Medicine*.

Implantable Device May Offer Better Pain Management: Patients with advanced cancer who used an implantable drug-delivery device to control their pain had better pain relief, fewer toxic side effects, and better survival than patients who received intensive medical pain management, researchers reported in the October 1, 2002 issue of the *Journal of Clinical Oncology* (reviewed March 23, 2005).

Stress Management Training for Cancer Patients: A self-administered stress management training program did a better job of helping patients cope with the adverse effects of chemotherapy than a one-hour program in which training was given by mental health professionals, according to the June 15, 2002 issue of the *Journal of Clinical Oncology* (reviewed March 23, 2005).

Zoledronic Acid Reduces Bone Complications of Advanced Prostate Cancer: In a study published in the October 2, 2002 issue of the *Journal of the National Cancer Institute*, patients with prostate cancer that had spread to the bones had fewer fractures and other bone complications when they took a new drug, zoledronic acid (also called zoledronate or Zometa®) than when they took a placebo (reviewed March 9, 2005).

Reducing Depression Does Not Reduce Fatigue: Cancer patients often experience both depression and fatigue, and physicians have had good reason to think that relieving depression might also reduce fatigue, but a new large randomized trial has disproved that theory and shifted researchers' attention to other possible strategies to fight cancer-related fatigue (March 23, 2005).

Part Three

Medical Decisions Surrounding the End of LIfe

Chapter 16

Preferences for Care at the End of Life

Patient Preferences Are Often Not Known

Predicting what treatments patients will want at the end of life is complicated by the patient's age, the nature of the illness, the ability of medicine to sustain life, and the emotions families endure when their loved ones are sick and possibly dying. When seriously ill patients are nearing the end of life, they and their families sometimes find it difficult to decide on whether to continue medical treatment, and if so, how much treatment is wanted and for how long. In these instances, patients rely on their physicians or other trusted health professionals for guidance.

In the best of circumstances, the patient, the family, and the physician have held discussions about treatment options including the length and invasiveness of treatment, chance of success, overall prognosis, and the patient's quality of life during and after the treatment. Ideally, these discussions would continue as the patient's condition changed. Frequently, however, such discussions are not held. If the patient becomes incapacitated due to illness, the patient's family and physician must make decisions based on what they think the patient would want.

Excerpts from "Advance Care Planning: Preferences for Care at the End of Life," by Barbara L. Kass-Bartelmes, M.P.H., C.H.E.S., and Ronda Hughes, Ph.D., *Research in Action*, Issue #12, March 2003, Agency for Healthcare Research and Quality (AHRQ), AHRQ Pub No. 03–0018.

Terms Patients Should Understand

Advance directives are also known as living wills. These are formal, legal documents specifically authorized by State laws that allow patients to continue their personal autonomy, and that provide instructions for care in case they become incapacitated and cannot make decisions. An advance directive may also be a durable power of attorney.

A **durable power of attorney** is also known as a health care proxy. This document allows the patient to designate a surrogate—a person who will make treatment decisions for the patient if the patient becomes too incapacitated to make such decisions.

Research Findings

The Agency for Healthcare Research and Quality (AHRQ) research indicates that most patients have not participated in advance care planning, yet many are willing to discuss end-of-life care. One way to determine patients' preferences for end-of-life care is to discuss hypothetical situations and find out their opinions on certain treatment patterns. These opinions can help clarify and predict the preferences they would be likely to have if they should become incapacitated and unable to make their own decisions.

Patients Need More Effective Advance Care Planning

Studies funded by AHRQ indicate that many patients have not participated in effective advance care planning. The Patient Self-Determination Act guarantees patients the right to accept or refuse treatment and to complete advance medical directives. However, despite patients' rights to determine their future care, AHRQ research reveals that:

- Less than 50 percent of the severely or terminally ill patients studied had an advance directive in their medical record.

- Only 12 percent of patients with an advance directive had received input from their physician in its development.

- Between 65 and 76 percent of physicians whose patients had an advance directive were not aware that it existed.

- Having an advance directive did not increase documentation in the medical chart regarding patient preferences.

- Advance directives helped make end-of-life decisions in less than half of the cases where a directive existed.

- Advance directives usually were not applicable until the patient became incapacitated and absolutely, hopelessly ill.

- Providers and patient surrogates had difficulty knowing when to stop treatment and often waited until the patient had crossed a threshold to actively dying before the advance directive was invoked.

- Language in advance directives was usually too nonspecific and general to provide clear instruction.

- Surrogates named in the advance directive often were not present to make decisions or were too emotionally overwrought to offer guidance.

- Physicians were only about 65 percent accurate in predicting patient preferences and tended to make errors of undertreatment, even after reviewing the patient's advance directive.

- Surrogates who were family members tended to make prediction errors of over-treatment, even if they had reviewed or discussed the advance directive with the patient or assisted in its development.

AHRQ research shows that care at the end of life sometimes appears to be inconsistent with the patients' preferences to forgo life-sustaining treatment, and patients may receive care they do not want. For example, one study found that patient preferences to decline cardiopulmonary resuscitation (CPR) were not translated into do-not-resuscitate (DNR) orders. DNR orders are requests from the patient or the patient's surrogate to the physician that certain forms of treatment or diagnostic testing not be performed. CPR is a procedure frequently addressed in DNR orders. Another study found that patients received life-sustaining treatment at the same rate regardless of their desire to limit treatment.

Patient Preferences for Treatment

Rank order of treatment preferences among patients age 64 and over who were admitted to a unit within the hospital's internal medicine department and were not acutely ill:[1]

1. Antibiotics (most preferred)

2. Blood transfusion

3.   Temporary tube feeding

4.   Temporary respirator

5.   Radiation

6.   Amputation

7.   Dialysis

8.   Chemotherapy

9.   Resuscitation

10.   Permanent respirator

11.   Permanent tube feeding (least preferred)

Patient Preference for Medical Care

- Patients are more likely to accept life-sustaining treatment for states they considered better than death than for states they considered worse than death (for example, patients were least likely to indicate they would want CPR if they were in a permanent coma).

- Patients were likely to accept or refuse treatment based on how invasive they perceive that treatment to be and how long the treatment is expected to last.

- Patients were more likely to accept treatment on a trial basis if the treatments were simple, such as receiving antibiotics.

- Patients are more likely to refuse treatment for a scenario with a worse prognosis (for example, more adult patients would refuse treatment if they had dementia with a terminal illness than if they only had dementia).

- Two-thirds of patients age 64 and over who were admitted to a hospital's internal medicine department but were not acutely ill desired less treatment if they were to become more cognitively impaired. For example, patients are far less likely to accept treatment if presented a hypothetical scenario for a cognitive impairment such as Alzheimer disease than for a physical impairment such as emphysema.

Patients with Chronic Illness Need Advance Planning

Because physicians are in the best position to know when to bring up the subject of end-of-life care, they are the ones who need to initiate and guide advance care planning discussions. Such discussions are usually reserved for people who are terminally ill or whose death is imminent, yet research indicates that people suffering from chronic illness also need advance care planning.

The majority of people who die in the United States (80 to 85 percent) are Medicare beneficiaries age 65 and over, and most die from chronic conditions such as heart disease, cerebrovascular disease, chronic obstructive pulmonary disease (COPD), diabetes, Alzheimer disease, and renal failure. Only about 22 percent of deaths in people age 65 and over are from cancer.

Patients Value Advance Care Planning Discussions

According to patients who are dying and their families who survive them, lack of communication with physicians and other health care providers causes confusion about medical treatments, conditions, prognoses, and the choices that patients and their families need to make. One AHRQ study indicated that about one-third of patients would discuss advance care planning if the physician brought up the subject, and about one-fourth of patients had been under the impression that advance care planning was only for people who were very ill or very old. Only five percent of patients stated that they found discussions about advance care planning too difficult.

AHRQ-funded studies have shown that discussing advance care planning and directives with their doctor increased patient satisfaction among patients age 65 years and over. Patients who talked with their families or physicians about their preferences for end-of-life care:

- had less fear and anxiety;
- felt they had more ability to influence and direct their medical care;
- believed that their physicians had a better understanding of their wishes; and
- indicated a greater understanding and comfort level than they had before the discussion.

Compared to surrogates of patients who did not have an advance directive, surrogates of patients with an advance directive who had discussed its content with the patient reported greater understanding, better confidence in their ability to predict the patient's preferences, and a stronger belief in the importance of having an advance directive.

Finally, patients who had advance planning discussions with their physicians continued to discuss and talk about these concerns with their families. Such discussions enabled patients and families to reconcile their differences about end-of-life care and could help the family and physician come to agreement if they should need to make decisions for the patient.

Advance Planning Helps Physicians Provide Care That Patients Want

Most people will eventually die from chronic conditions. These patients require the same kind of advance care planning as those suffering from predictably terminal conditions such as cancer. Understanding preferences for medical treatment in patients suffering from chronic illness requires that physicians and other health care providers consider patients' concerns about the severity of prospective health states, length and invasiveness of treatments, and prognosis.

By discussing advance care planning during routine outpatient visits, during hospitalization for exacerbation of illness, or when the patient or physician believes death is near, physicians can improve patient satisfaction with care and provide care at the end of life that is in accordance with the patient's wishes.

Reference

[1]Cohen-Mansfield J, Droge JA, Billib N. Factors influencing hospital patients' preferences in the utilization of life-sustaining treatments. *Gerontologist* 1992;32(1):89–95.

Chapter 17

Alzheimer Disease and End-of-Life Issues

Despite the best research efforts, Alzheimer disease (AD) remains incurable. Researchers are using sophisticated technologies to pinpoint how AD progressively steals memories and destroys personality; and yet, AD remains irreversible. Although one does not die of Alzheimer disease, during the course of the disease the body's defense mechanisms ultimately weaken increasing susceptibility to catastrophic infection and other causes of death related to frailty. At some point after the mind has been lost to this devastating disease, the body will be lost as well.

Families and caregivers of people with AD face many challenges as they cope with the steady loss of their loved one's mental and physical skills. As the disease moves to its end stages, certain steps can provide measures of comfort—both to the caregiver and to the person with AD. Health care professionals can help caregivers fill the last days with love and tenderness even through the wrenching turmoil of letting go.

Many caregivers are unaware that resources and health care professionals are available to provide comfort and help each AD patient end life with dignity. They face emotional conflict and unnecessary guilt.

"A lot of what we think about death and dying is based on the cancer model," says Dr. Stephen Post, professor in the department of bioethics at Case Western University School of Medicine. "Alzheimer's is a complicated and difficult disease." Late-stage AD is characterized

Excerpted from "Alzheimer's Disease and End-of-Life Issues," *Connections*, Volume 11, Numbers 1 and 2, National Institute on Aging (NIA), 2003.

by the inability to communicate by speech or recognize family members, the inability to move about without assistance, incontinence, loss of appetite, and loss of the ability to swallow, with death usually resulting from aspiration pneumonia, infection, or coronary arrest. On the average, the advanced stage of AD lasts 1.5 to 2 years, according to Dr. Post, though 20–30% of patients will live four, five, six, or even as long as ten years, he says.

Doctors, nurses, social workers, and other health care professionals can help caregivers understand the dying process and the role of palliative care for the AD patient. This is the purpose of palliative care—to provide comfort and symptom relief, without the use of aggressive treatments, such as tube feeding, mechanical respiration, dialysis, and cardiopulmonary resuscitation, which often only prolong the suffering of the patient. Community programs, such as hospice, can be of great service to family members and health care professionals by assisting with medications, patient physical care, and counseling. The objective in managing the advanced stages of Alzheimer disease should be to maximize comfort while preserving patient dignity and respect.

The Palliative Course

Experts agree that palliative care is the most appropriate course of action for advanced Alzheimer disease. Use of aggressive medical interventions in the advanced stage, such as CPR, feeding tubes, intravenous antibiotics, even dialysis, is considered by experts to be of little benefit and may impose a further burden of suffering on the patient. "The Alzheimer's Association firmly recommends palliative care and hospice approach in the advanced stages of the disease," says Dr. Post. "Family members should never be made to feel guilty in making a decision to allow a person with AD to die naturally."

"Health care professionals are duty-bound to do more than simply present technological options like items on a laundry list without clarifying the burdens that these technologies create for people with advanced dementia," Dr. Post says. Health care teams in these circumstances must be nonjudgmental and listen attentively to family wishes, while providing accurate facts on the adverse implications of prolonging end-of-life treatments.

Artificial Feeding and Hydration

Family members should be warned about the potential medical problems associated with artificial feeding and hydration. These include, in the case of nasogastric tubes, pain and discomfort related to the forceful introduction of physical devices in the esophagus, needed sedation, and infections often resulting from the procedure. "Many family members are not aware that no longer eating and drinking is part of the dying process, and it is normal," says Dr. Post.

"Our modern culture tends to treat dying as unnatural. Our technology allows us to forestall death, yet cannot prevent it. Family members need to be informed—with great compassion, sensitivity, and patience—about the dying process and how natural and inevitable it truly is. The body is shutting down. The natural process of dying means that the body no longer wants or needs food or fluids. This is often viewed as unnatural by caregivers and even some health care professionals. However, we need to explore our own feelings and attitudes toward death and dying before we can help families through this transitional process, this time of loss and change," comments Darby Morhardt, MSW, Social Worker, Northwestern University Alzheimer's Disease Center.

Cessation of food intake results in the release of endorphins which reduce pain. Feeding tubes and hydration block the release of endorphins and can result in weeks of "unnecessary suffering" Dr. Post said, with patients "uremic and bloated and unable to clear mucus from their lungs." Percutaneous endoscopic gastronomy (PEG) feeding can result in back-up to the esophagus, increasing the risk of aspiration pneumonia, while lack of ambulation—PEG feeding often requires physical restraint to prevent patients from pulling out their feeding tubes—increases the risk for bed ulcers and skin infections.

Artificial feeding also deprives a patient of taste, says Dr. Ladislav Volicer, clinical director of the Geriatric Research, Education and Clinical Center (GRECC) at the E.N.R.M. Veterans Hospital in Bedford, Massachusetts. "Alzheimer patients love sweets," Dr. Volicer says, "even in the later stages—things like milk shakes and ice cream." Artificial feeding also deprives patients and caregivers of personal contact which is a meaningful activity.

"We haven't had any tube feeding in the last 10 years," says Dr. Volicer, who often converts patients back to assisted feeding on arrival. "They can always eat to some degree," he says, "except during the actual dying process." Patients in the dying phase do not experience hunger and thirst, he adds.

Problems with choking can be addressed by substituting thick liquids, such as yogurt instead of milk, and by using commercial thickeners. "What we are trying to do is switch the emphasis of care from high tech to high touch," he says. "That also includes very aggressive management of pain. We use a lot of narcotics in the management of late-stage dementia."

Antibiotics may be useful for urinary tract infections, but they are not reliable against chest infections because of increasing resistance, says Dr. Post. Some physicians prefer to recommend acetaminophen (like Tylenol) for fever.

Hospital transfers should also be discouraged. "There is published evidence," says Dr. Volicer, "that the three month mortality rate is lower if patients are treated in a nursing home than if they are transferred to the hospital."

The End Draws Near

It is difficult to predict when an AD patient is going to die. "The average clinicians are not as good at this as they would be for cancer," says Dr. Jason Karlawish, of the University of Pennsylvania's Institute of Aging, "because there is a lack of clear understanding of this stage of AD." Dying for the AD patient is marked by little, if any, verbal output; complete dependency in all aspects of daily living; and the complications of brain failure which include episodes of aspiration, urinary tract infections, fevers, skin breakdowns, and more than 10% loss of body weight. "This is the typical profile of a patient who I would expect could die within a year," says Dr. Karlawish.

Working with Family Members

In the absence of advance directives, the health care team should work with family members to arrive at a consensus of care and abide by final decisions. There are often conflicts over the use of heroic efforts to prolong life. At odds are everything from the philosophies of individual providers and institutional caregivers to issues of patient competence in the absence of legal instruments. The solution—arrival at a plan by way of a narrative consensus. Health care workers can guide this effort by creating an environment of "equal standing," Dr. Karlawish says, in which all family members are encouraged to discuss how they perceive the patient's illness and arrive at a consensus that will provide the patient with the most comfort and the highest quality of remaining life. "You should be hearing yourself talking about half the time in the beginning," Dr. Karlawish says, "but if you've done it right, the caregiver should wind up doing most of the talking." Physicians should not be hesitant to recommend hospice as an option, he says.

End-of-Life Legal Instruments

What sets Alzheimer disease apart from many other terminal diseases is the progressive, irreversible loss of cognitive abilities, which begins early and becomes increasingly worse. The majority of patients arrive at the later stages of Alzheimer disease without advance directives. "In the mild stage, many patients are able to make decisions, but a substantial number, perhaps even 50%, will have difficulty with complex decisions like planning for the future," says Dr. Jason Karlawish, of the University of Pennsylvania's Institute of Aging.

By the advanced stage, the patient is no longer able to communicate pain or certain needs. "Once someone loses language," Dr. Karlawish says, "cognition becomes an interpretive act on the part of others." Pain is often related to immobility as well as constipation, osteoarthritis, and osteoporosis. The challenge to the physician "is to interpret the meaning of grunts, groans, and agitation—which are often misinterpreted by family members and the physician—and determine what the need is that is not being met."

Advance Directives: Durable Power of Attorney

Ideally, the health care team should initiate discussion of an end-of-life care plan while the patient is able to participate. The team should also be sensitive to the patient's and family's ability to tackle these issues. Some families will be quite capable of making orderly decisions about an impending death, but others may feel uncomfortable even thinking about what is going to happen to their loved one.

The durable power of attorney for health care, also referred to as the medical power of attorney, empowers one designated individual to make all medical decisions (if the patient lacks capacity) unless limited by other directives. The living will—also called instructions, directive to physicians, or declaration—states the patient's desires regarding life-sustaining or life-prolonging medical treatments.

The durable power of attorney for health care is superior to a living will, Dr. Post says, because it has "absolute legal clout" (not all States regard the living will as legally binding), and because of the prognostic uncertainty of the disease—"It's impossible to anticipate the incredible number of situations that might occur," he says.

Do Not Resuscitate Orders

Experts agree there is no question that do not resuscitate (DNR) orders should be standard procedure for advanced Alzheimer patients.

"Resuscitation is a horrendous experience for someone with Alzheimer disease," says Dr. Post. "Only 10% will survive the CPR effort, and almost all who do can be so severely injured by the application that they will not recover. And they will be even more compromised cognitively. Physicians should argue vehemently against any resuscitative efforts for advanced AD patients."

Additional Information

Alzheimer's Association
225 N. Michigan Ave., Suite 1700
Chicago, IL 60601
Toll-Free: 800-272-3900
Fax: 312-335-1110
Website: http://www.alz.org
E-mail: info@alz.org

Family Caregiver Alliance
180 Montgomery St., Suite 1100
San Francisco, CA 94104
Toll-Free: 800-445-8106
Phone: 415-434-3388
Website: http://caregiver.org
E-mail: info@caregiver.org

National Hospice and Palliative Care Organization
1700 Diagonal Road, Suite 625
Alexandria, VA 22314
Toll-Free: 800-658-8898
Phone: 703-837-1500
Fax: 703-837-1233
Website: http://www.nhpco.org
E-mail: nhpco_info@nhpco.org

Chapter 18

Advanced Cancer and End-of-Life Issues

When a patient's health care team determines that the cancer can no longer be controlled, medical testing and cancer treatment often stop, but the patient's care continues. The care focuses on making the patient comfortable. The patient receives medications and treatments to control pain and other symptoms, such as constipation, nausea, and shortness of breath. Some patients remain at home during this time, while others enter a hospital or other facility. Either way, services are available to help patients and their families with the medical, psychological, and spiritual issues surrounding dying. A hospice often provides such services.

The time at the end of life is different for each person. Each individual has unique needs for information and support. The patient's and family's questions and concerns about the end of life should be discussed with the health care team as they arise. The following information can help answer some of the questions that many patients, their family members, and caregivers have about the end of life.

How long is the patient expected to live?

Patients and their family members often want to know how long a person is expected to live. This is a hard question to answer. Factors such as where the cancer is located and whether the patient has other illnesses can affect what will happen. Although doctors may be able

"End-of-Life Care: Questions and Answers," Cancer Facts 8.15, National Cancer Institute (NCI), reviewed October 30, 2002.

to make an estimate based on what they know about the patient, they might be hesitant to do so. Doctors may be concerned about over- or underestimating the patient's lifespan. They also might be fearful of instilling false hope or destroying a person's hope.

When caring for the patient at home, when should the caregiver call for professional help?

A caregiver can contact the patient's doctor or nurse for help in any of the following situations:

- The patient is in pain that is not relieved by the prescribed dose of pain medication.
- The patient shows discomfort, such as grimacing or moaning.
- The patient is having trouble breathing and seems upset.
- The patient is unable to urinate or empty the bowels.
- The patient has fallen.
- The patient is very depressed or talking about committing suicide.
- The caregiver has difficulty giving medication to the patient.
- The caregiver is overwhelmed by caring for the patient, or is too grieved or afraid to be with the patient.
- At any time the caregiver does not know how to handle a situation.

What are some ways that caregivers can provide emotional comfort to the patient?

Everyone has different needs, but some emotions are common to most dying patients. These include fear of abandonment and fear of being a burden. They also have concerns about loss of dignity and loss of control. Some ways caregivers can provide comfort are as follows:

- Keep the person company—talk, watch movies, read, or just be with the person.
- Allow the person to express fears and concerns about dying, such as leaving family and friends behind. Be prepared to listen.
- Be willing to reminisce about the person's life.

- Avoid withholding difficult information. Most patients prefer to be included in discussions about issues that concern them.

- Reassure the patient that you will honor advance directives, such as living wills.

- Ask if there is anything you can do.

- Respect the person's need for privacy.

What are the signs that death is approaching? What can the caregiver do to make the patient comfortable?

Certain signs and symptoms can help a caregiver anticipate when death is near. It is important to remember that not every patient experiences each of the signs and symptoms. In addition, the presence of one or more of these symptoms does not necessarily indicate that the patient is close to death. A member of the patient's health care team can give family members and caregivers more information about what to expect.

Signs that death is approaching and suggestions for caregiving include:

Drowsiness, increased sleep, and/or unresponsiveness (caused by changes in the patient's metabolism). The caregiver and family members can plan visits and activities for times when the patient is alert. It is important to speak directly to the patient and talk as if the person can hear, even if there is no response. Most patients are still able to hear after they are no longer able to speak. Patients should not be shaken if they do not respond.

Confusion about time, place, and/or identity of loved ones; restlessness; visions of people and places that are not present; pulling at bed linens or clothing (caused in part by changes in the patient's metabolism). Gently remind the patient of the time, date, and people who are with them. If the patient is agitated, do not attempt to restrain the patient. Be calm and reassuring. Speaking calmly may help to reorient the patient.

Decreased socialization and withdrawal (caused by decreased oxygen to the brain, decreased blood flow, and mental preparation for dying). Speak to the patient directly. Let the patient know you are there for them. The patient may be aware and able to hear, but unable to respond. Professionals advise that giving the patient permission to let go can be helpful.

Decreased need for food and fluids, and loss of appetite (caused by the body's need to conserve energy, and its decreasing ability to use food and fluids properly). Allow the patient to choose if and when to eat or drink. Ice chips, water, or juice may be refreshing if the patient can swallow. Keep the patient's mouth and lips moist with products such as glycerin swabs and lip balm.

Loss of bladder or bowel control (caused by the relaxing of muscles in the pelvic area). Keep the patient as clean, dry, and comfortable as possible. Place disposable pads on the bed beneath the patient and remove them when they become soiled.

Darkened urine or decreased amount of urine (caused by slowing of kidney function and/or decreased fluid intake). Caregivers can consult a member of the patient's health care team about the need to insert a catheter to avoid blockage. A member of the health care team can teach the caregiver how to take care of the catheter if one is needed.

Skin becomes cool to the touch, particularly the hands and feet; skin may become bluish in color, especially on the underside of the body (caused by decreased circulation to the extremities). Blankets can be used to warm the patient. Although the skin may be cool, patients are usually not aware of feeling cold. Caregivers should avoid warming the patient with electric blankets or heating pads, which can cause burns.

Rattling or gurgling sounds while breathing, which may be loud; breathing that is irregular and shallow; decreased number of breaths per minute; breathing that alternates between rapid and slow (caused by congestion from decreased fluid consumption, a buildup of waste products in the body, and/or a decrease in circulation to the organs).

Breathing may be easier if the patient's body is turned to the side and pillows are placed beneath the head and behind the back. Although labored breathing can sound very distressing to the caregiver, gurgling and rattling sounds do not cause discomfort to the patient. An external source of oxygen may benefit some patients. If the patient is able to swallow, ice chips also may help. In addition, a cool mist humidifier may help make the patient's breathing more comfortable.

Turning the head toward a light source (caused by decreasing vision). Leave soft, indirect lights on in the room.

Increased difficulty controlling pain (caused by progression of the disease). It is important to provide pain medications as the patient's doctor has prescribed. The caregiver should contact the doctor if the prescribed dose does not seem adequate. With the help of the health care team, caregivers can also explore methods such as massage and relaxation techniques to help with pain.

Involuntary movements (called myoclonus), changes in heart rate, and loss of reflexes in the legs and arms are additional signs that the end of life is near.

What are the signs that the patient has died?

- There is no breathing or pulse.
- The eyes do not move or blink, and the pupils are dilated (enlarged). The eyelids may be slightly open.
- The jaw is relaxed and the mouth is slightly open.
- The body releases the bowel and bladder contents.
- The patient does not respond to being touched or spoken to.

What needs to be done after the patient has died?

After the patient has passed away, there is no need to hurry with arrangements. Family members and caregivers may wish to sit with the patient, talk, or pray. When the family is ready, the following steps can be taken.

- Place the body on its back with one pillow under the head. If necessary, caregivers or family members may wish to put the patient's dentures or other artificial parts in place.
- If the patient is in a hospice program, follow the guidelines provided by the program. A caregiver or family member can request a hospice nurse to verify the patient's death.
- Contact the appropriate authorities in accordance with local regulations. If the patient has requested not to be resuscitated through a do-not-resuscitate (DNR) order or other mechanism, do not call 911.
- Contact the patient's doctor and funeral home.
- When the patient's family is ready, call other family members, friends, and clergy.

143

• Provide or obtain emotional support for family members and friends to cope with their loss.

Additional Information

National Cancer Institute
6116 Executive Blvd.
Suite 3036A, MSC 8322
Bethesda, MD 20892-8322
Toll-Free: 800-4-CANCER (800-422-6237)
Toll-Free TTY: 800-332-8615
Website: http://www.cancer.gov
E-mail: cancergovstaff@mail.nih.gov

Chapter 19

Human Immunodeficiency Virus/Acquired Immune Deficiency Syndrome (HIV/ AIDS) and End-of-Life Issues

Dying in the Era of Highly Active Anti-Retroviral Therapy (HAART)

In the early days of the HIV epidemic, hospice referrals tended to follow a typical disease trajectory. A patient's clinical decline was most often marked by multiple hospitalizations, extensive muscle wasting and weight loss, desire to stop restorative therapies, and/or fatigue and resulting inability to cope with activities of daily living and problem-solving. Now, depending upon the patient's comorbidities and ability to adhere to combination therapies, there are multiple trajectories for end-stage HIV disease. Patients with active illicit substance use who are unable to adhere to treatment may have the course of illness complicated by recurrent skin abscesses, multiple episodes of endocarditis, and lack of medical follow-up resulting in antibiotic resistance and death from sepsis. These patients may also experience infections such as *Mycobacterium avium* complex (MAC), *Cryptococcal* meningitis, and *Pneumocystis carinii* pneumonia (PCP) as causes of death. For other patients, newer treatments may prolong survival time without much illness. In these cases, the cause of death has shifted from opportunistic infections to end-stage organ failure or other medical complications found with any chronic disease.

Excerpts from *A Clinical Guide to Supportive and Palliative Care for HIV/ AIDS*, 2003 Edition, U.S. Department of Health and Human Services (HHS).

Prognostic Indicators

Prognostication based upon a combination of signs and symptoms is crucial in determining the most appropriate clinical management strategy to alleviate suffering in persons near the end of life. For hospice programs in the U.S. to accept reimbursement from Medicare, patients must have a prognosis of six months or less if the disease were to run its normal course. Decisions to withdraw chronic therapies and introduce other treatments that might have been avoided earlier in the course of illness, such as steroids, must be based upon a reasonable assessment of the patient's life expectancy and goals.

Prognostication of time until death in HIV/AIDS is difficult. This is particularly true in young people because their basic cardiovascular health can sustain life longer than is possible in an older person with the same symptoms. Physicians tend to make overoptimistic prognostic predictions, particularly if they have had a long relationship with the patient.

With widespread use of HAART, predicting life expectancy is now more complex. Recent studies of patients with access to triple drug therapy suggest that disease progression to AIDS or death may be associated with timing of initial antiretroviral therapy. A recent Canadian study found that those starting therapy with a CD4 cell count lower than 200 cells/mm were three times more likely to die than those treated earlier in their course. The crude mortality rate for patients with access to HAART early in their trajectory (after 1997) is 6.7% at 28 months, much different from the statistic in the early epidemic. Viral load as a prognostic factor does not seem as important when patients have access to treatment. Previous studies may simply reflect that these patients were not treated soon enough to rescue a failing immune system.

Despite the development of multiple resistant strains, patients who are able to adhere to therapy seem to be living longer. Providers caring for people with long treatment histories often become frustrated with the lack of drug choices, but good supportive care can allow a patient to live until the next therapy is released. Liver failure, malignancies, and cardiovascular events are the issues facing patients with advanced disease; providers now need to be familiar with the palliative aspects of managing these problems.

In addition, providers must continually address the risks and benefits of continued antiretroviral therapy as patients approach the end of life. Just as patients may benefit from ongoing HAART therapy even in the face of resistant virus and declining immune function, there also may come a point where continued therapy will yield little benefit and the patient's quality of life may suffer due to medication toxicities. Providers need to be as familiar with the issues involved in stopping HAART as they are with the criteria for initiating HAART in treatment-eligible patients. HAART is also by definition future-oriented therapy, since the results are not expected in the short-term, but rather are seen in longer-term survival. This may confuse decision-making related to end-of-life care planning. Therefore, it is important for clinicians to work closely with patients through the complex decision-making that now surrounds HIV treatment in late-stage disease.

These issues have made end-stage HIV/AIDS more similar to other chronic diseases. Research must be pursued regarding what end-stage actually looks like to document the prognostic indicators and symptom management that can be useful. Without concrete knowledge, it is difficult to emotionally support patients near the end of life, and providers run the risk of again not recognizing this disease stage. Early recognition is absolutely critical for the kind of planning and closure patients need before death.

Setting Reasonable Goals and Maintaining Hope

Patients and providers in the era of HAART may be lulled into thinking that HIV/AIDS has been cured, without noting the larger picture that HIV/AIDS remains a fatal illness. If this perspective is lost, there is danger of reacting to every decline as something that can and must be fixed.

The provider must recognize how fear of death impacts management decisions (both by family and by provider). For some cultures, it is imperative to continue what may even appear to be futile therapy. In the face of even the bleakest situation, it is important to not insinuate that there is nothing more to be done. At these times, the patient and family should be helped to redefine hopes or goals.

When people are known to be dying, goals can be adjusted to fit the time they have left. For example, the new goal may be to live until an anniversary such as a birthday (within weeks) or a specific holiday. This could mean celebrating that event sooner to include the dying person (for example, holding a birthday party this week rather than trying to make it to the next month). Nature, poetry, and music may take on new meaning and can sustain one near the end of life as long as symptoms are controlled.

Clinical Management of Imminently Dying HIV/AIDS Patients

It is important that the family and patient understand normal landmarks in the dying process and overcome common misperceptions regarding imminent death. One such misperception is the belief that lack of appetite and diminished oral intake are causing profound disability and that fluid and nutrition are required. The normal dying process includes the following changes:

- loss of appetite
- decreased oral fluid intake, and decreased thirst
- increasing weakness and/or fatigue
- decreasing blood perfusion, including decreased urine output, peripheral cyanosis, and cool extremities
- neurologic dysfunction, including delirium, lethargy, coma, and changes in respiratory patterns
- loss of ability to close eyes
- noisy breathing as pharyngeal muscles relax

In particular, neurologic dysfunction can sometimes result in terminal delirium which can include a mounting syndrome of confusion, hallucinations, delirium, myoclonic jerks, and seizures prior to death. Recognized early, this can be treated with neuroleptics such as haloperidol or chlorpromazine.

When death occurs, the clinical signs include:

- absence of heartbeat and respirations
- fixed pupils
- skin color turns to a waxen pallor and extremities may darken
- body temperature drops
- muscles and sphincters relax, sometimes resulting in release of stool or urine

Preparation, which can involve the family, should include the following:

- creating a peaceful environment to the patient's liking
- preparing instructions about whom to call (usually not 911) when death occurs

- taking time to witness what is happening
- creating or using rituals that can help mark the occasion in a respectful way

When death occurs, families should be encouraged to take whatever time they need to feel what has happened, and say their goodbyes. There is no need to rush the body to a funeral home, and some families want to stay with the body for a period of time after death.

Considering Withdrawal of Nutrition and Hydration

In every culture, giving nourishment is seen as an act of caring as well as a method for improving health. As a person approaches death, eating and drinking become more difficult as one must have adequate strength to chew and to maintain an upright position. The palliative care team must find other ways for the family to offer support and care without forcing a dying person to take in more substance than they can handle. As the energy requirements diminish, forcing fluids in particular may cause more difficulty than withholding liquids might.

Ventilator Withdrawal for Intubated Patients

In instances like fatal *Pneumocystis carinii* pneumonia, mechanical ventilation may be withdrawn in order to discontinue futile and invasive medical treatment. These decisions are complex and involve ethical principles of withdrawing life-sustaining treatments that are well-established. It is important that clinicians establish with the family and, if possible, the patient that the goal of withdrawing ventilator support is to remove a treatment that is no longer desired or does not provide comfort to the patient. Clinicians need to work to develop a consensus among the health care team in order to withdraw ventilatory support; it is seldom an emergency decision, and time should be taken to resolve disagreements and concerns among the team and family. This procedure requires informed consent discussions, especially to inform family members that patients may not die immediately after ventilation is withdrawn.

After Death Care

It is important to respect the patient's and family's cultural, religious, and spiritual beliefs throughout the course of care, up to and including the time of death and beyond. Although 60% of people die in institutions in the U.S., most surveys show that most people prefer death in familiar surroundings. Every attempt should be made to allow the person to die where they feel most comfortable. Even in a clinical setting, being able to be with the person who is dying is very comforting to most family members. Every attempt should be made to remove unnecessary monitors such as pulse oximetry readers, intravenous lines, cardiac monitors, and even ventilators when possible.

At the time of death, those in attendance may appreciate a pastoral care provider who can lead them in prayer, or they may want to sing and to wait for the spirit to leave the room. Ritual cleansing, bathing with oils, or other cultural practices should be encouraged. Even after the family has gone and the body has been removed, it is advisable to leave a silk or plastic flower on the bed to allow hospital workers the opportunity to say goodbye and to grieve this death before they must go on to the care of another patient. Creating a memorial section in the intensive care unit or a busy ward gives health care workers permission to gain closure, especially when they are in an area where there are multiple deaths.

Chapter 20

Ethics and Legal Issues in Palliative Care

Ethics and Law

The ethics of care requires a delicate balance between the conventional practice of medicine and the wishes of the patient, appreciating that each human situation is unique. Not only should treatment options and likely outcomes be considered, but also patient values, hopes, and beliefs. Patients and families must be properly informed to make appropriate treatment decisions and help reset the goals of care at all stages of the illness.

Every palliative case presents its own ethical dimensions and dilemmas. The following case illustrates the diverse ethical and legal issues embedded in a common palliative care situation.

> Mr. W. was a 50-year-old construction worker, separated from his wife (though still legally married) and with a teenage child. He had a history of laryngeal carcinoma diagnosed one year before. He had a total laryngectomy and received radiation therapy, but the disease recurred. He was admitted to the hospital for what turned out to be a final seven weeks of hospitalization. His admission was initially prompted by increased shortness of breath and facial swelling following chemotherapy. His hospital stay was complicated by a left carotid erosion for which he had a bedside

Reprinted with permission from "Pain Medicine and Palliative Care: Ethics and Legal Issues," StopPain.org, Beth Israel Medical Center, New York, NY, © 2000–2005 Continuum Health Partners, Inc.

carotid ligation. He spent two weeks in the medical intensive care unit (MICU) for stabilization and treatment of pneumonia. Mr. W. had elected the do not resuscitate (DNR) option.

His hospital course was marked by increased pain, facial swelling, periodic seizures, a second pneumonia, and progressive weakness. At all times, he was bed-bound and artificially fed. His pain was relatively well-controlled, but the facial swelling was uncontrollable. Communication was possible to some extent through hand signals. Decisions were made after lengthy explanations to the patient and his wife—his designated health care agent.

In the final weeks of life, Mr. W.'s condition further deteriorated. His ability to communicate markedly decreased. In response to his enormous suffering, palliative care staff recommended sedation for Mr. W. Although his wife supported the decision, several nurses and house officers were concerned that such an intervention would go beyond the boundaries of appropriate symptom management. Mr. W.'s feeding tube was withdrawn, in accord with symptom control, comfort measures, and the patient's wishes. The patient, completely unresponsive in the last five days of his life, died very peacefully.

In this complex case, many questions can be raised:

- What are the ethical issues?
- What constitutes an ethical problem?
- Are ethical questions different from legal questions?
- Who decides?
- How do we define consent?
- Are advance directives necessary?
- What does DNR mean?
- Is withholding and withdrawal of treatment identical? Are they ever acceptable?
- Can we ever stop artificial nutrition and hydration?
- Is sedation an option at the end of life? How does sedation differ from physician-assisted suicide (PAS) or euthanasia?

This case suggests many more questions than answers. Although the following overview might simplify the understanding of the multiple issues embedded in a clinical case, one should remember that ethics cannot be equated with an easy recipe for solving problems. Ethics is a complex domain and needs ongoing learning, discussion, and reflection essential to the practice of good medicine.

Since ethical decisions are sometimes complex and difficult, in most major hospitals an ethics committee is available to guide the medical team in the decision-making process. The modalities of access vary according to the facility. Most ethics committees are accessible to families, patients, and medical teams.

Cardinal Principles

What is ethics?

Ethics is a generic term for different ways to examine moral life. Clinical ethics is a "practical discipline that provides a structural approach to decision-making that can assist health professionals to identify, analyze, and resolve ethical issues in clinical medicine" (Jonsen AR, Siegler M, Winsdale WJ. *Clinical Ethics. 3rd ed*. McGraw-Hill, NY, 1992). The ethics of a case arises out of the facts and values embedded in the case itself. Ethics in palliative care is a matter of practical reasoning about individual patients. Although there are many approaches proposed by ethicists for the analysis and resolution of difficult situations, the most commonly used are organized around principles, such as respect for autonomy, beneficence, non-maleficence, and justice. The principles are balanced and weighed in any particular ethical situation. Sometimes they come into conflict and create an ethical dilemma.

What are the basic ethical principles?

Respect for autonomy recognizes the right and ability of an individual to decide for himself or herself based on his or her own values, beliefs, and life span. This implies that the patient may choose a treatment that might differ from the advised course of care. The patient's decision should be informed and well-considered, reflecting his/her values. It is acceptable that a patient refuse certain therapy according to his own religious beliefs. Many factors interfere with the expression and appreciation of the patient's preferences including compromised competence of the patient, stress of illness, and comprehension difficulty. Respect for autonomy implies truth-telling and exchange of accurate information about status, goals of care, options, and expectations.

153

Beneficence requires that the physician prevent or remove harm, while doing or promoting good. It is the most commonly used principle in the application of care. It implies that the health care team should do positive acts in maximizing the benefits of treatment. Examples include delivering effective and beneficial treatments for pain or other symptoms, providing sensitive support, and assisting patients and families in any way possible.

Non-maleficence supposes that one ought not to inflict harm deliberately. Violation of this concept may include offering information in an insensitive way, providing inappropriate treatment of pain or other symptoms, continuing aggressive treatment not suitable to the patient's condition, providing unwanted sedation, or withholding or withdrawing treatment.

Justice relates to fairness in the application of care. It implies that patients receive care to which they are entitled medically and legally. Justice can be translated into "give to each equally," or "to each according to need," or to "each his due." Different theories of justice debate the terms due, equally, and priority. Organ transplantation, selection in the emergency room, or admission to the inpatient or outpatient hospice unit, are applications of this principle. Who should have priority? The principle of justice implies a consideration for the common good and societal considerations.

How Law Differs from Ethics

In the administration of care, one cannot ignore the different legal requirements relevant to each situation. Although some cases might be defensible under ethical principles, they might not be permissible under legal provisions. Law is defined as minimal ethics, in the sense that it is based on the values of a society. It is also the reflection of a societal consensus on particular issues. It varies from society to society, from state to state. In the U.S., law is divided into two systems: federal (across the states) and state (within the state). It can be made by:

- Judges (common law). Example: Supreme Court of the United States recognition for the right to refuse medical care

- Legislatures (statutory law). Example: Uniform Definition of Death Act

- Executive agencies (regulatory law). Example: Regulations for Protection of Human Subjects of Research

Most end-of-life issues fall under common law (case by case decided by the tribunals, such as consent/withholding or withdrawal of treatment) or statutory law (different state law, for example, physician-assisted suicide/do-not-resuscitate law).

Legal provisions impose limits on decisions that might be ethically sound but nevertheless risky. They provide a framework to guide certain decisions or practices. This framework is defined in terms of requirements that need to be fulfilled in order to avoid liability.

Chapter 21

Life Support Choices

Understanding Life Support Measures

Life support replaces or supports a failing bodily function. In treatable or curable conditions, life support is used temporarily until the body can resume normal functioning. But, in situations where a cure is not possible, life support may prolong suffering. This chapter is meant to explain various life support terminology and measures the health care team may need to address while your loved one is in the intensive care unit.

A treatment may be beneficial if it relieves suffering, restores functioning, or enhances the quality of life. The same treatment can be considered detrimental if it causes pain or prolongs the dying process without offering benefit. That treatment may diminish a person's quality of life.

The decision to forego life support is a personal one. It is important to talk to your physician regarding the risk and benefit of each therapy. All life support measures are optional treatments.

Commonly Used Life Support Terminology

Do-Not-Resuscitate Order (DNR)

A DNR order is an order written by your physician instructing health care providers not to attempt cardiopulmonary resuscitation

(CPR) in case of cardiac (heart stops beating) or respiratory arrest (breathing stops). A person with a valid DNR order will not be given CPR under these circumstances.

Do-Not-Resuscitate/Full Care

Remember: Do-not-resuscitate does not mean do not treat. Patients have the right to receive any and all treatments. When cure is not possible, your physician may decide that the use of CPR may not be medically appropriate. It is a choice to say no to CPR, but yes to all other medically appropriate treatments.

Palliative Care: Comfort Care/Hospice Care

Palliative care is a comprehensive approach to treating the symptoms of illness when cure is not possible. Comfort care focuses on the physical, psychological, and spiritual needs of the patient. The goal is to achieve the best quality of life available by relieving suffering, controlling pain, and achieving maximum independence. Respect for the patient's culture, beliefs, and values, is an essential component. Pain and discomfort associated with terminal illness can always be treated.

Commonly Used Life Support Measures

Cardiopulmonary Resuscitation/Advanced Cardiac Life Support (CPR/ACLS)

CPR/ACLS are a group of treatments used when someone's heart and/or breathing stops. CPR is used in an attempt to restart the heart and breathing. It may consist of artificial breathing, and it can include pressing on the chest to mimic the heart's function to restart circulation. Electric shocks (defibrillation) and drugs can also be used to stimulate the heart.

Defibrillation

Defibrillation is the sending of a powerful electric shock through the heart. It is used when the heart stops beating effectively on its own.

Does defibrillation always restart the heart?

If the heart has lost all of its electrical activity or is so damaged that it no longer has enough muscle to pump blood through the body, defibrillation may not be successful in restarting the heart. If you do not wish to receive CPR, your physician must write a do-not-resuscitate (DNR) order on the chart. This order can be revoked at any time for any reason.

Vasopressors

Vasopressors are a group of powerful drugs that cause blood vessels to get smaller and tighter, thereby raising blood pressure. This therapy is only given in the intensive care unit.

Artificial Nutrition and Hydration (Tube Feeding)

Tube feeding is the administration of a chemically balanced mix of nutrients and fluids through a feeding tube. Most commonly, a feeding tube is inserted into the stomach via the nasal passage (nasogastric or NG tube) or through the wall of the abdomen (gastronomy tube or PEG) by means of a surgical procedure. Another type of feeding tube is inserted surgically through the abdominal wall into the small intestine (jejunostomy tube).

Intravenous Feeding

Intravenous (IV) feedings are given to patients who are unable to tolerate tube feedings. Similar to tube feedings, the IV feeding provides the patient with the needed amount of protein, carbohydrate, fat, vitamins, and minerals. Nutrition and hydration may be supplied temporarily, until the patient recovers adequate ability to eat and drink, or it can be supplied indefinitely. Although potentially valuable and life saving in many situations, artificial nutrition and hydration do not provide comfort care for dying patients. Available scientific evidence has shown that death without artificial nutrition or hydration may cause less suffering.

Mechanical Ventilation

Mechanical ventilation is used to support or replace the function of the lungs. A machine called a ventilator (or respirator) forces air into the lungs. The ventilator is attached to a tube inserted in the nose or mouth and down into the windpipe (trachea). MV may be used short term (for example, to treat pneumonia), or it may be needed indefinitely for permanent lung disease or trauma to the brain. Some patients on long-term MV live a quality of life that is acceptable to them. For some patients, MV may only prolong the dying process.

Dialysis

Dialysis does the work of the kidneys which remove waste from the blood and manage fluid levels. This procedure requires a special central venous catheter. Blood circulates from the body through the dialysis machine where it is filtered and then returned. Dialysis can be performed in the ICU or in the dialysis unit, depending upon the condition of the patient. Some patients may live on dialysis for years, but dialysis for the chronically ill, dying patient may only prolong the dying process.

Pacemakers

A pacemaker is a device that produces a low electrical current that stimulates the heart muscle to beat. The heart can be paced temporarily until healing occurs. A surgical procedure to insert a permanent pacer may be required. Patients with incurable heart disease may choose not to have a pacemaker.

Additional Information

National Hospice and Palliative Care Organization
1700 Diagonal Rd., Suite 625
Alexandria, VA 22314
Toll-Free: 800-658-8898
Phone: 703-837-1500
Fax: 703-837-1233
Website: http://www.nhpco.org
E-mail: nhpco_info@nhpco.org

Society of Critical Care Medicine
701 Lee St., Suite 200
Des Plaines, IL 60016
Phone: 847-827-6888
Fax: 847-827-6886
Website: http://www.sccm.org
E-mail: info@sccm.org

Chapter 22

Termination of Life-Sustaining Treatment

On the medicine wards, there are patients who are receiving treatments or interventions that keep them alive, and doctors face the decision to discontinue these treatments. Examples include dialysis for acute or chronic renal failure and mechanical ventilation for respiratory failure. In some circumstances, these treatments are no longer of benefit, and in others the patient or family no longer wants them.

When is it justifiable to discontinue life-sustaining treatments?

- If the patient has the ability to make decisions, fully understands the consequences of their decision, and states they no longer want a treatment, it is justifiable to withdraw the treatment.

- Treatment withdrawal is also justifiable if the treatment no longer offers benefit to the patient.

How do I know if the treatment is no longer of benefit?

In some cases, the treatment may be futile; that is, it may no longer fulfill any of the goals of medicine. In general, these goals are to cure if possible, or to palliate symptoms, prevent disease or disease complications, or improve functional status. For example, patients with severe head trauma judged to have no chance for recovery of brain function can no longer benefit from being maintained on a mechanical ventilator. All that continuation would achieve in such a case is maintenance of biologic function. In such a case, it would be justifiable to withdraw mechanical ventilation.

Do different standards apply to withholding and withdrawing care?

Many clinicians feel that it is easier to not start (withhold) a treatment, such as mechanical ventilation, than to stop (withdraw) it. While there is a natural tendency to believe this, there is no ethical distinction between withholding and withdrawing treatment. In numerous legal cases, courts have found that it is equally justifiable to withdraw as to withhold life-sustaining treatments. Also, most bioethicists, including the President's Commission, are of the same opinion.

Does the patient have to be terminally ill to refuse treatment?

Though in most cases of withholding or withdrawing treatment the patient has a serious illness with limited life expectancy; the patient does not have to be terminally ill in order for treatment withdrawal or withholding to be justifiable. Most states have laws that guarantee the right to refuse treatment to terminally ill patients, usually defined as those having less than 6 months to live. These laws do not forbid other patients from exercising the same right. Many court cases have affirmed the right of competent patient to refuse medical treatments.

What if the patient is not competent?

In some cases, the patient is clearly unable to voice a wish to have treatment withheld or withdrawn. As with DNR orders, there are two general approaches to this dilemma—advance directives and surrogate decision makers.

Advance Directive

An advance directive is a document which indicates with some specificity the kinds of decisions the patient would like made should he/she be unable to participate. In some cases, the document may spell out specific decisions (for example, a living will); while in others it will designate a specific person to make health care decisions for them (for example, a durable power of attorney for health care). There is some controversy over how literally living wills should be interpreted. In some cases, the document may have been drafted in the distant past, and the patient's views may have changed. Similarly, some patients do change their minds about end-of-life decisions when they actually face them. In general, preferences expressed in a living will are most compelling when they reflect long held, consistently stable views of the patient. This can often be determined by conversations with family members, close friends, or health care providers with long-term relationships with the patient.

Surrogate Decision Maker

In the absence of a written document, people close to the patient and familiar with their wishes may be very helpful. The law recognizes a hierarchy of family relationships in determining which family member should be the official spokesperson, though generally all close family members and significant others should be involved in the discussion and reach some consensus. The hierarchy is as follows:

1. Legal guardian with health care decision making authority

2. Individual given durable power of attorney for health care decisions

3. Spouse

4. Adult children of patient (all in agreement)

5. Parents of patient

6. Adult siblings of patient (all in agreement)

Deciding If the Patient Is Competent

Sometimes the patient is awake, alert, and conversant, but their decisions seem questionable or irrational. First, it is important to distinguish an irrational decision from simple disagreement. If you feel strongly that a certain course of action is what's best for the patient, it can seem irrational for them to disagree. In these situations, it is critical to talk with the patient and find out why they disagree.

Patients are presumed to be competent to make a treatment decisions. Often it's better to say they have decision making capacity to avoid confusion with legal determinations of competence. In the courts, someone's competence is evaluated in a formal, standardized way. These court decisions do not necessarily imply anything about capacity for making treatment decisions. For example, an elderly grandfather may be found incompetent to manage a large estate, but may still have intact capacity to make treatment decisions.

In general, the capacity to make treatment decisions, including to withhold or withdraw treatment, is considered intact if the patient:

- understands the clinical information presented

- appreciates his/her situation, including consequences with treatment refusal

- is able to display reason in deliberating about their choices

- is able to clearly communicate their choice

If the patient does not meet these criteria, then their decision to refuse treatment should be questioned and handled in much the same way as discussed for the clearly incompetent patient. When in doubt, an ethics consultation may prove helpful.

Is a psychiatry consult required to determine decision making capacity?

A psychiatry consult is not required, but can be helpful in some cases. Psychiatrists are trained in interviewing people about very personal, sensitive issues, and thus can be helpful when patients are facing difficult choices with fears or concerns that are difficult to talk about. Similarly, if decision making capacity is clouded by mental illness, a psychiatrist's skill at diagnosis and potential treatment of such disorders can be helpful.

Does depression or other history of mental illness mean a patient has impaired decision making capacity?

Patients with active mental illness including depression should have their decision making capacity evaluated carefully. They should not be presumed to be unable to make treatment decision. In several studies, patients voiced similar preferences for life-sustaining treatments when depressed as they did after treatment of their depression. Depression and other mental disorders should prompt careful evaluation which may often be helped by psychiatry consultation.

Is it justifiable to withhold or withdraw food or fluids?

This question underscores the importance of clarifying the goals of medical treatment. Any medical intervention can be withheld or withdrawn, including nutrition and IV fluids. At all times, patients must be given basic humane, compassionate care. They should be given a comfortable bed, human contact, warmth, and be kept as free from pain and suffering as possible. While some believe that food and fluids are part of the bare minimum of humane treatment, both are still considered medical treatments. Several court cases have established that it is justifiable to withhold or withdraw food and fluids.

Is it justifiable to withhold or withdraw care because of costs?

It is rarely justifiable to discontinue life-sustaining treatment for cost reasons alone. While we should always try to avoid costly treatments that offer little or no benefit, our obligation to the patient outweighs our obligation to save money for health care institutions. There are rare situations in which costs expended on one terminally ill patient could be clearly better used on another, more viable patient. For instance, a terminally ill patient with metastatic cancer and septic shock is in the last ICU bed. Another patient, young and previously healthy, now with a self-limited but life-threatening illness, is in the emergency room. In such cases, it may be justifiable to withdraw ICU treatment from the terminally ill patient in favor of the more viable one. Even so, such decisions must be carefully considered and made with the full knowledge of patients and their surrogate decision makers.

Chapter 23

Organ or Tissue Donation

Organ Donation and Transplantation

In recent years, the science of organ transplantation has made great strides. In 2004, there were more than 20,000 transplant operations utilizing organs from more than 7,000 deceased donors, an increase of close to 11 percent over the 2003 total.[1] However, there still is a critical shortage of organs. Here are some statistics:

- The number of people waiting to receive an organ transplant in the United States is rising. There are now more than 90,000 people on the national organ transplantation waiting list.[2]

- Each day, 74 people receive an organ transplant, but another 18 people on the waiting list die because organs are not available.[2]

- As of August 2003, in the United States there were over:

  - 55,000 people waiting for a kidney transplant

  - 17,000 people waiting for a liver transplant

  - 3,000 people waiting for a heart and lung transplant

- Experts suggest that each of us could save or help as many as 50 people by being an organ donor.

This chapter includes excerpts from: "Organ Donation and Transplantation," National Women's Health Information Center, August 2003; and excerpts from "Organ Donation: FAQ," U.S. Department of Health and Human Services (HHS).

Who can be an organ donor?

It you are 18 years or older, you can show you want to be an organ donor by signing a donor card or telling your family members. If you are under age 18, you must have a parent's or guardian's consent. There are no age limits on who can donate.

What organs and tissues can be donated?

- Organs: heart, kidneys, pancreas, lungs, liver, and intestines
- Tissue: cornea, skin, bone marrow, heart valves, and connective tissue

How does a person become a donor candidate?

- State your intent to be an organ donor on your driver's license.
- Fill out a donor card and carry it in your wallet.
- Tell your family and loved ones that you want to be a donor after you die.
- You may also want to tell your family health care provider, lawyer, and your religious leader that you would like to be a donor.

Does the donor's family have to pay for the cost of organ donation?

No. The donor's family neither pays for, nor receives payment for organ and tissue donation. The transplant recipient's health insurance policy (or Medicare or Medicaid) usually covers the cost of transplant.

If I am a donor, will that affect the quality of my medical care?

No. A transplant team does not become involved with the patient until doctors have determined that all possible efforts to save the patient's life have failed.

Does organ donation disfigure the body?

No. Donation does not change the appearance of the body. Organs are removed surgically in a routine operation. It does not interfere with having a funeral, including open casket services.

Who manages the distribution of organs?

The United Network for Organ Sharing (UNOS) maintains the national Organ Procurement and Transplantation Network (OPTN). Through the UNOS Organ Center, organ donors are matched to waiting recipients 24 hours a day, 365 days a year.

How are minority women affected by organ transplants?

Minority women suffer more from diseases like diabetes, kidney disease, and high blood pressure—diseases that can lead to organ failure. Finding organ donors can be challenging for minority women. Members of different racial and ethnic groups are usually more genetically similar and more likely to find organ donors within their own ethnic groups. For example, the most likely match for a kidney transplant is between a donor and patient of similar ancestry. Therefore, more donations by minority women increase the likelihood that a good match can be found.

Frequently Asked Questions about Organ Donation

Are there age limits for donors?

There are no age limitations on who can donate. The deciding factor on whether a person can donate is the person's physical condition, not the person's age. Newborns as well as senior citizens have been organ donors. Persons younger than 18 years of age must have a parent's or guardian's consent.

If I sign a donor card or indicate my donation preferences on my driver's license, will my wishes be carried out?

Even if you sign a donor card it is essential that your family know your wishes. Your family may be asked to sign a consent form in order for your donation to occur. If you wish to learn how organ donation preferences are documented and honored where you live, contact your local organ procurement organization (OPO). The OPO can advise you of specific local procedures, such as joining donor registries that are available to residents in your area.

Can I sell my organs?

No! The National Organ Transplant Act (Public Law 98-507) makes it illegal to sell human organs and tissues. Violators are subject to fines and imprisonment. Among the reasons for this rule is the concern of Congress that buying and selling of organs might lead to inequitable access to donor organs with the wealthy having an unfair advantage.

How are organs distributed?

Patients are matched to organs based on a number of factors including blood and tissue typing, medical urgency, time on the waiting list, and geographical location.

Can I be an organ and tissue donor and also donate my body to medical science?

Total body donation is an option, but not if you choose to be an organ and tissue donor. If you wish to donate your entire body, you should directly contact the facility of your choice to make arrangements. Medical schools, research facilities and other agencies need to study bodies to gain greater understanding of disease mechanisms in humans. This research is vital to saving and improving lives.

Can non-resident aliens donate and receive organs?

Non-resident aliens can both donate and receive organs in the United States. During 2002 and 2003, 513 of the 26,090 organ donors were non-resident aliens, or less than two per cent. Policies developed by the Organ Procurement and Transplantation Network (OPTN) allow up to 5% of recipients at a transplant center to be from other countries. From 1995 to 2002, non-resident aliens accounted for only about one per cent of more than 20,000 transplants performed annually. Organ allocation is based on the principles of equity and medical utility with the concept of justice applied to both access (consideration) as well as allocation (distribution).

If I have a previous medical condition, can I still donate?

Regardless of any pre-existing medical circumstances or conditions, determination of suitability to donate organs or tissue may be based on a combination of factors that take into account the donor's general health and the urgency of need of the recipient. This determination is usually done by the medical staff that recovers the organs or by the transplant team that reviews all of the data about the organ(s) or tissue that have been recovered from the donor.

References

1. News Release, March 29, 2005, U.S. Department of Health and Human Services (HHS), available at http://www.hhs.gov/news/press/2005pres/20050329.html, accessed March 1, 2006.

2. "Organ and Tissue Donation/Transplantation," HHS, available at http://www.organdonor.gov, accessed March 1, 2006.

Additional Information

United Network for Organ Sharing (UNOS)
P.O. Box 2482
Richmond, VA 23218
Toll-Free: 888-894-6361
Website: http://www.unos.org
E-mail: webmaster@unos.org

Eye Bank Association of America
1015 18th St. N.W., Suite 1010
Washington, DC 20036
Phone: 202-775-4999
Fax: 202-429-6036
Website: http://www.restoresight.org
E-mail: info@restoresight.org

American Association of Tissue Banks
1320 Old Chain Bridge Rd., Suite 450
McLean, VA 22101
Phone: 703-827-9582
Fax: 703-356-2198
Website: http://www.aatb.org
E-mail: aatb@aatb.org

Chapter 24

Physician-Assisted Suicide

Physician-assisted suicide (PAS) generally refers to a practice in which the physician provides a patient with a lethal dose of medication, upon the patient's request, which the patient intends to use to end his or her own life.

Is physician-assisted suicide the same as euthanasia?

No. Physician-assisted suicide refers to the physician providing the means for death, most often with a prescription. The patient, not the physician, will ultimately administer the lethal medication. Euthanasia generally means that the physician would act directly, for instance by giving a lethal injection, to end the patient's life. Some other practices that should be distinguished from PAS are:

- Terminal sedation: This refers to the practice of sedating a terminally ill competent patient to the point of unconsciousness, then allowing the patient to die of her disease, starvation, or dehydration.

"Physician-Assisted Suicide," by Clarence H. Braddock III, M.D., MPH; Project Director, Bioethics Education Project; Faculty, Departments of Medicine and Medical History and Ethics; and Mark R. Tonelli, M.D., MA; Assistant Professor, Pulmonary and Critical Care Medicine. © 2001 University of Washington. All Rights Reserved. Reprinted with permission. For additional information, visit http://depts.washington.edu/bioethx. Reviewed in December 2005 by Dr. David A. Cooke, M.D., Diplomate, American Board of Internal Medicine.

- Withholding/withdrawing life-sustaining treatments: When a competent patient makes an informed decision to refuse life-sustaining treatment, there is virtual unanimity in state law and in the medical profession that this wish should be respected.

- Pain medication that may hasten death: Often, a terminally ill, suffering patient may require dosages of pain medication that impair respiration or have other effects that may hasten death. It is generally held by most professional societies, and supported in court decisions, that this is justifiable so long as the primary intent is to relieve suffering.

Is physician-assisted suicide ethical?

The ethics of PAS continue to be debated. Some argue that PAS is ethical. Often this is argued on the grounds that PAS may be a rational choice for a person who is choosing to die to escape unbearable suffering. Furthermore, the physician's duty to alleviate suffering may, at times, justify the act of providing assistance with suicide. These arguments rely a great deal on the notion of individual autonomy, recognizing the right of competent people to choose for themselves the course of their life, including how it will end.

Others have argued that PAS is unethical. Often these opponents argue that PAS runs directly counter to the traditional duty of the physician to preserve life. Furthermore, many argue if PAS were legal, abuses would take place. For instance, the poor or elderly might be covertly pressured to choose PAS over more complex and expensive palliative care options.

What are the arguments in favor of PAS?

Those who argue that PAS is ethically justifiable offer the following sorts of arguments:

1. **Respect for autonomy:** Decisions about time and circumstances of death are very personal. A competent person should have the right to choose death.

2. **Justice:** Justice requires that we "treat like cases alike." Competent, terminally ill patients are allowed to hasten death by treatment refusal. For some patients, treatment refusal will not suffice to hasten death; their only option is suicide. Justice requires that we should allow assisted death for these patients.

174

3. **Compassion:** Suffering means more than pain; there are other physical and psychological burdens. It is not always possible to relieve suffering. Thus PAS may be a compassionate response to unbearable suffering.

4. **Individual liberty versus state interest:** Though society has strong interest in preserving life, that interest lessens when a person is terminally ill and has a strong desire to end their life. A complete prohibition on assisted death excessively limits personal liberty. Therefore, PAS should be allowed in certain cases.

5. **Openness of discussion:** Some would argue that assisted death already occurs, albeit in secret. For example, morphine drips ostensibly used for pain relief may be a covert form of assisted death or euthanasia. That PAS is illegal prevents open discussion in which patients and physicians could engage. Legalization of PAS would promote open discussion.

What are the arguments against PAS?

Those that argue that PAS should remain illegal often offer arguments such as these:

1. **Sanctity of life:** This argument points out strong religious and secular traditions against taking human life. It is argued that assisted suicide is morally wrong because it contradicts these beliefs.

2. **Passive versus active distinction:** The argument here holds that there is an important difference between passively letting die and actively killing. It is argued that treatment refusal or withholding treatment equates to letting die (passive) and is justifiable, whereas PAS equates to killing (active) and is not justifiable.

3. **Potential for abuse:** Here the argument is that certain groups of people, lacking access to care and support, may be pushed into assisted death. Furthermore, assisted death may become a cost-containment strategy. Burdened family members and health care providers may encourage the option of assisted death. To protect against these abuses, it is argued PAS should remain illegal.

4. **Professional integrity:** Here opponents point to the historical, ethical traditions of medicine that are strongly opposed to

taking life. For instance, the Hippocratic oath states, "I will not administer poison to anyone where asked," and "Be of benefit, or at least do no harm." Furthermore, major professional groups (American Medical Association, American Geriatrics Society) oppose assisted death. The overall concern is that linking PAS to the practice of medicine could harm the public's image of the profession.

5. **Fallibility of the profession:** The concern raised here is that physicians will make mistakes. For instance, there may be uncertainty in diagnosis and prognosis; there may be errors in diagnosis and treatment of depression; or inadequate treatment of pain. Thus the State has an obligation to protect lives from these inevitable mistakes.

Is PAS illegal?

In most states, aiding in a suicide is a crime, while suicide or attempted suicide itself is not illegal. The state of Oregon is the only state that currently has legalized PAS.

However, several major court decisions have been made regarding PAS. In the case of Compassion in Dying versus Washington, the Ninth U.S. Circuit Court of Appeals held that individuals have a right to choose how and when they die. Later, the Second Circuit Court found a New York law on PAS in conflict with the 14th amendment, which says that no state shall "deny to any person within its jurisdiction the equal protection of the laws." The Court held that competent patients were being treated differently than incompetent patients. The U.S. Supreme Court has ruled that there is no constitutional right to assisted suicide, and made a legal distinction between refusal of treatment and PAS. However, the Court also left the decision of whether to legalize PAS up to each individual state.

There have also been a couple of high-profile cases related to specific PAS incidents. Dr. Timothy Quill was investigated, but not indicted for his participation in the suicide of a patient after he published his account of the incident. In November of 1998, *60 Minutes* aired a tape of Dr. Jack Kevorkian administering a lethal injection. His patient, 52 year-old Thomas Youk, suffered from amyotrophic lateral sclerosis (ALS), otherwise known as Lou Gehrig disease. As a result of the show, Kevorkian was tried for first degree murder in Oakland County, Michigan. Prosecutors argued that in giving a lethal injection Kevorkian stepped over the line of PAS into euthanasia, and that his actions amounted to murder. Kevorkian was convicted of second degree murder and is currently serving a 10 to 25 year prison sentence.

What does the medical profession think of PAS?

Surveys of individual physicians show that half believe that PAS is ethically justifiable in certain cases. However, professional organizations such as the American Medical Association have generally argued against PAS on the grounds that it undermines the integrity of the profession.

Surveys of physicians in practice show that about one in five will receive a request for PAS sometime in their career. Somewhere between 5–20% of those requests are eventually honored.

What do patients and the general public think of PAS?

Surveys of patients and members of the general public find that the vast majority think that PAS is ethically justifiable in certain cases, most often those cases involving unrelenting suffering.

What should I do if a patient asks me for assistance in suicide?

One of the most important aspects of responding to a request for PAS is to be respectful and caring. Virtually every request represents a profound event for the patient, who may have agonized over his situation and the possible ways out. The patient's request should be explored, to better understand its origin, and to determine if there are other interventions that may help ameliorate the motive for the request. In particular, one should address:

- Motive and degree of suffering: Are there physical or emotional symptoms that can be treated?

- Psychosocial support: Does the patient have a system of psychosocial support, and has she discussed the plan with them?

- Accuracy of prognosis: Every consideration should be given to acquiring a second opinion to verify the diagnosis and prognosis.

- Degree of patient understanding: The patient must understand the disease state and expected course of the disease. This is critical since patient may misunderstand clinical information. For instance, it is common for patients to confuse incurable cancer with terminal cancer.

What if the request persists?

If a patient's request for aid-in-dying persists, each individual clinician must decide his or her own position and choose a course of action that is ethically justifiable. Careful reflection ahead of time can prepare one to openly discuss your position with the patient, acknowledging and respecting difference of opinion when it occurs. Organizations exist which can provide counseling and guidance for terminally ill patients. No physician, however, should feel forced to supply assistance if he or she is morally opposed to PAS.

Chapter 25

Autopsies

Autopsy: Questions and Answers

What is an autopsy?

An autopsy is an exam of the body of a person who has died. The purpose of an autopsy is to answer questions about the person's illness or the cause of death. In addition, autopsies provide valuable information that helps doctors save the lives of others. Autopsies are performed by specially trained physicians called pathologists.

Who may request an autopsy?

You can request an autopsy if you are the person's next of kin or the legally responsible party. Your doctor will ask you to sign a consent form to give permission for the autopsy. You may limit the autopsy in any manner you wish. If the cause of death is unclear, the pathologist may perform an autopsy without the family's permission.

What is the procedure for an autopsy?

First, the pathologist looks at the body for clues about the cause of death. Next, he or she examines the internal organs, taking samples as needed to look at under a microscope. The autopsy takes from two to four hours. The autopsy room looks like an operating room. An atmosphere of dignity and respect is maintained at all times.

What does an autopsy cost?

Because autopsies help doctors learn more about illness and ways to improve medical care, autopsies are usually performed without charge.

Will an autopsy interfere with funeral arrangements?

No. Pathologists perform autopsies in a way that does not interfere with burial or cremation. Once the autopsy is completed, the hospital tells the funeral home. An autopsy will not delay funeral services.

When will the results of an autopsy be known?

The first findings from an autopsy are usually ready in two to three days. The doctor can review these results with you. A final report may take many weeks because of the detailed studies performed on tissue samples. The doctor will also review the final report with you.

New Evidence Report Finds Autopsies Help to Uncover Medical Diagnostic Discrepancies

Autopsies continue to detect clinically important diagnostic discrepancies, according to an evidence report released by the Agency for Healthcare Research and Quality. Based on an analysis of more than 50 studies spanning 40 years, researchers estimate that in U.S. hospitals in the year 2000 the correct cause of death escaped clinical detection in 8–23% of cases, with as many as 4–8% of all deaths having a diagnostic discrepancy that may have harmed the patient. In addition to clinically missed diagnoses, up to five percent of autopsies disclosed clinically unsuspected complications of care.

These diagnostic discrepancy rates do not simply reflect selection by clinicians of diagnostically challenging cases, according to the study authors. In fact, considerable evidence suggests that clinicians have trouble predicting which autopsies are likely to yield important new information. The researchers note that, although often referred to as diagnostic errors, these findings refer to discrepancies between clinical diagnoses and autopsy diagnoses and not necessarily to medical mistakes. While diagnostic discrepancies can result from a clinician's failure to consider an appropriately broad listing of alternative diagnoses or misinterpretation of test results, there are also situations with atypical symptoms or limited diagnostic test information, they explained. These discrepancies, regardless of source, create inaccuracies in death certificates and hospital discharge data, both of which play important roles in epidemiologic research and health care policy decisions, the study authors said.

The evidence report examined the benefits of the autopsy as a tool in health care performance measurement and improvement. However, the researchers did not attempt to address other roles of the autopsy in medical education, furthering medical research, quality control within the medical specialty of pathology, verification of second opinion consultations, and legal documentation of findings, or the bereavement process for surviving family members. The focus of the report on the autopsy's role in detecting quality problems reflected an objectively quantifiable area to evaluate the potential negative effects of the trend toward fewer autopsies during the past 40 years.

In 1994, the last year for which national data exist, the autopsy rate for all non-forensic deaths fell below 6 percent, from a high of 50 percent in the 1960s. This decline is probably due to lack of reimbursement for autopsies, the attitudes of clinicians regarding the utility of autopsies in light of other diagnostic advances, and general unfamiliarity with the autopsy and techniques for requesting one, especially among physicians in medical training, according to the study authors. The evidence report was requested by the College of American Pathologists.

Part Four

End-of-Life Care Facilities

Chapter 26

Hospice Care: At Home or in a Nursing Facility

Hospice Facts

What is hospice?

Hospice care involves a core interdisciplinary team of professionals and volunteers who provide medical, psychological, and spiritual support to the terminally ill, as well as support for the patient's family. The care is primarily based in the home, enabling families to remain together in peace, comfort, and dignity.

What are the advantages of hospice care?

Hospice care is a cost-effective alternative to the high costs associated with hospitals and traditional institutional care. Hospice care allows terminally ill patients and their families to remain together in the comfort and dignity of their home. Hospice care relies on the combined knowledge and skill of an interdisciplinary team of professionals, including physicians, nurses, home care aides, social workers,

This chapter includes: "Hospice Fact Sheet," and "Fact or Fiction: Learning the Truth about Hospice," © 2005 Hospice Association of America. All rights reserved. Reprinted with permission. And, "Families and Caregivers," © 2004 Indiana Association for Home & Hospice Care, Inc. All rights reserved. Reprinted with permission. Also, "Helping You Choose Quality Home Care and Hospice Services," © Joint Commission on Accreditation of Healthcare Organizations, 2006. Reprinted with permission.

counselors, and volunteers. Hospice is the preferred choice of health care delivery for the terminally ill and their families. Hospice treats the person, not the disease; focuses on the family, not the individual; and emphasizes the quality of life, not the duration.

When was the first hospice established?

While the hospice concept dates back to ancient times, the American hospice movement did not begin until the 1960s. The first hospice in this country—The Connecticut Hospice, Inc.—began providing in-home services in March 1974. It was funded by the National Cancer Institute for its first three years.

How many hospices exist today?

Medicare hospice participation has grown at a dramatic rate, largely as a result of a 1989 Congressional mandate (PL 101-239, §6005) to increase reimbursement rates by 20%. The number of hospices participating in Medicare increased from 31 in 1984 to 2,273 in 2000. This number consists of 739 home health agency-based hospices, 554 hospital-based hospices, 20 skilled nursing facility-based hospices, and 960 freestanding hospices.

What is the future of hospice care?

The need for hospices will continue to rise due to the growing aging population, the increasing number of persons with acquired immune deficiency syndrome (AIDS), and the rising health care costs. More importantly, medical professionals, as well as the general public are choosing hospice over other forms of health care delivery because of its holistic, patient-family, in-home centered philosophy.

Who pays for hospice care?

Hospice services are covered under Medicare, and currently 45 states offer hospice care as an option under their Medicaid programs. In addition, hospice care is a covered benefit under most private insurance plans, HMOs, and other managed care organizations. Military personnel and their dependents are covered for hospice under CHAMPUS. Hospices continue to rely heavily on grants and community support to fund care and hospice service that is not reimbursed for patients with little or no insurance.

Families and Caregivers: Hospice Services and Capabilities

Hospice programs make it possible for terminally ill patients to spend the final stages of their lives at home or in home-like settings with an emphasis on palliative and supportive care that will enable them and their families to cope with this difficult transition.

Hospice is a comprehensive, medically-directed, team-oriented program of care that seeks to treat and comfort terminally ill patients and their families, establishing pain management and symptom control as clinical goals, and understanding that psychological and spiritual pain are as significant as physical pain.

Hospice is a philosophy of care that accepts death as a natural part of life, seeking neither to hasten nor to prolong the dying process. Hospice is caring that strives to help patients truly live until they die.

The philosophy of hospice care is central to the delivery and effectiveness of its services. The basic elements of hospice care include:

- care of the patient and family as one unit
- pain and symptom management
- staff availability all day and night
- medical and nursing care
- social work services
- counseling, including bereavement counseling for up to one year after the patient's death
- coordination of medications, medical supplies, and durable medical equipment
- physical, occupational, and speech therapy
- specially trained hospice volunteer support

Hospice care is most often provided at home. However, patients who have accepted hospice care can continue to receive that same approach to care should an inpatient stay become necessary. Inpatient general care is available when symptoms cannot be managed in the home. Inpatient respite care is available on a limited basis to provide short-term relief for the caregiver. Private pay or Medicaid room and board nursing home patients are also eligible for hospice care if the facility has made arrangements with a local hospice provider.

With increasing pressure to reduce hospital stays, the dependence on hospice programs will grow. In fact, through hospice support at home, many patients with end-stage illnesses can avoid costly emergency room visits and inpatient admissions.

Many people, even those who may have been a little reluctant to seek hospice services, are surprised by the full spectrum of physical, emotional, social, and spiritual support hospice provides. Most families say, "we don't know how we would have coped without the help of hospice."

Each hospice patient and family has special needs; therefore, each patient/family care program is unique. Hospice is responsible for the coordination of all aspects of the terminal care. Services are provided by an interdisciplinary team of professionals and volunteers. The composition of the hospice team depends on the patient's and family's needs. The team can include:

- patient
- patient's family
- patient's attending (primary) physician who is responsible for the medical care plan
- hospice medical director who serves as a consultant or, if patient selects, may be the attending physician
- nurses who direct care and comfort
- home health aides/homemakers for personal care and light housekeeping
- physical, occupational, or speech therapists as needed
- social workers for counseling and coordination
- hospice volunteers specially trained to provide support, companionship, and to be a special friend to the patient and family
- hospice volunteer coordinator
- pastoral/spiritual care counselor who provides direct counseling when patient/family do not have access to their own spiritual resource, and serves as a consultant to the hospice team and to area clergy who provide direct service
- bereavement coordinator/counselor who offers grief counseling for the patient and survivors (available for up to one year after patient's death for family)
- nutritional counselor, as needed

Early intervention by the hospice team promotes the most integrated and effective array of services for patients and families. Hospice services are not solely for the final days of a patient's life. Hospice care is most effective when there are several weeks, if not months, of interaction to establish trust between the patient/family and the hospice team as well as to create the infrastructure of support for the patient and family at home.

The majority of hospice patients probably receive care under the Medicare Hospice Benefit which has specific eligibility criteria. Indiana Medicaid recipients may also receive hospice care under the Medicaid Hospice Benefit. Most private insurers and managed care programs offer a hospice benefit but the aspects and criteria for eligibility for it vary from program to program. If you have a patient you think would benefit from a hospice program, contact your local hospice agency.

Helping You Choose Quality Home Care and Hospice Services

Choosing home care or hospice services can be an emotional and difficult decision. But gathering the right information can help make your decision easier. First of all, be sure to understand the needs of the patient—whether that is you or a loved one. Next, know what to ask when you talk to representatives from the home care or hospice program. the Joint Commission on Accreditation of Healthcare Organizations (JCAHO) has put together a list of questions to help you get the information you need.

There are many different types of health care services provided in the home:

- Home medical equipment companies deliver and maintain equipment and instruct patients and/or family members on how to use it.

- Home health professional services include nursing, medical, social work, and speech, physical, and occupational therapies.

- Personnel care and support services assist with activities such as bathing and light housekeeping.

- Pharmaceutical services provide medications and check the patient's response to medications.

Hospice programs provide support for terminally ill patients and their families. Ask your doctor or the hospital discharge planner or social worker to recommend a few local home care or hospice programs. Talk with representatives from each one, and use the following questions to help you get the information you need to choose the best organization for you.

General Questions to Ask before Choosing Home Care or Hospice Services

- What types of services does the home care or hospice provide? Does it offer services for children?

- How long has the home care or hospice been in business?

- Does the home care or hospice accept payment from Medicare and Medicaid? Does it have a list of its fees and services? Can the home care or hospice help you find financial help if you need it?

- How does the home care or hospice train and manage its staff? Does a supervisor come to the patient's home to review the care being given? Are the home care workers licensed and bonded?

- Is the home care or hospice prepared in case of an emergency like a power failure or a natural disaster? Will it still be able to deliver the services you need?

Questions about Quality Care

- Does the home care or hospice have volunteers who visit the patient at home?

- Does an independent group like the Joint Commission on Accreditation of Healthcare Organizations review the home care or hospice? Accreditation means that the home care or hospice has met national standards for patient care and safety.

- Will the home care or hospice create a care plan just for you or your loved one? You and your home care professional should agree on the services the patient will receive, how often the visits will take place, and how long treatment will last.

- Does a nurse or therapist conduct an initial visit and review the type of care the patient needs at home? Are family members, doctors, or other health care professionals involved in this review?

- If medical equipment like a suction machine, oxygen, or wheel chair is needed, will the home care or hospice teach the patient or responsible family members how to use the equipment in the home?

- How often is medical equipment checked? Are replacements included?

- Does the home care or hospice explain the patient's rights and responsibilities? Will you receive a copy of a Patient Bill of Rights?

- How does the home care or hospice make sure that each patient's treatment remains confidential?

- Does the home care or hospice have a 24-hour telephone number you can call when you have questions or complaints?

- Does the home care or hospice have a list of references, such as doctors, patients, and their family members that you can contact?

Founded in 1951, the Joint Commission on Accreditation of Healthcare Organizations is an independent, not-for-profit organization that evaluates more than 15,000 health care facilities in the United States, including hospitals, nursing homes, outpatient clinics, laboratories, behavioral health care organizations, health plans, and home care organizations.

To find out if the home care organization or hospice you are considering is accredited by the Joint Commission, see Quality Check® on the Internet. Quality Check® is a guide to all Joint Commission accredited health care organizations and programs, and also has reports that include information on the organization's performance and how it compares to other organizations nationwide and statewide.

Fact or Fiction: Learning the Truth about Hospice

Fiction: Hospice is a place where the terminally ill go to die.

Fact: Hospice is not a place, but a concept of care. More than 90% of the hospice services provided in the U.S. are based in the home. Care provided in the home allows families to be together when they need it most sharing the final days in peace, comfort, and dignity. However, when home care is not an option, in-patient care can be available through a contracting hospital, skilled nursing facility, or the hospice's own in-patient facility (if available). In addition, in-patient care is available to those receiving home care in emergency situations or when family members need respite care.

Fiction: Hospice only serves persons diagnosed with cancer.

Fact: Although 71% of the patients who were admitted to hospice agencies in 1996 had conditions related to cancer, there were other frequent admission diagnoses including diseases of the circulatory system; infectious and parasitic diseases, which includes human immunodeficiency virus (HIV); diseases of the nervous system and sense organs, such as Alzheimer disease, Parkinson disease, and meningitis; and diseases of the respiratory system.

Fiction: A patient needs Medicare or Medicaid to afford hospice services.

Fact: Although insurance coverage for hospice is available through Medicare and in 44 states under Medicaid, most private insurance plans, HMOs, and other managed care organizations include hospice care as a benefit. In addition, through community contributions, memorial donations, and foundation gifts many hospices are able to provide patients who lack sufficient payment with free services. Other programs charge patients in accordance with their ability to pay.

Fiction: A physician decides whether a patient should receive hospice care and which agency should provide that care.

Fact: The role of the physician is to recommend care, whether hospice or traditional curative care. It is the patient's right and decision to determine when hospice is appropriate and which program suits his or her needs. Before entering a hospice, however, a physician must certify that a patient has been diagnosed with a terminal illness and has a life expectancy of six months or less.

Fiction: Hospice services are very expensive because 24-hour on-call services are provided.

Fact: Generally hospice costs less than care in hospitals, nursing homes, or other institutional settings for one basic reason: in those facilities a patient is charged each day for all general services such as food services and basic medical supplies. With hospice, a patient pays only for the services he or she or the family cannot provide and that are not covered by insurance. In 1997 the charges per hospital day were estimated at $2,121 or $454 in a skilled nursing facility. In 1997 hospice care cost approximately $108 per covered day of care. It is also estimated that Medicare's hospice program saves $1.68 for every dollar spent for Part A benefits in the last month of life.

Fiction: To be eligible for hospice care, a patient must already be bedridden.

Fact: Hospice care is appropriate at the time of the terminal prognosis, regardless of the patient's physical condition. Many of the patients served through hospice continue to lead productive and rewarding lives. Together, the patient, family, and physician determine when hospice services should begin.

Fiction: After six months, patients are no longer eligible to receive hospice care through Medicare and other insurances.

Fact: According to the Medicare hospice program, services may be provided to terminally ill Medicare beneficiaries with a life expectancy of six months or less. However, if the patient lives beyond the initial six months, he or she can continue receiving hospice care as long as the attending physician recertifies that the patient is terminally ill. Medicare, Medicaid, and many private and commercial insurances will continue to cover hospice services as long as the patient meets hospice criteria of having a terminal prognosis and is recertified with a limited life expectancy of six months or less.

Fiction: Once a patient elects hospice, he or she can no longer receive care from the primary care physician.

Fact: Hospice reinforces the patient-primary physician relationship by advocating either office or home visits, according to the physician preference. Hospices work closely with the primary physician and consider the continuation of the patient-physician relationship to be of the highest priority.

Fiction: Once a patient elects hospice care, he or she cannot return to traditional medical treatment.

Fact: Patients always have the right to reinstate traditional care at any time, for any reason. If a patient's condition improves or the disease goes into remission, he or she can be discharged from a hospice and return to aggressive, curative measures if so desired. If a discharged patient wants to return to hospice care, Medicare, Medicaid, and most private insurance companies and HMOs will allow readmission.

Fiction: Hospice means giving up hope.

Fact: When faced with a terminal illness, many patients and family members tend to dwell on the imminent loss of life rather than on making the most of the life that remains. Hospice helps patients reclaim the spirit of life. It helps them understand that even though death can lead to sadness, anger, and pain, it can also lead to opportunities for reminiscence, laughter, reunion, and hope—hope that hospice will enable a patient to live his or her life to its fullest.

Additional Information

Joint Commission on Accreditation of Healthcare Organizations
One Renaissance Blvd.
Oakbrook Terrace, IL 60181
Phone: 630-792-5800
Website: http://www.jcaho.org
Quality Check® Website: http://www.qualitycheck.org
E-mail: customerservice@jcaho.org

Chapter 27

Types of Long-Term Care

Assess Your Needs

There are many different kinds of long-term care. Long-term care can take place at home, in senior centers, at community centers, in assisted living and special retirement communities, as well as in nursing homes. Long-term care service is not only nursing home care.

Medicare does not pay for most long-term care. Medicare pays only for medically necessary skilled nursing facility or home health care. You must meet certain conditions for Medicare to pay for these types of care when you get out of the hospital. Most long-term care is to assist people with support services such as dressing, bathing, and using the bathroom. Medicare does not pay for this type of care which is often called custodial care. Custodial care is care that helps you with activities of daily living. It may also include care that most people do for themselves.

Following are some of the many kinds of custodial care people often need, like help with activities of daily living or care most people do themselves. Think about whether you need these services now, or if you may need them in the future. Note the services you think you may need. You may need help with only one or two types of activities of daily living, like help with eating or bathing. Or, you may need help with many activities of daily living or with care needs, like diabetes

This chapter includes: "Steps to Choosing Long-Term Care: Steps 1 and 3," and "Types of Long-Term Care: Overview and Nursing Homes," from the Centers for Medicare and Medicaid Services (CMS), March 2005.

monitoring or oxygen if you have breathing problems. Also, your needs may change over time. It is important to make a list of the kinds of services you need and revise this list as your needs change.

Will I need help with the following activities of daily living?

- bathing
- dressing
- eating
- using the bathroom, including caring for a catheter or colostomy bag if needed
- moving into or out of a bed, chair, or wheelchair
- other_____

Will I need help with additional services?

- preparing meals
- shopping
- housework and laundry
- getting to appointments
- paying bills and other money matters
- home maintenance and repairs
- using the telephone
- other_____

Will I need help with personal care?

- remembering to take medicine
- diabetes monitoring
- using eye drops
- getting oxygen
- taking care of colostomy or bladder catheters
- other_____

Types of Long-Term Care: Overview

The cost of long-term care can vary quite a bit depending on what kind of care you need, where you get the care, and where you live. Table 27.1 shows how these costs generally compare with each other.

Nursing Homes

Nursing homes provide care to people who cannot be cared for at home or in the community. These facilities provide a wide range of personal care and health services. This care generally is to assist people with support services such as dressing, bathing, and using the bathroom when people cannot take care of themselves due to physical, emotional, or mental problems. Medicare does not pay for this type of care and does not pay for most nursing home care. The cost for nursing homes varies depending on where you live and what type of care you need.

Some nursing homes may provide skilled care after an injury or hospital stay. Medicare pays for skilled nursing facility care for a limited period of time if you meet certain criteria.

Nursing Home: Checklist

It is important for you and your family members to visit the nursing home to make sure that it can accommodate your needs, as well

Table 27.1. Comparison of Long-Term Care Facilities, Services, and Cost

Type of Care	Help with activities of daily living	Help with additional services	Help with care needs	Range of costs
Community-Based Services	Yes	Yes	No	Low to medium
Home Health Care	Yes	Yes	Yes	Low to high
In-Law Apartments	Yes	Yes	Yes	Low to high
Housing for Aging and Disabled Individuals	Yes	Yes	No	Low to high
Board and Care Homes	Yes	Yes	Yes	Low to high
Assisted Living	Yes	Yes	Yes	Medium to high
Continuing Care Retirement Communities	Yes	Yes	Yes	High
Nursing Homes	Yes	Yes	Yes	High

as those of your family. A few things to consider when choosing a nursing home are:

- Is the nursing home accepting new residents?

- Is the nursing home easy to visit for family and friends?

- Does the nursing home use hospitals where my doctor practices?

- Does the nursing home have the services I need?

- Does the nursing home have a variety of activities I might enjoy?

- Do residents appear clean and well-groomed?

- Do the residents have the same staff on a daily basis?

- Is there enough staff available to assist residents?

- Does the staff respond quickly to residents' calls for help?

- Does the nursing home have an active resident and/or family council?

- Is the nursing home clean and pleasant?

- Is the nursing home certified by Medicare and Medicaid?

- Are the nursing home and its current administrator licensed?

- How much is the cost of care in this nursing home?

- What services are included in this price?

- What additional costs will I have to pay?

Ask to see the nursing home's last annual state inspection report. Did the report find any problems? Ask how the problems were fixed.

Find What Is Right for You

Quality care means doing the right thing, at the right time, in the right way, for the right person and producing the best possible results. The Medicare program regulates and enforces rules to ensure that nursing homes, home health agencies, and hospitals comply with federal standards for patient health and safety and quality of care. However, the quality of long-term care programs, services, and facilities may vary.

Here are some ways to learn about how long-term care programs and services in your area rate in quality:

- Ask friends and other people you know who use different kinds of long-term care services if they are happy with the services they get.

- Call your State or local long-term care ombudsman. Ombudsmen visit nursing homes and other long-term care facilities regularly to visit residents and take care of complaints. Your local area ombudsman can also give you information on the most recent State inspection survey for long-term care facilities in your area.

- Look at the Nursing Home Compare and Home Health Compare sections on the Medicare website. You can also find out if a continuing care retirement community is accredited from the Commission on Accreditation of Rehabilitation Facilities.

- Call your State health department. Ask if you can get information on the quality of nursing homes and other long-term care facilities and services in your area. You can get the telephone number of your State health department by looking in the blue pages of your local telephone book.

Additional Information

Centers for Medicare and Medicaid Services
Toll-Free: 800-MEDICARE (800-633-4227)
Toll-Free TTY: 877-486-2048
Websites: http://www.medicare.gov or http://www.cms.hhs.gov

Joint Commission on Accreditation of Healthcare Organizations
One Renaissance Blvd.
Oakbrook Terrace, IL 60181
Phone: 630-792-5800
Website: http://www.jcaho.org
Quality Check® Website: http://www.qualitycheck.org
E-mail: customerservice@jcaho.org

Commission on Accreditation of Rehabilitation Facilities
4891 E. Grant Road
Tucson, AZ 85712
Toll-Free Voice/TTY: 888-281-6531
Phone: 520-325-1044
Fax: 520-318-1129
Website: http://www.carf.org

Chapter 28

Long-Term Care:
Choosing the Right Place

Many of us hope to stay in our homes as we grow older. Often we are able to do that. But later in life—usually by our 80s and 90s—some of us need a hand with everyday activities like shopping, cooking, or bathing. A few of us need more help on a regular basis. Maybe that means it is time to move to a place where expert care is available around-the-clock.

Where to Start

Do you think that your family member cannot live at home any longer? It might be your husband or wife, a parent, aunt or uncle, or even a grandparent. You have added a hand rail on the front steps and grab bars in the bathroom. You made plans for a home health aide to come to the house every day. You arranged for help with meals, and you visit every day. But now you wonder if staying at home is the best choice. Where do you go for help? Here are some answers to that and other questions that you might have as you look for the best place for you or a relative to live.

Sometimes the need for help grows over time. For example, Bob is 87 years old. He has lived alone since his wife died ten years ago. For the last few years, he has needed more and more help doing things for himself. First, he had trouble making meals. So, he ate a big lunch at the local senior center until last year when he gave up driving. Now sometimes his daughter drops off meals. Other times meals are

National Institute on Aging (NIA), September 2003.

delivered by a local program. The stairs in his house are getting too hard to climb. Bob also forgets more and more things. He often forgets to take his blood pressure medicine. He has also left the burner on the stove turned on several times. He does not want to move in with his daughter and her family, so Bob and his daughter are looking for a new place for him to live.

Over the last year, Bob's daughter has been thinking this time might come. She knows what is available. She has looked into how they will pay for the care her dad needs. Bob too has been doing some planning. He is sad about leaving his home, but he has been preparing for the time when he would need more help. He even put his name on a waiting list for a nearby retirement community that he liked. Now they have an opening there. The admission coordinator at the community will help him decide if he can live in one of their apartments or needs to be in their assisted living facility.

Bob and his daughter were fortunate. Sometimes you need to make a choice quickly. If you have not planned ahead, then making a decision might not be so easy. For example, Alice and her husband have lived in their house for 50 years. At 84, she still loves to cook and work in her garden every day. Last week she slipped in her bathroom, fell, and broke her hip. Now after an operation to fix her hip, she needs to go somewhere for nursing care and rehabilitation. Her doctors do not know if she will ever recover enough to go home again. Her children live hundreds of miles away. But her husband and family only have a few days to find a place.

Alice and her family were not prepared like Bob and his family. The social worker and discharge planner at the hospital will help them find a place for Alice to go for therapy after she leaves the hospital. But if she is too frail to go home after her hip heals, she and her family will have to choose a place for her to live permanently.

What Are the Choices?

There are two kinds of long-term care, senior living facilities based on how much help is needed:

- assisted living facilities
- skilled nursing facilities or nursing homes

You should think about an assisted living facility if you or a relative do not need a lot of medical care but do need more help than can easily be gotten at home. Assisted living homes can give someone as much help as needed with daily living, but offer only some nursing care or none at all. People often live independently in their own unit. The place provides meals and house cleaning, offers interesting things to do, and may take residents wherever they need to go, like the doctor or the shopping mall. They can also provide help with bathing, dressing, and taking medicines, if needed.

Some assisted living facilities are part of a continuing care retirement community or life-care community. These communities offer independent living and skilled nursing facilities as well as assisted living. Sometimes assisted living help is set up in a home with only a few residents. These are often called board and care homes.

If your relative becomes very frail or suffers from the later stages of dementia, more care could be needed. A nursing home or skilled nursing facility may be necessary if someone:

- needs round-the-clock nursing care
- might wander away without supervision
- needs help with meals, bathing, personal care, medications, and moving around
- needs more help than the current caregiver can possibly give, or cannot live alone

A nursing home or skilled nursing facility will supply 24-hour services and supervision, including medical care and some physical, speech, and occupational therapy to people living there. They might also offer other services such as social activities and transportation. As a rule, the rooms are for one or two people. Some facilities want residents to bring some special items from home to make their rooms more familiar. Some even allow a pet or make it possible for couples to stay together.

Both assisted living and skilled nursing facilities sometimes offer special areas for people with dementia. These areas are designed to meet the specific needs of these people and to keep them safe from wandering.

How to Choose

Ask Questions: Find out about what is available in your area. Is there any place close enough for family and friends to visit easily? Ask doctors, friends, relatives, local hospital discharge planners and social workers, and religious organizations about local facilities.

Also, each State has long-term care ombudsmen. They have information and may be able to answer questions about a place you are considering. The ombudsman is also available to help solve problems that might come up between a nursing home and the resident or the family. To find your State long-term care ombudsman, call the Administration on Aging Eldercare Locator at 800-677-1116 or visit the website at http://www.eldercare.gov.

Is the person in need of long-term care a military veteran? They might be able to get help through the Department of Veterans Affairs programs. You can check by going to http://www.va.gov, calling the VA Health Care Benefits number, 877-222-8387, or contacting the VA medical center nearest you.

Call: Once you have a list of possible places, get in touch with each one. Ask basic questions about openings and waiting lists, number of residents, costs and methods of payment, and their link to Medicare and Medicaid. Take a few minutes to think about what is important to you or your relative, such as transportation, meals, activities, connection to a certain religion, or special units for Alzheimer disease.

Visit: Make plans to meet with the director of nursing and director of social services. Medicare offers a nursing home checklist to use when visiting. Some of the things to look for include certification for Medicare and Medicaid, handicap access, no strong odors (either bad or good ones), contact between staff and current residents, volunteers, and the appearance of residents. If the nursing home is a member of the Joint Committee on Accreditation of Healthcare Organizations, ask to see that group's review of the home. Ask yourself if you would feel reassured leaving your loved one there.

Visit Again: Make a second visit without an appointment, maybe on another day of the week or time of day, so you will meet other staff members. See if your first thoughts are still the same.

Understand: Once you or your relative have made a choice, be sure to understand the facility's contract and payment plan. If you do not understand it, you could have a lawyer review it before signing.

How to Pay

There are several ways to pay for nursing facility care for people over age 65 including:

- Medicare
- private pay
- Medicaid
- long-term care insurance

Let's see what happened after Alice left the hospital. She went directly to a skilled nursing facility. It had a rehabilitation unit where she began to receive physical therapy. Medicare covered most of her costs for the first few weeks as she got better. Then she had a stroke which left her unable to move her left arm and leg. While she was in the hospital for the stroke, her doctors decided Alice should probably not return home. She no longer qualified for Medicare to pay for her nursing home care.

- Many people believe that Medicare will pay for long stays in a nursing home, but it does not. The Federal Medicare program and private Medigap (Medicare supplemental) insurance only cover short times of home health or nursing home care. They pay for a short stay in a nursing home for someone who is getting better after leaving the hospital, but still needs nursing care and therapy.

Alice's husband started to pay for her care on his own, but they did not have a lot of savings. When they had used most of their savings, her husband arranged for her to apply for Medicaid. The good news about Medicaid is that her husband did not have to sell their home for her to qualify for this support.

- Many people start paying for long-term care with their own money (private pay). Later they may become eligible for state-run Medicaid. Each state decides who qualifies for this program. Contact your state government to learn more. Keep in mind that applying for Medicaid takes at least three months.

Alice's children are now looking into buying long-term care insurance for themselves. They do not want to have the same worries if they need nursing care when they are older.

- Long-term care insurance is a private insurance policy you can buy years before you think you might need it. Each policy is different. Your State insurance commission can tell you more about private long-term care policies. They can also offer tips on how to buy long-term care insurance. These agencies are listed in your telephone book, under Government.

Making a Smooth Transition

Moving to a care facility can be a big change for the whole family. Some facilities or community groups have a social worker who can help you prepare for the change. Allow some time to adjust after the move has taken place.

Regular visits by family and friends can make this move easier. This reassures and comforts the person getting used to a new place. Visits are good, too, for keeping an eye on the care that is being given. They also help family to develop a good relationship with the staff caring for their loved one.

Additional Information

Eldercare Locator
Administration on Aging
330 Independence Ave., S.W.
Washington, DC 20201
Toll-Free: 800-677-1116
Phone: 202-619-7501
Website: http://www.eldercare.gov
E-mail:
eldercarelocator@spherix.com

Centers for Medicare and Medicaid Services
Toll-Free: 800-MEDICARE (800-633-4227)
Toll-Free TTY: 877-486-2048
Websites: http://www.medicare.gov or http://www.cms.hhs.gov

Joint Commission on Accreditation of Healthcare Organizations
One Renaissance Blvd.
Oakbrook Terrace, IL 60181
Phone: 630-792-5800
Website: http://www.jcaho.org
Quality Check® Website: http://www.qualitycheck.org
E-mail:
customerservice@jcaho.org

Commission on Accreditation of Rehabilitation Facilities
4891 E. Grant Road
Tucson, AZ 85712
Toll-Free (Voice/TTY): 888-281-6531
Phone: 520-325-1044
Fax: 520-318-1129
Website: http://www.carf.org

National Institute on Aging (NIA)
Information Center
P.O. Box 8057
Gaithersburg, MD 20898-8057
Toll-Free: 800-222-2225
Toll-Free TTY: 800-222-4225
Website: http://www.nia.nih.gov

Chapter 29

Alternatives to Nursing Home Care

Other Alternatives

The following alternatives to nursing home care may work for people who require less than skilled care, or who require skilled care for only brief periods of time. Many people with long-term skilled care needs require a level and amount of care that cannot be easily handled outside of a nursing home.

Home and Community Care

A person who is ill or disabled may be able to get help from a variety of home services that might make moving into a nursing home unnecessary. Home services include Meals on Wheels programs, friendly visiting and shopper services, and adult day care. These programs are found in most communities.

If you are considering home care, discuss this option with family members to learn if they are able to help provide your care or help arrange for other care providers to come to your home. Some nursing homes may provide respite care and admit a person in need of care for a short period of time to give the home caregivers a break. Depending on the case, Medicare, private insurance, and Medicaid may pay some home care costs that are related to medical care.

This chapter includes information from Centers for Medicare and Medicaid Services documents: "Other Options," "About Social Managed Care Plan," and "About PACE," from *Alternatives to Nursing Home Care*, July 2005.

Subsidized Senior Housing (Non-Medical)

There are Federal and State programs that help pay for housing for older people with low to moderate incomes. Some of these subsidized facilities offer assistance to residents who need help with certain tasks such as shopping and laundry. Residents generally live independently in an apartment within the senior housing complex.

Assisted Living (Non-Medical Senior Housing)

If you only need help with a small number of tasks such as cooking and laundry, or reminders to take medications, assisted living facilities maybe an option worth considering. Assisted living is a general term for living arrangements in which some services are available to residents who still live independently within the assisted living complex. In most cases, assisted living residents pay a regular monthly rent and then pay additional fees for the services that they require.

Board and Care Homes

Board and Care homes are group living arrangements designed to meet the needs of people who cannot live independently, but do not require nursing home services. These homes offer a wider range of services than independent living options. Most provide help with some of the activities of daily living including eating, walking, bathing, and toileting. In some cases, private, long-term care insurance and medical assistance programs will help pay for this type of living arrangement. Keep in mind that many of these homes do not get payment from Medicare or Medicaid and are not strictly monitored.

Continuing Care Retirement Communities (CCRCs)

CCRCs are housing communities that provide different levels of care based on the residents' needs—from independent living apartments to skilled nursing care in an affiliated nursing home. Residents move from one setting to another based on their needs, but continue to remain a part of their CCRC community. Be sure to check the record of the CCRC's nursing home. Your CCRC contract usually will require you to use it. Many CCRCs require a large payment prior to admission and also charge monthly fees. For this reason, many CCRCs may be too expensive for older people with modest incomes.

Social Managed Care Plan

A social managed care plan is an organization that provides the full range of Medicare benefits offered by standard managed care plans, plus additional services which include care coordination, prescription drug benefits, chronic care benefits covering short-term nursing home care, a full range of home and community based services such as homemaker, personal care services, adult day care, respite care, and medical transportation. Other services that may be provided include eyeglasses, hearing aids, and dental benefits. These plans offer the full range of medical benefits that are offered by standard managed care plans plus chronic care/extended care services. Membership offers other health benefits that are not provided through Medicare alone or most other senior health plans.

Current Social Managed Care Plan Sites

There are currently four social managed care plans participating in Medicare and each social managed care plan has eligibility criteria. These social managed care plans are located in: Portland, Oregon; Long Beach, California; Brooklyn, New York; and Las Vegas, Nevada. Listed below are the four plans and the criteria for joining each plan.

Kaiser Permanente in Portland, Oregon

The enrollee must be 65 years of age or older, must have Medicare Part A and Part B, must continue to pay the Part B premium, and must live in Kaiser Permanente's social managed care plan service area. The enrollee cannot have end-stage renal disease, or reside in an institutional setting. In order to receive the long-term care benefit, an expanded care resource coordinator will visit you at home to determine if you qualify for nursing home certification based on criteria established by the State of Oregon Senior and Disabled Services. These criteria may include needing daily ongoing assistance from another person with one of the following activities of daily living: walking or transferring indoors, eating, managing medications, controlling difficult or dangerous behavior, controlling your bowels or bladder, or the need for protection and supervision because of confusion or frailty.

SCAN, Long Beach, California

The enrollee must be 65 years of age or older, must have Medicare Part A and Part B, must continue to pay the Part B premium, and must live in SCAN's service area. The enrollee cannot have end-stage renal disease. In addition, in order to receive extended home care services, members must have a Nursing Home Certificate which indicates that the member's informal support system, such as a family member or caregiver, is not sufficient to keep the member out of a nursing home.

Elderplan, Brooklyn, New York

The enrollee must be 65 years of age or older, must have Medicare Part A and Part B, must continue to pay the Part B premium, and must live in Elderplan's service area. The enrollee cannot have end-stage renal disease. In order to receive chronic care benefits, the enrollee must meet state nursing home certifiable criteria.

Health Plan of Nevada, Las Vegas, Nevada

The enrollee must be at least 65 years of age, or may be under 65 if they are disabled. The enrollee must have Medicare Part A and Part B, must continue to pay the Part B premium, and must live in Health Plan of Nevada's service area. The enrollee cannot have end-stage renal disease. For the long-term care benefit, the beneficiary must meet certain criteria based on established medical, psychological, functional, and social criteria as well as needing to be medically necessary.

Your Cost

Each plan has different requirements for premiums. All plans have co-payments for certain services. Before making any health plan decisions, you should contact the plan directly.

Program of All Inclusive Care for the Elderly (PACE)

PACE is unique. It is an optional benefit under both Medicare and Medicaid that focuses entirely on older people who are frail enough to meet their State's standards for nursing home care. It features comprehensive medical and social services that can be provided at an adult day health center, home, and/or inpatient facilities. For most patients, the comprehensive service package permits them to continue living at home while receiving services, rather than be institutionalized. A team of doctors, nurses, and other health professionals assess participant needs, develop care plans, and deliver all services which are integrated into a complete health care plan. PACE is available only in States which have chosen to offer PACE under Medicaid.

Eligibility

Eligible individuals who wish to participate must voluntarily enroll. PACE enrollees also must:

- be at least 55 years of age;
- live in the PACE service area;
- be screened by a team of doctors, nurses, and other health professionals as meeting that state's nursing facility level of care; and
- be able to safely live in a community setting at the time of enrollment.

Services

PACE offers and manages all of the medical, social, and rehabilitative services their enrollees need to preserve or restore their independence, to remain in their homes and communities, and to maintain their quality of life. The PACE service package must include all Medicare and Medicaid services provided by that State. In addition, the PACE organization provides any service determined necessary by the interdisciplinary team. Minimum services that must be provided in the PACE center include primary care services, social services, restorative therapies, personal care and supportive services, nutritional counseling, recreational therapy, and meals. Services are available 24 hours a day, 7 days a week, 365 days a year.

Generally, these services are provided in an adult day health center setting, but may also include in-home and other referral services that enrollees may need. This includes such services as medical specialists, laboratory and other diagnostic services, and hospital and nursing home care. An enrollee's need is determined by PACE's medical team of care providers. PACE teams include:

- primary care physicians and nurses
- physical, occupational, and recreational therapists
- social workers
- personal care attendants
- dietitians
- drivers

The PACE team has frequent contact with their enrollees. This helps them to detect subtle changes in their enrollee's condition, and

211

they can react quickly to changing medical, functional, and psycho-social problems.

Payment

PACE receives a fixed monthly payment per enrollee from Medicare and Medicaid. The amounts are the same during the contract year, regardless of the services an enrollee may need. Persons enrolled in PACE may have to pay a monthly premium depending on their eligibility for Medicare and Medicaid.

PACE Provider Organizations

AltaMed Senior Buena Care
5425 E. Pomona Blvd.
Los Angeles, CA 90022-1716
Phone: 323-728-0411

**Center for Elders
Independence**
510 17th St., Suite 400
Oakland, CA 94612-1367
Phone: 510-433-1150

Sutter Senior Care
1234 U Street
Sacramento, CA 95818-1433
Phone: 916-446-3100

Total Long-Term Care
200 East 9th Ave.
Denver, CO 80203-2903
Phone: 303-869-4664

Florida PACE Centers, Inc.
5200 N.E. Second Ave.
Miami, FL 33137-2706
Phone: 305-751-7223

ViaChristi HOPE, Inc.
935 S. Glendale
Wichita, KS 67218-3002
Phone: 316-858-1111

Hopkins ElderPlus
4940 Eastern Ave.
Baltimore, MD 21224-2780
Phone: 410-550-7044

**Elder Service Plan of
the Cambridge Health
Alliance**
270 Green St.
Cambridge, MA 02139-3312
Phone: 617-381-7100

**Elder Service Plan of the
East Boston Neighborhood
Health Center**
10 Gove St.
East Boston, MA 02128-1920
Phone: 617-568-4602

Summit ElderCare
277 E. Mountain St.
Worcester, MA 01608-2898
Phone: 508-852-2026

**Elder Service Plan of Harbor
Health Services, Inc.**
2216 Dorchester Ave.
Dorchester, MA 02124-5607
Phone: 617-296-5100

Elder Service Plan of the North Shore
20 School St.
Lynn, MA 01901-2952
Phone: 781-581-7565

Uphams Elder Service Plan
1140 Dorchester Ave.
Boston, MA 02125-3305
Phone: 617-288-0970

Center for Senior Independence
7800 W. Outer Dr.
Suite 240
Detroit, MI 48235-3458
Phone: 313-653-2020

Total Community Care
904-A Las Lomas Rd. N.E.
Albuquerque, NM 87102-2633
Phone: 505-924-2650

Comprehensive Care Management
612 Allerton Ave.
Bronx, NY 10467-7404
Toll-Free: 877-226-8500 (member services)
Website: http://www.ccmny.org
Service Sites: Manhattan, Bronx, Brooklyn, Queens, and Westchester Counties

Eddy Senior Care
504 State St.
Schenectady, NY 12305-2414
Phone: 518-382-3290

Independent Living for Seniors
2066 Hudson Ave.
Rochester, NY 14617-4300
Phone: 585-922-2800

PACE CNY
100 Malta Lane
North Syracuse, NY 13212-2375
Phone: 315-452-5800

Concordia Care
2373 Euclid Heights Blvd.
Cleveland Heights, OH 44106-2705
Phone: 216-791-3580

TriHealth Senior Link
4750 Wesley Ave.
Suite J
Cincinnati, OH 45212-2244
Phone: 513-531-5110

Providence ElderPlace–Portland
13007 N.E. Glisan St.
Portland, OR 97230-2545
Phone: 503-215-6556

Community LIFE
2400 Ardmore Blvd., Suite 700
Pittsburgh, PA 15221-5238
Phone: 412-436-1320

LIFE–Pittsburgh, Inc.
One Parkway Center
875 Greentree Rd., Suite 200
Pittsburgh, PA 15220-3508
Phone: 412-388-8042

LIFE–University of Pennsylvania School of Nursing
4101 Woodland Ave.
Philadelphia, PA 19104-4510
Phone: 215-573-7200

LIFE St. Agnes
1500 S. Columbus Blvd.
Philadelphia, PA 19147
Phone: 215-339-4747

PACE Organization of Rhode Island
225 Chapman St.
Providence, RI 02905
Phone: 401-490-6566

Palmetto Senior Care
15 Richland Memorial Park
Suite 203
Columbia, SC 29203-6843
Phone: 803-434-3770

Alexian Brothers Community Services
425 Cumberland St., Suite 110
Chattanooga, TN 37404-1905
Phone: 423-698-0802

Bienvivir Senior Health Services
2300 McKinley Ave.
El Paso, TX 79930-2240
Phone: 915-562-3444

Basics at Jan Werner
3108 S. Fillmore St.
Amarillo, TX 79110-1026
Phone: 806-374-5516

Providence ElderPlace–Seattle
4515 Martin Luther King Jr. Way S., Suite 100
Seattle, WA 98108-2174
Phone: 206-320-5325

Additional Information

Eldercare Locator
Administration on Aging
330 Independence Ave., S.W.
Washington, DC 20201
Toll-Free: 800-677-1116
Phone: 202-619-7501
Website: http://www.eldercare.gov
E-mail: eldercarelocator@spherix.com

The Elder Care Locator can help you find necessary and convenient services that serve the elderly in their community.

Chapter 30

Home Care for Critically Ill Patients

Chapter Contents

Section 30.1

Selecting Quality Home Health Care

"Home Health Care: A Guide for Families,"
Administration on Aging, August 27, 2003.

Home Health Care

- There are 1.4 million home health care patients.

- Average length of home health care service is 69 days.

- Heart disease is the most common primary diagnosis—13% of discharges.

Source: U.S. 2000 data, from "Home Health Care," *Health, United States, 2004*, National Center for Health Statistics, Centers for Disease Control and Prevention (CDC).

A Guide for Families

How do I make sure that home health care is quality care?

As with any important purchase, it is always a good idea to talk with friends, neighbors, and your local area agency on aging to learn more about the home health care agencies in your community. In looking for a home health care agency, the following 20 questions can be used to help guide your search.

1. How long has the agency been serving this community?

2. Does the agency have any printed brochures describing the services it offers and how much do they cost? If so, get one.

3. Is the agency an approved Medicare provider?

4. Is the quality of care certified by a national accrediting body such as the Joint Commission for the Accreditation of Healthcare Organizations?

5. Does the agency have a current license to practice (if required in the state where you live)?

6. Does the agency offer seniors a Patients' Bill of Rights that describes the rights and responsibilities of both the agency and the senior being cared for?

7. Does the agency write a plan of care for the patient (with input from the patient, his or her doctor, and family) and update the plan as necessary?

8. Does the care plan outline the patient's course of treatment describing the specific tasks to be performed by each caregiver?

9. How closely do supervisors oversee care to ensure quality?

10. Will agency caregivers keep family members informed about the kind of care their loved one is getting?

11. Are agency staff members available around the clock, seven days a week, if necessary?

12. Does the agency have a nursing supervisor available to provide on-call assistance 24 hours a day?

13. How does the agency ensure patient confidentiality?

14. How are agency caregivers hired and trained?

15. What is the procedure for resolving problems when they occur, and who can I call with questions or complaints?

16. How does the agency handle billing?

17. Is there a sliding fee schedule based on ability to pay, and is financial assistance available to pay for services?

18. Will the agency provide a list of references for its caregivers?

19. Who does the agency call if the home health care worker cannot come when scheduled?

20. What type of employee screening is done?

Screening Process

When purchasing home health care directly from an individual provider (instead of through an agency), it is even more important to screen the person thoroughly. This should include an interview with the home health caregiver to make sure that he or she is qualified for the job. You should request references. Also, prepare for the interview by making a list of any special needs the senior might have. For example, you would want to note whether the elderly patient needs help getting into or out of a wheelchair. Clearly, if this is the case, the home health caregiver must be able to provide that assistance. The screening process will go easier if you have a better idea of what you are looking for first.

Another thing to remember is that it always helps to look ahead, anticipate changing needs, and have a backup plan for special situations. Since every employee occasionally needs time off (or a vacation), it is unrealistic to assume that one home health care worker will always be around to provide care. Seniors or family members who hire home health workers directly may want to consider interviewing a second part-time or on-call person who can be available when the primary caregiver is unavailable. Calling an agency for temporary respite care may help to solve this problem.

In any event, whether you arrange for home health care through an agency or hire an independent home health care aide on an individual basis, it helps to spend some time preparing for the person who will be doing the work. Tell the home health care provider (both verbally and in writing) the following things that he or she should know about the senior:

- illnesses/injuries, and signs of an emergency medical situation
- likes and dislikes
- medications: how and when they should be taken
- need for dentures, eyeglasses, canes, walkers, etc.
- possible behavior problems and how best to deal with them
- problems getting around (in or out of a wheelchair, for example, or difficulty walking)
- special diets or nutritional needs
- therapeutic exercises

In addition, you should give the home health care provider more information about:

- clothing the person may need (if/when it gets too hot or too cold);

- how you can be contacted (and who else should be contacted in an emergency);
- how to find and use medical supplies and medications;
- when to lock up the apartment/house and where to find the keys;
- where to find food, cooking utensils, and serving items;
- where to find cleaning supplies;
- where to find light bulbs and flash lights, and where the fuse box is located (in case of a power failure);
- where to find the washer, dryer, and other household appliances (as well as instructions for how to use them).

A Word of Caution

Although most states require that home health care agencies perform criminal background checks on their workers and carefully screen job applicants for these positions, the actual regulations will vary depending on where you live. Therefore, before contacting a home health care agency, you may want to call your local area agency on aging or department of public health to learn what laws apply in your state.

How can I apply for home health care?

The cost of home health care varies across states and within states. In addition, costs will fluctuate depending on the type of health care professional required. Home care services can be paid for directly by the patient and his or her family members or through a variety of public and private sources. Sources for home health care funding include Medicare, Medicaid, the Older Americans Act, the Veterans' Administration, and private insurance. Medicare is the largest single payer of home care services. The Medicare program will pay for home health care if all of the following conditions are met:

- The patient must be homebound and under a doctor's care.
- The patient must need skilled nursing care, or occupational, physical, or speech therapy on at least an intermittent basis (that is, regularly but not continuously).
- The services provided must be under a doctor's supervision and performed as part of a home health care plan written specifically for that patient.

219

- The patient must be eligible for the Medicare program and the services ordered must be medically reasonable and necessary.

- The home health care agency providing the services must be certified by the Medicare program.

Section 30.2

Assistive Technology: Help for Patients with Chronic Conditions

"Assistive Technology," Administration on Aging, August 27, 2003.

Assistive technology is any service or tool that helps the elderly or disabled do the activities they have always done but must now do differently. These tools are also sometimes called adaptive devices.

Such technology may be something as simple as a walker to make moving around easier or an amplification device to make sounds easier to hear (for talking on the telephone or watching television, for instance). It could also include a magnifying glass that helps someone who has poor vision read the newspaper or a small motor scooter that makes it possible to travel over distances that are too far to walk. In short, anything that helps the elderly continue to participate in daily activities is considered assistive technology.

Just as older people may have many different types of disabilities, many different categories of assistive devices and services are available to help overcome those disabilities including:

- **Adaptive switches:** Modified switches that seniors can use to adjust air conditioners, computers, telephone answering machines, power wheelchairs, and other types of equipment. The tongue or the voice might activate these switches.

- **Communication equipment:** Anything that enables a person to send and receive messages, such as a telephone amplifier.

- **Computer access:** Special software that helps a senior access the Internet, or basic hardware, such as a modified keyboard or mouse, which makes the computer more user friendly.

- **Education:** Audio books or Braille writing tools for the blind come under this category, along with resources that allow people to get additional vocational training.

- **Home modifications:** Construction or remodeling work, such as building a ramp for wheelchair access, which allows a senior to overcome physical barriers and live more comfortably with a disability or recover from an accident or injury.

- **Tools for independent living:** Anything that empowers the elderly to enjoy the normal activities of daily living without assistance from others, such as a handicapped-accessible bathroom with grab bars in the bathtub.

- **Job-related items:** Any device or process that a person needs to do his or her job better or easier. Examples might include a special type of chair or pillow for someone who works at a desk or a back brace for someone who does physical labor.

- **Mobility aids:** Any piece of equipment that helps a senior get around more easily, such as a power wheelchair, wheelchair lift, or stair elevator.

- **Orthotic or prosthetic equipment:** A device that compensates for a missing or disabled body part. This could range from orthopedic shoe inserts for someone who has fallen arches to an artificial arm for someone whose limb has been amputated.

- **Recreational assistance:** New methods and tools to enable people who have disabilities to enjoy a wide range of fun activities. Examples include swimming lessons provided by recreational therapists or specially equipped skis for seniors who have lost a limb as a result of accident or illness.

- **Seating aids:** Any modifications to regular chairs, wheelchairs, or motor scooters that help a person stay upright or get up and down unaided or that help to reduce pressure on the skin. This could be something as simple as an extra pillow or as complex as a motorized seat.

- **Sensory enhancements:** Anything that makes it easier for those who are partially or fully blind or deaf to better appreciate the world around them. For instance, a television caption decoder would be an assistive device for a senior who is hard of hearing.

- **Therapy:** Equipment or processes that help someone recover as much as possible from an illness or injury. Therapy might involve a combination of services and technology, such as having a physical therapist use a special massage unit to restore a wider range of motion to stiff muscles.

- **Transportation assistance:** Devices for elderly individuals that make it easier for them to get into and out of their cars or trucks and drive more safely, such as adjustable mirrors, seats, and steering wheels. Services that help the elderly maintain and register their vehicles, such as a drive-up window at the department of motor vehicles, would also fall into this category.

What are the benefits of assistive technology?

For many seniors, assistive technology makes the difference between being able to live independently and having to get long-term nursing or home health care. For others, assistive technology is critical to the ability to perform simple activities of daily living, such as bathing and going to the bathroom.

According to a 1993 study conducted by the National Council on Disability, 80 percent of the elderly persons who used assistive technology were able to reduce their dependence on others. In addition, half of those surveyed reduced their dependence on paid helpers, and half were able to avoid entering nursing homes. Assistive technology can also reduce the costs of care for the elderly and their families. Although families may need to make monthly payments for some pieces of equipment, for many this cost is much less than the cost of home health or nursing home care.

Is assistive technology right for me?

Whether you are conducting a needs assessment or trying to make a decision after such an assessment, it is always a good idea to ask the following questions about assistive technology:

- Does a more advanced device meet more than one of my needs?

- Does the manufacturer of the assistive technology have a preview policy that will let me try out a device and return it for credit if it does not work as expected?

- How are my needs likely to change over the next six months? How about over the next six years or longer?

- How up-to-date is this piece of assistive equipment? Is it likely to become obsolete in the immediate future?

- What are the tasks that I need help with, and how often do I need help with these tasks?

- What types of assistive technology are available to meet my needs?

- What, if any, types of assistive technology have I used before, and how did that equipment work?

- What type of assistive technology will give me the greatest personal independence?

- Will I always need help with this task? If so, can I adjust this device and continue to use it as my condition changes?

How can I pay for assistive technology?

Right now, no single private insurance plan or public program will pay for all types of assistive technology under any circumstances. However, Medicare Part B will cover up to 80 percent of the cost of assistive technology if the items being purchased meet the definition of durable medical equipment.

Depending on where you live, the state-run Medicaid program may pay for part of the cost of some assistive technology.

Seniors who are eligible for veterans' benefits should definitely look into whether they can receive assistance from the Department of Veterans Affairs (DVA).

Private health insurance and out-of-pocket payment are two other options for purchasing assistive technology.

Subsidy programs provide some types of assistive technology at a reduced cost or for free. Many businesses and not-for-profit groups have set up subsidy programs that include discounts, grants, or rebates to get consumers to try a specific product.

Section 30.3

Respiratory Home Health Care

Respiratory care at home can contribute to improved quality of life and significant cost savings. Your respiratory care practitioner can help you with your treatment, answer questions you may have, provide instructions, and offer suggestions. Here are some tips to ensure that you get the greatest benefit from your respiratory home care.

Get Involved

It is important for you to exercise your rights as a patient. Ask questions of your physician, your respiratory care practitioner, your discharge planner, and if necessary, your home medical equipment supplier. If training is necessary, make sure that you and a family caregiver participate.

Discuss all the options that are available to you regarding your care plan, renting versus buying equipment, and insurance coverage. Provide all the information that is requested about your family and home situation to help your health care provider plan for your care after you are discharged from the hospital.

Safety

Safety for you, your caregivers, and visitors is very important. If you have been prescribed oxygen therapy, you should not smoke while using oxygen, and no one near you should smoke either. Put up no smoking signs in your home where you will be using oxygen.

Because oxygen is flammable, you should stay at least five feet away from gas stoves, lighted fireplaces, candles, or any other open flame. Do not use flammable products like aerosol sprays, paint thinner, or rubbing alcohol. Keep an all-purpose fire extinguisher nearby, and let the fire department know that you have oxygen in the house.

If you have a cylinder of oxygen, make sure it is in a stand or secured to something solid. The tank is heavy, and if it gets knocked over and damaged, the gas could escape making the cylinder act like a rocket. If you have long tubing that lets you move about the house, warn visitors so they won't trip on it. If you have a vessel of liquid oxygen, keep it upright. If it falls on its side, the oxygen will pour out, and it is so cold it could hurt your skin.

Make sure your electrical system does not overload because of the equipment you are using. Use only grounded electrical outlets. Avoid extension cords. Notify the electric company that you have a ventilator or oxygen concentrator in your home so your house will get priority attention if the power fails.

Infection Control

Preventing infections can help the respiratory home care patient stay as healthy as possible. Hand washing is the single most important action for patients and caregivers to perform on a routine basis. Use a liquid soap and lots of warm running water. Work up a good lather and scrub for at least 15 seconds (including fingernails). Rinse well, with your hands pointed down to keep the dirty water from running up your arms. Dry your hands with a clean paper or cloth towel. Even if the caregiver wears gloves in caring for the patient, hand washing is required before putting the gloves on and after taking them off. If you have to use a moisturizer on your hands, avoid a petroleum-based product if you wear latex gloves.

Your respiratory care equipment should be cleaned on a regular basis. Besides washing with a mild detergent and rinsing carefully, it is necessary to sanitize your equipment in a vinegar solution of one part vinegar to three parts distilled water. Rinse carefully and let the parts air dry on a clean cloth or towel.

If you use oxygen and there is a humidifier in the system, you need to wash the bottle in warm, soapy water daily and sanitize it once or twice a week. If you have an oxygen concentrator, it is necessary to clean the air filter and compressor filter on a scheduled basis. If you use a metered-dose inhaler or a nebulizer, the mouthpiece should be rinsed with warm water after each use and sanitized as directed by your health care provider.

These are only guidelines, and the specific directions for cleaning and sanitizing your home medical equipment should be part of the instructions you get from your health care provider or your home medical equipment company.

Section 30.4

Home Care for Cancer Patients

This section includes an excerpt from "Home Care for Cancer Patients," Cancer Facts 8.5, National Cancer Institute (NCI), June 9, 2003; and an excerpt from PDQ® Cancer Information Summary. National Cancer Institute; Bethesda, MD. Transitional Care Planning: Supportive Care–Professional (PDQ®). Updated June 2005, available at http://cancer.gov. Accessed March 1, 2006.

Cancer patients often feel more comfortable and secure being cared for at home. Many patients want to stay at home so that they will not be separated from family, friends, and familiar surroundings. Home care can help patients achieve this desire. It often involves a team approach that includes doctors, nurses, social workers, physical therapists, family members, and others. Home care can be both rewarding and demanding for patients and caregivers. It can change relationships and require families to address new issues and cope with all aspects of patient care. To help prepare for these changes, patients and caregivers are encouraged to ask questions and get as much information as possible from the home care team or organizations devoted to home care. A doctor, nurse, or social worker can provide information about patients' specific needs, the availability of home care services, and a list of local home care agencies.

Services provided by home care agencies may include access to medical equipment; visits from registered nurses, physical therapists, and social workers; help with running errands, meal preparation, and personal hygiene; and delivery of medication. The state or local health department is another important resource in finding home care services. The health department should have a registry of licensed home care agencies.

Transitional Care Planning: Special Considerations

Caring for a patient at home places increased technical and emotional demands on the family. Many families have numerous out-of-home responsibilities. In addition, family members might be physically or psychosocially compromised and thus unable to assume the primary care role. The following factors need to be assessed when determining whether a spouse or caregiver can handle home care:

- the caregiver's age, health, motivation, and sex (women are more likely to provide home care)

- the length of hospital stay (prolonged stay may complicate transition to home care)

- other demands on the caregiver

- the degree of patient distress (particularly pain)

- the technical nature of care

- decision-making skills required for care delivery

Some patient groups are at a higher risk (for instance, older black women who are alone and poor and who have multiple chronic illnesses are at risk for difficulties after they leave the hospital). Rural patients are also at risk for home care complications, particularly if the terminal phase of disease is prolonged and physical debilitation increases. Access to available health care may be limited.

The importance of assessing the family's motivation and ability to provide care for the patient cannot be stressed enough. Assessment must be broad and include psychological, spiritual, social, physical, and legal considerations, and where appropriate, must also include the level of pre-existing interpersonal conflicts, and the family's beliefs and values with regard to home care, dying, and the use of opioids for pain control.

Adequate pain and symptom management is a key component to successful home management, but this can only be accomplished if the family and primary caregiver understand the need for the control of pain and other symptoms. Health care providers and caregivers need to understand that uncontrolled symptoms, particularly poorly controlled pain, can dramatically increase the physical and psychological burdens of caregiving.

There should be an understanding of who to call for support or advice regarding problems that may arise. As an illness progresses, the need for consistent personnel who know the ill person's situation becomes the key component of successful delivery of care in the home. The central role of family caregivers in cancer management is increasingly recognized. Family caregivers play an essential role in promoting compliance with medical treatment, managing side effects, performing practical tasks, and providing emotional and social support.

It is also noteworthy that caregivers often function as proxies for patients in reporting symptoms and psychological distress; however, studies show that family caregivers tend to overestimate the psychosocial distress of patients which may be a result of their own underreported burden and distress.

Insurance and Financial Considerations

Other important issues for assessment in transitional care planning include insurance coverage, the availability of community resources, legal concerns, and advanced directives. Most insurance companies cover home care, but some policies limit services to specified settings, for example, payment may be dependent on the patient having had a preceding hospitalization or having need for skilled nursing services.

It is important to ascertain insurance limits on specific services as well as lifetime limitations. Primary care physicians, nurses, and social workers may need to assume the role of patient advocate when dealing with third-party insurers, case managers, and managed care companies.

For these reasons it is important to design a home care plan that provides adequate safety to the patient, is least distressing to the family, and utilizes resources appropriately. It is often helpful to explore other resources that do not require insurance or patient payment including sectarian as well as nonsectarian family agencies which may provide limited unskilled services.

Nursing assistants and aides (unskilled nursing services) are usually not covered by insurance; however, hospice care may cover this expense. Proprietary home care services provide this care at the expense of the patient and family.

Additional Information

Centers for Medicare and Medicaid Services
Toll-Free: 800-MEDICARE (800-633-4227)
Toll-Free TTY: 877-486-2048
Websites: http://www.medicare.gov or http://www.cms.hhs.gov

The National Association for Home Care
228 7th St., S.E.
Washington, DC 20003
Phone: 202-547-7424

Fax: 202-547-3540
Website: http://www.nahc.org

The Visiting Nurse Associations of America
99 Summer St., Suite 1700
Boston, MA 02110
Phone: 617-737-3200
Fax: 617-737-1144
Website: http://www.vnaa.org
E-mail: vnaa@vnaa.org

Eldercare Locator
Administration on Aging
330 Independence Ave., S.W.
Washington, DC 20201
Toll-Free: 800-677-1116
Phone: 202-619-7501
Website: http://www.eldercare.gov
E-mail: eldercarelocator@spherix.com

Part Five

End-of-Life Caregiving

Chapter 31

Communications among Patients, Families, and Providers

The Time to Discuss Your Views about End-of-Life Care

When it comes to creating memories and sharing in significant life events, the family is the focal point for commemoration and celebration. We plan for weddings, the birth of a child, going off to college, and retirement. Despite the conversations we have for these life events, rarely, if ever, do we have conversations about how we want to live in the final phase of our lives—until a crisis hits.

Death and dying—once-taboo subjects—are becoming increasingly relevant for baby boomers and their aging parents. We know from research that Americans are more likely to talk to their children about safe sex and drugs than to talk to their terminally ill parents about end-of-life care options and preferences.

With approximately 2.4 million Americans dying each year and the number growing—it is important that thoughtful, serious, personal conversations take place about the kinds of experiences Americans want for themselves or their loved ones as the inevitable end-of-life draws near. Often such conversations are avoided out of an understandable desire to spare each other's feelings. They need not be.

Hospice Care: Comfort and Compassion When It's Needed Most

Experts agree that the time to discuss your views about end-of-life care and to learn about the end-of-life options available is before a life-threatening illness occurs or a crisis hits. This greatly reduces the stress of making decisions about end-of-life care under duress. By preparing in advance, you can avoid some of the uncertainty and anxiety associated with not knowing what your loved ones want. Instead, you can make an educated decision that includes the advice and input of loved ones.

Plan Ahead

Let your loved ones know now—when you are still able to effectively communicate—what your preferences for treatment would be if you were confronting a terminal illness. For example, you may want to indicate that if you ever become terminally ill, your preference is to receive hospice care.

These are a few simple steps you can take to ensure that your end-of-life wishes are followed when the need arises:

- Draw up a living will of written instructions to make known what you want done if, for example, you are seriously ill and the only way you can be kept alive is by artificial means.

- Have an advance directive in place that authorizes a person of your choosing (usually a spouse or close relative) to make decisions if you become unable to do so for yourself. Make sure to communicate your wishes to this person and make sure this person agrees to assume the responsibility. Because every state has different laws, it is in your best interest to consult a lawyer about these documents.

These documents can be useful tools for making known your end-of-life care wishes. However, they should not be used as stand alone documents. It is also important to have detailed, personal conversations with your family and loved ones about these issues.

Discuss Your Wishes Early

Discuss your end-of-life wishes with your family and loved ones now—before a crisis hits. This is essential to ensuring that your end-of-life care wishes are met. You may want to use the following occasions as opportunities for having this conversation:

- around significant life events, such as marriage, birth of a child, death of a loved one, retirement, birthdays, anniversaries, and college graduation

- while you are drawing up your will or doing other estate and financial planning

- before and after annual medical checkups

- when major illness requires that you or a family member move out of your home and into a retirement community, nursing home, or other long-term care facility

- during holiday gatherings, such as Thanksgiving, when family members are present

Discussions might also be prompted by:

- newspaper articles about illness and funerals
- movies
- sermons
- television talk shows, dramas and comedies
- magazines and books

When appropriate, include your children in these conversations, not just your parents. It is never too early to start thinking about these issues. Have regular discussions about your views on end-of-life since they may change over time. And do not forget to discuss your end-of-life wishes with your doctor.

Take the Initiative

Even if you have done everything to communicate your wishes, you may find yourself in a situation where you need to take the initiative and have the discussion with family members or loved ones who have not shared their thoughts with you. Here are a few helpful pointers to keep in mind as you plan for having this conversation.

Do your homework. Before initiating the discussion, learn about end-of-life care services available in your community. Become familiar with what each option offers so you can determine which ones meet your own, or your loved one's, end-of-life needs and desires.

Select an appropriate setting. Plan for the conversation since this is not a discussion to have on the spur of the moment. Find a quiet, comfortable place that is free from distraction to hold a one-on-one discussion. Usually, a private setting is best.

Ask permission. People cope with end-of-life issues in many ways. Asking permission to discuss this topic assures your loved one that you will respect his or her wishes and honor them. Some ways of asking permission are:

- "I'd like to talk about how you would like to be cared for if you got really sick. Is that okay?"

- "If you ever got sick, I would be afraid of not knowing the kind of care you would like. Could we talk about this now? I'd feel better if we did."

As mentioned, another method of initiating the conversation is to share with your loved one an article, magazine, or story about the topic. Even watching a television show or movie on the topic together can encourage the conversation. If you think your loved one would be more comfortable with someone else present, you may want to invite a social worker or spiritual advisor to help in this regard.

Know what to expect. Keep in mind that you have initiated this conversation because you care about your loved one's well-being—especially during difficult times. Try to focus on maintaining a warm and caring manner throughout the conversation by using nonverbal communication to offer support. Allow your loved one to set the pace. Nodding your head in agreement, holding your loved one's hand, and reaching out to offer a hug or comforting touch are ways that you can show your love and concern. Understand that it is normal to encounter resistance the first time you bring up this topic. Do not be surprised or discouraged; instead, plan to try again at another time. Questions to ask your loved one about his or her end-of-life care include:

- How would you like your choices honored at the end-of-life?

- Would you like to spend your final days at home or in a home-like setting?

- Do you think it is important to have medical attention and pain control tailored to fit your needs?

- Is it important for you—and your family—to have emotional and spiritual support?

If your loved one responds yes in answer to these questions, he or she may want the kind of end-of-life care that hospice provides.

Be a good listener. Keep in mind that this is a conversation, not a debate. Sometimes, just having someone to talk to is a big help. Be sure to make an effort to hear and understand what the person is saying. These moments, although difficult, are important and special to both of you. Some important things to do:

- Listen for the wants and needs that your loved one expresses.
- Make clear that what your loved one is sharing with you is important.
- Show empathy and respect by addressing these wants and needs in a truthful and open way.
- Verbally acknowledge your loved one's rights to make life choices—even if you do not agree with them.

The true objective of family conversation is more than a simple package of papers with advance directives and estate details. Those things matter because they will guide final actions. But, what matters most is to talk with the people you love about decisions near the end of life, to come to terms with inevitable loss, and thus to honor the cycle of life.

How to Talk about Your End-of-Life Care Wishes

It is all about talking—talking with your loved ones about your health care preferences; talking with your doctor about your options so that you can make informed decisions; and talking with your health care agent so your wishes are honored if you can not make decisions yourself. Talking before a crisis can help you and your loved ones prepare for any difficult decisions related to health care at the end of life.

How to Talk with Your Loved Ones about End-of-Life Care Issues

Remember, it is up to you to take the initiative and express your wishes. Your family or loved ones are not likely to raise the issue for you. Talking about end-of-life issues can be difficult for anyone. One way to approach the subject is to talk about why you have decided to talk about these issues. For example:

- Did a particular event cause you to make the decision?

- Did a case you read about in the newspaper or something that happened to a family member make you think about it?

- Is the decision part of a broader effort on your part to prepare for the end of life, for instance making your last will and testament for distribution of your property?

- What is motivating you to take these actions now?

Sometimes sharing your personal concerns and values, spiritual beliefs, or views about what makes life worth living can be as helpful as talking about specific treatments and circumstances. For example:

- How important is it to be to be physically independent and to stay in your own home? (Independence can be extremely important to some and is less so to others.)

- What aspects of your life give it the most meaning?

- How important would it be for you to be able to recognize people or interact with them?

- What are your particular concerns about dying? About death?

- How do your religious or spiritual beliefs affect your attitudes toward dying and death?

- Would you want your health care agent to take into account the effect of your illness on any other people?

- Should financial concerns enter into decisions about your treatment?

- Would you prefer to die at home if possible?

One final point: Reassess your decisions over time. These are not simple questions and your views may change. It is important that you review these issues and discuss your choices as your personal health or circumstances change in your life.

How to Talk with Your Health Care Agent about Your End-of-Life Care Wishes

Your health care agent needs to know about the quality of life that is important to you and when and how aggressively you would want medical treatments provided. Talking to your agent means discussing values and quality-of-life issues as well as treatments and medical situations. Because situations could occur that you might not anticipate, your agent may need to base a decision on what he or she knows about your values and your views of what makes life worth living. These are not simple questions, and your views may change. For this reason, you need to talk to your agent in depth and over time.

The following questions may help you discuss these issues with your health care agent:

- How do you want to be treated at the end of your life?

- Are there treatments you particularly want to receive or refuse?

- What are you afraid might happen if you cannot make decisions for yourself?

- Do you have any particular fears or concerns about the medical treatments that you might receive? Under what circumstances?

- What makes those things frightening?

- What do phrases like no heroic measures, or dying with dignity actually mean to you? (People often use these expressions with different meanings.)

For example, if you had a massive stroke:

- Would you want to receive aggressive treatments (such as mechanical ventilation, antibiotics, or tube feeding) for a time, but have them stopped if there were no improvement in your condition?

- What kind of treatment would you want if you were in a state of prolonged unconsciousness and were not expected to recover?

- Would you want life support or would you rather receive palliative (comfort) care only?

- What are your views about artificial nutrition and hydration (tube feeding)?

- Do you want to receive these types of treatment no matter what your medical condition? On a trial basis? Never?

- If your heart stopped, under what circumstances would you want doctors to use cardio-pulmonary resuscitation (CPR) to try to resuscitate you?

How to Talk with Your Doctor about Your End-of-Life Care Wishes

Do not wait until a crisis occurs before discussing concerns about end-of-life treatments with your doctor. Chances are that he or she is waiting for you to start the conversation. When you discuss your concerns and choices:

1. Let your doctor know that you are completing directives.

2. Ask your doctor to explain treatments and procedures that may seem confusing before you complete your directives.

3. Talk about what to expect from pain and what may be your pain management options.

4. Make sure your doctor knows the quality of life that is important to you.

5. Make sure your doctor is willing to follow your directives. The law does not force physicians to follow directives if they disagree with your wishes for moral or ethical reasons.

6. Give your doctor a copy of your completed directives. Make sure your doctor knows the name and telephone number of your appointed health care agent.

7. Assure your doctor that your family and your appointed health care agent know your wishes.

You may ask your doctor specifically:

*   Will you talk openly and candidly with me and my family about my illness?

*   What decisions will my family and I have to make, and what kinds of recommendations will you give to help us make these decisions?

*   Will you go to bat for me with my insurance provider or health plan if you believe that their decisions are not in my best interest?

*   What will you do if I have a lot of pain or other uncomfortable symptoms?

*   How will you help us find excellent professionals with special training when we need them (for example, medical, surgical and palliative care specialists, faith leader, or social workers)?

- Will you let me know if treatment stops working so that my family and I can make appropriate decisions?

- Will you support me in getting hospice care?

- If I reach a point where I am too sick to speak for myself, how will you make decisions about my care?

- Will you still be available to me even when I am sick and close to the end of my life?

How to Talk with a Doctor If You Are a Health Care Agent for a Loved One

Establish open communication with the doctor. Identify the attending physician. Make an appointment to speak about your loved one's care. Be assertive in expressing your wishes. Clearly state the reasons behind your requests without being hostile.

Ask questions. To be effective and to make informed decisions, learn as much as possible about your loved one's condition and prognosis. If you don't ask, the physician might not tell you everything you need to know to make an informed decision.

Ask about the goals of the treatment plan—often. A physician's definition of recovery can be different from what is acceptable to you or your loved one. Some providers may have a hard time withholding or withdrawing treatments.

Seek the assistance of a social worker or patient representative if necessary. Such professionals can help improve communication between you and the physician. Don't be afraid to speak to the facility's administration. If the physician is unresponsive, go directly to his or her superiors including the chief of medicine, risk manager, hospital lawyer, or administrator.

How to Talk with Your Faith Leader about Your End-of-Life Care Wishes

It may also be helpful to talk with your faith leader about your wishes and care at the end of life from a spiritual perspective. The following are questions to help guide your discussion:

- In what ways is your spirituality/religion meaningful for you?

- How is your spirituality/religion important to you in daily life?

- What specific practices do you carry out as part of your religious and spiritual life (for example, prayer, meditation, service. etc.)

- How do your religious or spiritual beliefs affect your attitudes toward dying and death?

- Are there religious or spiritual practices or rituals that you would like to have available in the hospital or at home?

- Are there religious or spiritual practices that you wish to plan for at the time of death, or following death?

- From what sources do you draw strength in order to cope with this illness?

- For what in your life do you still feel gratitude even though ill?

- When you are afraid or in pain, how do you find comfort?

You may want to ask your faith leader specifically:

- Will you understand and support my need for my spiritual self to be nourished and to grow, even as my physical being deteriorates?

- If I have negative feelings like frustration, sadness, despair, anger at God or life, will you listen empathetically?

- Will you help me if I have problems communicating with my family or friends?

- Will you continue to visit me even if I get very sick or it is difficult to talk with me?

- Will you visit with my family and help them with their spiritual concerns about my illness?

- Will you just sit and be with me, even if I don't want to talk?

What to Do If Family Members Disagree with Your End-of-Life Care Wishes

To ensure that your wishes are followed, be certain that the person you appoint to be your agent understands your wishes and will abide by them. Your agent has the legal right to make decisions for you even if close family members disagree. However, if close family members express strong disagreement, your agent and your health care professional may find it extremely difficult and unpleasant to carry out the decisions you would want.

If you foresee that your agent may encounter serious resistance, the following steps can help forestall interference from others:

- Communicate with family members you anticipate may object to your decisions.

- Tell them in writing whom you have appointed to be your health care agent and explain why you have done so.

- Let them know that you do not wish them to be involved with decisions about your medical care and give a copy of these communications to your agent as well.

Give your primary care physician, if you have one, copies of written communications you have made. Prepare a more specific, written living will than normally would be necessary. Make it clear in your documents that you want your agent to resolve any uncertainties that could arise when interpreting the living will. A way to say this is: "My agent should make any decisions about how to interpret or when to apply my living will."

Additional Information

National Hospice and Palliative Care Organization
1700 Diagonal Rd., Suite 625
Alexandria, VA 22314
Toll-Free: 800-658-8898
Phone: 703-837-1500
Fax: 703-837-1233
Website: http://www.nhpco.org
E-mail: nhpco_info@nhpco.org

Chapter 32

Holding On, Letting Go

Our culture tells us that we should fight hard against age, illness, and death: "Do not go gentle into that good night," the Dylan Thomas poem says. "Rage, rage against the dying of the light." And holding on, to life, to our loved ones, is indeed a basic human instinct. However, as the end of life approaches, "raging against the dying of the light," often begins to lose importance, and letting go may instead feel like the right thing to do.

This chapter discusses the shifting emotions and considerations involved in holding on or letting go. Addressing these sensitive issues ahead of time will allow a person with a chronic illness to have some choice or control over his or her care, help families with the process of making difficult decisions, and may make this profound transition a little easier for everyone concerned.

The opinions of the dying person are important, and it is often impossible to know what those beliefs are unless we discuss the issues ahead of time. Planning ahead gives the caregiver and loved ones choices in care and is kinder to the person who will have to make decisions.

Holding On

As people, we have an instinctive desire to go on living. We experience this as desires for food, activity, learning, etc. We also feel attachments to loved ones, such as family members, friends, and even pets, and we do not want to leave them. We do not so much decide to go on living, as find ourselves doing it automatically. Robert Frost said once, "In three words, I can sum up everything I have learned about life: It goes on." Even in difficult times, it is our nature to hold on for better times.

When we realize that the end of life may be approaching, other thoughts and feelings arise. The person who is ill will want to be with loved ones, and may also feel a sense of responsibility towards them, not wanting to fail them nor cause them grief. He/she may have unfinished business. For example, the person may want to reconcile with estranged family members or friends and will find it both easier and more important to do. Fears arise and may be so strong that they are hard to think about or even admit: fear of change, of the dying process, of what happens after death, of losing control, of dependency, and so on. Both the person who is ill and the caregiver might also experience resentment, sadness, and anger at having to do what neither wants to do—namely face death and dying.

In one way or another, hope remains. The object of hope may change. As death comes closer, the family may hope for a restful night, or another visit with a particular friend, or just a quiet passing from this life to whatever we hope follows it. Often, as the end of life nears, we keep two incompatible ideas in our minds at the same time. The Jewish prayer of the gravely ill puts it well for both the person who is ill and the loved ones caring for him/her: "I do not choose to die. May it come to pass that I may be healed. But if death is my fate, then I accept it with dignity."

Letting Go

As death nears, most people feel a lessening of their desire to live longer. This is not a matter of depression. Instead, they sense it is time to let go, perhaps as in other times in life when one senses it is time for a major change. Examples might be leaving home, getting married, divorcing, or changing jobs. Some people describe a sense of profound tiredness, of a tiredness that no longer goes away with rest. Others, who may have overcome many adversities in their lives, reach a point where they feel they have struggled as much as they have been called upon to do and will struggle no more. Refusing to let go can prolong dying, but it cannot prevent it. Dying, thus prolonged, can become more a time of suffering than of living.

Family members and friends who love the dying person may experience a similar change. At first, one refuses to admit the possibility of a loved one dying. Then one refuses to accept the death happening.

246

Lastly, one may see that dying is the better of two bad choices, and be ready to give the loved one permission to die. As mentioned, the dying are distressed at causing grief for those who love them, and receiving permission to die can relieve their distress. There is a time for this to happen. Before that, it feels wrong to accept a loss, but after that it can be an act of great kindness to say, "You may go when you feel it is time. I will be okay."

Other Concerns

Letting go gets mixed up in our minds with a person wanting to die, although these are really separate situations. There are various reasons a person may want to die, reasons quite separate from those for letting go. Depression is one response to finding life too painful in some way. Some people cannot tolerate losing control, so they want to take control of dying. It can be unpleasant to be disabled, or in a place one does not want to be, or isolated from the important people and things in one's life. Very often, a severely ill person feels like a burden to family and friends, and may wish to die rather than let this continue. Fears of the future, even of dying, may be so great that a person wants to die to get away from that future. Inadequately controlled pain or other symptoms can make life seem unbearable. For many of these problems, the right sort of help can make a great improvement, and replace the desire to die with a willingness to live out this last part of one's life.

Chronic Illness

So far, this chapter has been about the very end of life. Many, or even most, people go through a period of chronic illness before they die. Along the way, there are numerous choices to make. Caregivers and people they care for have to decide whether or not to get a particular treatment or procedure. How long can one keep trying to do usual activities, including work, and when must they admit that that phase of their lives is over? Most of us have things we have dreamed of doing, but never got to do. Now may be the time to do that thing, no matter how difficult, or it may be time to let it be just a beautiful dream. Chronic illness brings up one situation after another where caregivers and care receivers must decide either to hold on or to let go.

Planning Ahead

Planning ahead means thinking about what is important, and what is not. It also means talking about this with those close to us. Even though we think we know what someone else thinks and believes, we really do not know until we ask. You cannot read other people's minds.

When we think about the last part of our own or someone else's life, consider these questions: What makes life worth living? What would make it definitely not worth living? What might at first seem like too much to put up with, but then might seem manageable after getting used to the situation and learning how to deal with it? If I knew life was coming to an end, what would be comforting and make dying feel safe? What, in that situation, would I most want to avoid? Some matters to consider would be: being able to talk with people, activity, physical comfort, alertness, the burden of care on others, being at home (or not being there), how much distress it would be worth in order to live another month, what medical procedures are not worth enduring, what I think is the best way for a person to die, how important it is to be in control of how one lives and how one dies, whose opinion should be sought in making choices about end-of-life care. One especially important matter is to complete the Advance Health Care Directive for both the person who is ill and the caregiver, so that there is an official spokesperson when the person who is ill is too sick or too confused to speak.

If, as caregivers, we have not had the necessary conversations—whether due to reluctance, dementia, or a crisis—we might have to think about the issues without the benefit of much information. Some questions that might help in thinking about this are: What has that person actually told me? How can I find out for sure about her or his wishes? Turning now to myself as the caregiver, what would be important to me? What would I especially like to know about that person's wishes? What would be the limits of what I could do? Could I take time off work? How much? What physical limitations do I have? What kinds of care would be just too much emotionally for me? Am I willing to accept the responsibility of being someone's official spokesperson? If that person has relatives who would be especially difficult to deal with, how would I manage being the official maker of decisions?

All of these questions may sound very difficult to discuss now, when the time for decisions is still in the future. However, they are harder to discuss when someone is really sick, emotions are high, and decisions must be made quickly. Dementia soon takes away the ability to discuss complicated issues. The earlier everyone sits down to talk, the better. The best way to start is simply to start. Arrange a time to talk. Someone else's death or illness may offer a good opportunity to bring up thoughts you had about their choices. Perhaps you could say you want to talk about things that might happen in the future, in case of serious illness. Have some ideas to bring up. Be prepared to listen a lot, and to ask questions. Do your best not to criticize what the other person says. If you know the other person will not want to talk much about this topic, have just one or two important things to say or to ask. Be prepared to break off the conversation, and to come back to it another time. Write down the important things people say. Eventually, you can use your notes to prepare a statement of wishes and make this statement part of an advance directive about health care decisions, whether or not the formal document has been completed.

Making the Decision

Is it time to let go? Or time to give a loved one permission to die? There are three ways to help decide.

1. **Look at the medical situation.** Has the illness really reached its final stages? When it has, the body is usually moving on its own toward dying, with strength declining, appetite poor, and often the mind becoming sleepier and more confused. Treatments are no longer working as well as before, and everyday activities are becoming more and more burdensome. In a sense, life is disappearing.

2. **Talk with people you trust.** Discuss the situation with the family members and friends who seem to be able to see things as they are. You might also talk with people who are not personally involved. Choose the people whose judgment you trust, not just those with an official role of giving advice. Most importantly, what does the dying person think?

3. **Listen to your heart.** Try to see beyond your fears and wishes, to what love and caring are saying to you. What is really best for the one who is dying, and for the others around? Given that death is unavoidable, what is the kindest thing to do? It might be holding on. It might be letting go.

Resources

Family Caregiver Alliance
180 Montgomery St., Suite 1100
San Francisco, CA 94104
Toll-Free: 800-445-8106
Phone: 415-434-3388
Website: http://caregiver.org
E-mail: info@caregiver.org

Compassion & Choices
P.O. Box 101810
Denver, CO 80250-1810
Toll-Free: 800-247-7421
Fax: 303-639-1224
Website: http://www.compassionindying.org

Hospice Foundation of America
1621 Connecticut Ave., N.W., Suite 300
Washington, DC 20009
Toll-Free: 800-854-3402
Fax: 202-638-5312
Website: http://www.hospicefoundation.org
E-mail: info@hospicefoundation.org

National Hospice and Palliative Care Organization
1700 Diagonal Road, Suite 625
Alexandria, VA 22314
Toll-Free: 800-658-8898
Phone: 703-837-1500
Fax: 703-837-1233
Website: http://www.nhpco.org
E-mail: nhpco_info@nhpco.org

Chapter 33

Information for Caregivers

Chapter Contents

Section 33.1

Self-Care Tips for Caregivers

First, Care for Yourself

On an airplane, an oxygen mask descends in front of you. What do you do? As we all know, the first rule is to put on your own oxygen mask before you assist anyone else. Only when we first help ourselves can we effectively help others. Caring for yourself is one of the most important—and one of the most often forgotten—things you can do as a caregiver. When your needs are taken care of, the person you care for will benefit, too.

Effects of Caregiving on Health and Well-Being

We hear this often: "My husband is the person with Alzheimer's, but now I'm the one in the hospital." Such a situation is all too common. Researchers know a lot about the effects of caregiving on health and well-being. For example, if you are a caregiving spouse between the ages of 66 and 96 and are experiencing mental or emotional strain, you have a risk of dying that is 63 percent higher than that of people your age who are not caregivers.[1] The combination of loss, prolonged stress, the physical demands of caregiving, and the biological vulnerabilities that come with age place you at risk for significant health problems as well as an earlier death.

Older caregivers are not the only ones who put their health and well-being at risk. If you are a baby boomer who has assumed a caregiver role for your parents while simultaneously juggling work and raising adolescent children, you face an increased risk for depression, chronic illness, and a possible decline in quality of life.

But despite these risks, family caregivers of any age are less likely than non-caregivers to practice preventive health care and self-care behavior. Regardless of age, sex, and race or ethnicity, caregivers report problems attending to their own health and well-being while managing caregiving responsibilities. They report:

- sleep deprivation;
- poor eating habits;
- failure to exercise;
- failure to stay in bed when ill;
- postponement of, or failure to make, medical appointments.

Family caregivers are also at increased risk for excessive use of alcohol, tobacco, and other drugs—and for depression. Caregiving can be an emotional roller coaster. On the one hand, caring for your family member demonstrates love and commitment and can be a very rewarding personal experience. On the other hand, exhaustion, worry, inadequate resources, and continuous care demands are enormously stressful. Studies show that an estimated 46 percent to 59 percent of caregivers are clinically depressed.

Taking Responsibility for Your Own Care

You cannot stop the impact of a chronic or progressive illness or a debilitating injury on someone for whom you care. But, there is a great deal that you can do to take responsibility for your personal well-being and to meet your own needs.

Identifying Personal Barriers

Many times, attitudes and beliefs form personal barriers that stand in the way of caring for yourself. Not taking care of yourself may be a lifelong pattern, with taking care of others an easier option. However, as a family caregiver you must ask yourself, "What good will I be to the person I care for if I become ill? If I die?" Breaking old patterns and overcoming obstacles is not an easy proposition, but it can be done—regardless of your age or situation. The first task in removing personal barriers to self-care is to identify what is in your way. For example,

- Do you feel you have to prove that you are worthy of the care recipient's affection?
- Do you think you are being selfish if you put your needs first?

253

- Is it frightening to think of your own needs? What is the fear about?

- Do you have trouble asking for what you need? Do you feel inadequate if you ask for help? Why?

Sometimes caregivers have misconceptions that increase their stress and get in the way of good self-care. Here are some of the most commonly expressed:

- I am responsible for my parent's health.

- If I don't do it, no one will.

- If I do it right, I will get the love, attention, and respect I deserve.

"I never do anything right," or "There's no way I could find the time to exercise," are examples of negative self-talk, another possible barrier that can cause unnecessary anxiety. Instead, try positive statements: "I'm good at giving John a bath." "I can exercise for 15 minutes a day." Remember, your mind believes what you tell it.

Basing behavior on thoughts, beliefs, attitudes, and misconceptions like those noted can cause caregivers to continually attempt to do what cannot be done, to control what cannot be controlled. The result is a feeling of continued failure and frustration, and often, an inclination to ignore your own needs. Ask yourself what might be getting in your way and keeping you from taking care of yourself.

Moving Forward

Once you've started to identify any personal barriers to good self-care, you can begin to change your behavior, moving forward one small step at a time. Following are some effective tools for self-care that can start you on your way.

Tool #1: Reducing Personal Stress

Perception and response to an event is a significant factor in how we adjust and cope with it. The stress you feel is not only the result of your caregiving situation, but also the result of your perception of it—whether you see the glass as half full or half empty. It is important to remember that you are not alone in your experiences.

Your level of stress is influenced by many factors, including:

- Whether your caregiving is voluntary. If you feel you had no choice in taking on the responsibilities, the chances are greater that you will experience strain, distress, and resentment.

- Your relationship with the care recipient. Sometimes people care for another with the hope of healing a relationship. If healing does not occur, you may feel regret and discouragement.

- Your coping abilities. How you coped with stress in the past predicts how you will cope now. Identify your current coping strengths so that you can build on them.

- Your caregiving situation. Some caregiving situations are more stressful than others. For example, caring for a person with dementia is often more stressful than caring for someone with a physical limitation.

- Whether support is available.

Steps to Managing Stress

1. **Recognize warning signs early.** These might include irritability, sleep problems, and forgetfulness. Know your own warning signs, and act to make changes. Don't wait until you are overwhelmed.

2. **Identify sources of stress.** Ask yourself, "What is causing stress for me?" Sources of stress might be too much to do, family disagreements, feelings of inadequacy, inability to say no.

3. **Identify what you can and cannot change.** Remember, we can only change ourselves; we cannot change another person. When you try to change things over which you have no control, you will only increase your sense of frustration. Ask yourself, "What do I have some control over? What can I change?" Even a small change can make a big difference. The challenge we face as caregivers is well expressed in words from the Serenity Prayer: "Grant me the serenity to accept the things I cannot change, courage to change the things I can, and the wisdom to know the difference."

4. **Take action.** Taking some action to reduce stress gives us a sense of control. Stress reducers can be simple activities like walking and other forms of exercise, gardening, meditation, or having coffee with a friend. Identify some stress reducers that work for you.

Tool #2: Setting Goals

Setting goals or deciding what you would like to accomplish in the next three to six months is an important tool for taking care of yourself. Here are some sample goals you might set:

- take a break from caregiving
- get help with caregiving tasks like bathing and preparing meals
- feel more healthy

Goals are generally too big to work on all at once. We are more likely to reach a goal if we break it down into smaller action steps. Once you've set a goal, ask yourself, "What steps do I take to reach my goal?" Make an action plan by deciding which step you will take first, and when. Then get started!

Example: Goal and Action Steps

Goal: Feel more healthy. Possible action steps:

1. Make an appointment for a physical check-up.

2. Take a half-hour break once during the week.

3. Walk three times a week for 10 minutes.

Tool #3: Seeking Solutions

Seeking solutions to difficult situations is, of course, one of the most important tools in caregiving. Once you've identified a problem, taking action to solve it can change the situation and also change your attitude to a more positive one, giving you more confidence in your abilities.

Steps for Seeking Solutions

1. **Identify the problem.** Look at the situation with an open mind. The real problem might not be what first comes to mind. For example, you think that the problem is simply that you are tired all the time, when the more basic difficulty is your belief that "no one can care for John like I can." The problem? Thinking that you have to do everything yourself.

2. **List possible solutions.** One idea is to try a different perspective: "Even though someone else provides help to John in a

different way than I do, it can be just as good." Ask a friend to help. Call Family Caregiver Alliance or the Eldercare Locator and ask about agencies in your area that could help provide care.

3. **Select one solution from the list.** Then try it!

4. **Evaluate the results.** Ask yourself how well your choice worked.

5. **Try a second solution.** If your first idea didn't work, select another. But don't give up on the first; sometimes an idea just needs fine tuning.

6. **Use other resources.** Ask friends, family members, and professionals for suggestions.

7. **If nothing seems to help,** accept that the problem may not be solvable now. You can revisit it at another time.

Note: All too often, we jump from step one to step seven and then feel defeated and stuck. Concentrate on keeping an open mind while listing and experimenting with possible solutions.

Tool #4: Communicating Constructively

Being able to communicate constructively is one of a caregiver's most important tools. When you communicate in ways that are clear, assertive, and constructive, you will be heard and get the help and support you need.

Communication Guidelines

- Use "I" messages rather than "you" messages. Saying "I feel angry" rather than "You made me angry" enables you to express your feelings without blaming others or causing them to become defensive.

- Respect the rights and feelings of others. Do not say something that will violate another person's rights or intentionally hurt the person's feelings. Recognize that the other person has the right to express feelings.

- Be clear and specific. Speak directly to the person. Don't hint or hope the person will guess what you need. Other people are not mind readers. When you speak directly about what you need or feel, you are taking the risk that the other person might disagree or say no to your request, but that action also shows respect for the other person's opinion. When both parties speak directly, the chances of reaching understanding are greater.

- Be a good listener. Listening is the most important aspect of communication.

Tool #5: Asking for and Accepting Help

When people have asked if they can be of help to you, how often have you replied, "Thank you, but I'm fine." Many caregivers don't know how to marshal the goodwill of others and are reluctant to ask for help. You may not wish to burden others or admit that you can't handle everything yourself.

Be prepared with a mental list of ways that others could help you. For example, someone could take the person you care for on a 15-minute walk a couple of times a week. Your neighbor could pick-up a few things for you at the grocery store. A relative could fill out some insurance papers. When you break down the jobs into very simple tasks, it is easier for people to help. People do want to help—it is up to you to tell them how.

Help can come from community resources, family, friends, and professionals. Ask them. Don't wait until you are overwhelmed, exhausted, or your health fails. Reaching out for help when you need it is a sign of personal strength.

Tips on How to Ask

- Consider the person's special abilities and interests. If you know a friend enjoys cooking but dislikes driving, your chances of getting help improve if you ask for help with meal preparation.

- Resist asking the same person repeatedly. Do you keep asking the same person because she has trouble saying no?

- Pick the best time to make a request. Timing is important. A person who is tired and stressed might not be available to help out. Wait for a better time.

- Prepare a list of things that need doing. The list might include errands, yard work, visiting with your loved one. Let the helper choose what he or she would like to do.

- Be prepared for hesitance or refusal. It can be upsetting for the caregiver when a person is unable or unwilling to help. But in the long run, it would do more harm to the relationship if the person helps only because he or she doesn't want to upset you. To the person who seems hesitant, simply say, "Why don't you think about it." Try not to take it personally when a request is turned down. The person is turning down the task, not you. Try not to let a refusal prevent you from asking for help again. The person who refused today may be happy to help at another time.

- Avoid weakening your request. "It's only a thought, but would you consider staying with Grandma while I go to church?" This request sounds like it's not very important to you. Use "I" statements to make specific requests: "I would like to go to church on Sunday. Would you stay with Grandma from 9 a.m. until noon?"

Tool #6: Talking to the Physician

In addition to taking on the household chores, shopping, transportation, and personal care, 37 percent of caregivers also administer medications, injections, and medical treatment to the person for whom they care. Some 77 percent of those caregivers report the need to ask for advice about the medications and medical treatments. The person they usually turn to is their physician.

But while caregivers will discuss their loved one's care with the physician, caregivers seldom talk about their own health which is equally important. Building a partnership with a physician that addresses the health needs of the care recipient and the caregiver is crucial. The responsibility of this partnership ideally is shared between you as caregiver, the physician, and other health care staff. However, it will often fall to you to be assertive, using good communication skills, to ensure that everyone's needs are met—including your own.

Tips on Communicating with Your Physician

- **Prepare questions ahead of time.** Make a list of your most important concerns and problems. Issues you might want to discuss with the physician are changes in symptoms, medications, or general health of the care recipient, your own comfort in your caregiving situation, or specific help you need to provide care.

- **Enlist the help of the nurse.** Many caregiving questions relate more to nursing than to medicine. In particular, the nurse can answer questions about various tests and examinations, preparing for surgical procedures, providing personal care, and managing medications at home.

- **Make sure your appointment meets your needs.** For example, the first appointment in the morning or after lunch and the last appointment in the day are the best times to reduce your waiting time or accommodate numerous questions. When you schedule your appointment, be sure you convey clearly the reasons for your visit so that enough time is allowed.

- **Call ahead.** Before the appointment, check to see if the doctor is on schedule. Remind the receptionist of special needs when you arrive at the office.

- **Take someone with you.** A companion can ask questions you feel uncomfortable asking and can help you remember what the physician and nurse said.

- **Use assertive communication and "I" messages.** Enlist the medical care team as partners in care. Present what you need, what your concerns are, and how the doctor and/or nurse can help. Use specific, clear "I" statements like the following: "I need to know more about the diagnosis; I will feel better prepared for the future if I know what's in store for me." Or, "I am feeling rundown. I'd like to make an appointment for myself and my husband next week."

Tool #7: Starting to Exercise

You may be reluctant to start exercising, even though you've heard it's one of the healthiest things you can do. Perhaps you think that physical exercise might harm you, or that it is only for people who are young and able to do things like jogging. Fortunately, research suggests that you can maintain or at least partly restore endurance, balance, strength, and flexibility through everyday physical activities like walking and gardening. Even household chores can improve your health. The key is to increase your physical activity by exercising and using your own muscle power.

Exercise promotes better sleep, reduces tension and depression, and increases energy and alertness. If finding time for exercise is a problem, incorporate it into your daily activity. Perhaps the care recipient can walk or do stretching exercise with you. If necessary, do frequent short exercises instead of those that require large blocks of time. Find activities you enjoy.

Walking, one of the best and easiest exercises, is a great way to get started. Besides its physical benefits, walking helps to reduce psychological tension. Walking 20 minutes a day, three times a week, is very beneficial. If you can't get away for that long, try to walk for as long as you can on however many days you can. Work walking into your life. Walk around the mall, to the store, or a nearby park. Walk around the block with a friend.

Tool #8: Learning from Emotions

It is a strength to recognize when your emotions are controlling you (instead of you controlling your emotions). Our emotions are messages to which we need to listen. They exist for a reason. However negative or painful, our feelings are useful tools for understanding what is happening to us.

Even feelings such as guilt, anger, and resentment contain important messages. Learn from them, and then take appropriate action. For example, when you cannot enjoy activities you previously enjoyed, and your emotional pain overshadows all pleasure, it is time to seek treatment for depression—especially if you are having thoughts of suicide. Speaking with your physician is the first step.

Caregiving often involves a range of emotions. Some feelings are more comfortable than others. When you find that your emotions are intense, they might mean the following:

- You need to make a change in your caregiving situation.
- You are grieving a loss.
- You are experiencing increased stress.
- You need to be assertive and ask for what you need.

Summing Up

Remember, it is not selfish to focus on your own needs and desires when you are a caregiver—it's an important part of the job. You are responsible for your own self-care. Focus on the following self-care practices:

- learn and use stress-reduction techniques
- attend to your own health care needs
- get proper rest and nutrition
- exercise regularly

- take time off without feeling guilty
- participate in pleasant, nurturing activities
- seek and accept the support of others
- seek supportive counseling when you need it, or talk to a trusted counselor or friend
- identify and acknowledge your feelings
- change the negative ways you view situations
- set goals

Reference

[1]Shultz, Richard and Beach, Scott (1999). Caregiving as A Risk for Mortality: The Caregiver Health Effects Study. *JAMA*, December 15, 1999, Vol. 282, No.23.

Additional Information

Family Caregiver Alliance
180 Montgomery St., Suite 1100
San Francisco, CA 94104
Toll-Free: 800-445-8106
Phone: 415-434-3388
Website: http://caregiver.org
E-mail: info@caregiver.org

Eldercare Locator
Administration on Aging
330 Independence Ave., S.W.
Washington, DC 20201
Toll-Free: 800-677-1116
Phone: 202-619-7501
Website: http://www.eldercare.gov
E-mail: eldercarelocator@spherix.com

Section 33.2

Who Is Providing Care?

Reprinted from "Caregiving Statistics," with permission of the National Family Caregivers Association, Kensington, MD, the nation's only organization for all family caregivers. 1-800-896-3650, www.nfcacares.org.

The following statistics have been compiled from a wide variety of sources. The original source follows each statement or group of statements. Note: Survey statistics sometimes seem to contradict each other. That's because each study or survey has its own methodology, its own set of variables, data sources, etc. It doesn't mean one is right and the other wrong. It does mean you need to understand how the survey was developed and constructed.

Caregiving Population

- More than 50 million people provide care for a chronically ill, disabled, or aged family member or friend during any given year.

- Caregiving is no longer predominantly a women's issue. Men now make up 44% of the caregiving population. (Source: National Family Caregivers Association (NFCA) *Random Sample Survey of Family Caregivers*, Summer 2000, Unpublished.)

- Caregivers providing care for a family member over the age of 50 routinely underestimate the length of time they will spend as caregivers—only 46% expected to be caregivers longer than two years. In fact, the average length of time spent on caregiving was about eight years, with approximately one-third of respondents providing care for 10 years or more. (Source: *Met Life Juggling Act Study, Balancing Caregiving with Work and the Costs of Caregiving*, Met Life Mature Market Institute, November 1999.)

- Most women will spend 17 years caring for children and 18 years helping an elderly parent. (Source: *101 Facts on the Status of Working Women* produced by Business and Professional Women's Foundation.)

Economics of Caregiving

- The value of the services family caregivers provide for free is esti-mated to be $257 billion a year. That is twice as much as is actu-ally spent on home care and nursing home services. (Source: Peter S. Arno, *Economic Value of Informal Caregiving*, presented at the American Association of Geriatric Psychiatry, February 24, 2002.)

- Caregiving families tend to have lower incomes than non-caregiving families. Thirty-five percent of average American households have incomes of under $30,000. Among caregiving families the percent-age is 43%. (Source: National Family Caregivers Association (NFCA) *Random Sample Survey of Family Caregivers*, Summer 2000.)

- Of the estimated 2.5 million Americans who need assistive tech-nology such as wheelchairs, 61% can't afford it. (Source: Lisa I. Iezzoni, M.D., M.Sc., *When Walking Fails: Personal and Health Policy Considerations*, Research in Profile, a National Program of the Robert Wood Johnson Foundation, March 2002.)

- Out-of-pocket medical expenses for a family that has a disabled member who needs help with activities of daily living (eating, toi-leting, etc.) are more than 2.5% greater (11.2% of income compared to 4.1%) than for a family without a disabled member. (Source: Drs. Altman, Cooper and Cunningham, The Case of Disability in the Family: Impact on Health Care Utilization and Expenditures for Non-disabled Members, *Milbank Quarterly* 77 (1) pages 39–75, 1999.)

Impact of Caregiving

- Elderly spousal caregivers with a history of chronic illness them-selves who are experiencing caregiving-related stress have a 63% higher mortality rate than their non-caregiving peers. (Source: Schulz, R. and Beach, S. R. Caregiving as a Risk Factor for Mortal-ity: The Caregiver Health Effects Study, *Journal of the American Medical Association*, December 15, 1999, Vol. 282, No. 23.)

- The stress of family caregiving for persons with dementia has been shown to impact a person's immune system for up to three years after their caregiving ends thus increasing their chances of developing a chronic illness themselves. (Source: Drs. Janice-Kiecolt Glaser and Ronald Glaser, *Chronic stress and age-related increases in the proinflammatory cytokine IL-6*, Proceedings of the National Academy of Sciences, June 30, 2003.)

- Family caregivers who provide care 36 or more hours weekly are more likely than non-caregivers to experience symptoms of depression or anxiety. For spouses, the rate is six times higher; for those caring for a parent, the rate is twice as high. (Source: Cannuscio, CC, C Jones, I Kawachi, GA Colditz, L Berkman, and F Rimm, Reverberation of family illness: A longitudinal assessment of informal caregiver and mental health status in the nurses' health study. *American Journal of Public Health 2002*; 92:305-1311.)

- Family caregivers providing high levels of care have a 51% incidence of sleeplessness and a 41% incidence of back pain. (Source: National Family Caregivers Association, *Caregiving Across the Life Cycle*, 1998.)

Caregiving and Work

- Thirty-seven percent of employees don't believe that their organizations provide a real and ongoing effort to inform employees of the family-friendly programs that are available. (Source: Families and Work Institute.)

- Forty-two percent of parents of special needs children lack basic workplace supports, such as paid sick leave and vacation time. (Source: Ellen Galinsky and James Bond, *The 1998 Business Work-Life Study–A Source Book*, Families and Work Institute.)

- Women average 11.5 years out of the paid labor force, primarily because of caregiving responsibilities; men average 1.3 years. (Source: *101 Facts on the Status of Working Women* produced by Business and Professional Women's Foundation.)

- American businesses lose between $11 billion and $29 billion each year due to employees' need to care for loved ones 50 years of age and older. (Source: National Alliance for Caregiving/Met Life, *Met Life Study of Employer Costs for Working Caregivers*.)

- Both male and female children of aging parents make changes at work in order to accommodate caregiving responsibilities. Both have modified their schedules (men 54%, women 56%). Both have come in late and/or left early (men 78%, women 84%), and both have altered their work-related travel (men 38%, women 27%). (Source: *Sons at Work: Balancing Employment and Eldercare*, Met Life Mature Market Institute, June 2003.)

Caregiving and Health Care

- Over 40% of U.S. primary care physicians think they don't have enough time to spend with patients. (Source: *The Commonwealth Fund Quarterly Report*, Fall 2000, Volume 6, Issue 3.)

- Family caregivers provide the overwhelming majority of home care services in the U.S., approximately 80%. (Source: *Long-term Care Users Range in Age and Most Do Not Live in Nursing Homes*, November 8, 2000, U.S. Agency for Healthcare Research and Quality.)

- In 2000, 50 percent of caregivers reported that different providers gave different diagnoses for the same set of symptoms, and 62 percent reported that different providers gave other conflicting information. Another recent survey found that 44 percent of physicians believe that poor care coordination leads to unnecessary hospitalization, and 24 percent stated it can lead to otherwise unnecessary nursing home stays. (Source: *Partnership for Solutions, Chronic Conditions: Making the Case for Ongoing Care*, Johns Hopkins University, December 2002.)

- By the year 2030, nearly 150 million Americans will have some type of chronic illness, a 50% increase since 1995. (Source: *Partnership for Solutions: Harris Survey*, Johns Hopkins University, data presented at March 2003 conference, Washington, DC. And, *Partnership for Solutions: Chronic Conditions: Making the Case for Ongoing Care*, Johns Hopkins University, December 2002.)

- Family caregivers who acknowledge their role are more proactive in reaching out for resources and talking with their loved one's doctor than non-acknowledged caregivers. (Source: National Family Caregivers Association, *Survey of Self-Identified Family Caregivers*, 2001.)

- Over 40 percent of family caregivers provide some type of nursing care for their loved ones, such as giving medications, changing bandages, managing machinery, and monitoring vital signs. (Source: National Family Caregivers Association (NFCA) *Random Sample Survey of Family Caregivers*, Summer 2000 and C. Levine, *Rough Crossings: Family Caregivers' Odysseys through the Health Care System*. New York: United Hospital Fund, 1998.)

- One-third of family caregivers who change dressings and manage machines, receive no instructions. (Source: Henry J. Kaiser Family Foundation, *Wide Circle of Caregiving*, 1998.)

Chapter 34

How to Help during the Final Weeks of Life

Understanding the Problem

The end of life cannot be predicted for any of us. We do not know when it will happen, who will be with us, how it will occur, or what we will feel. We do know more about the answers to these questions for people living with advanced cancer, however. Cancer is a chronic illness, which means that it takes time for it to grow worse. Dying with a chronic illness is very different from dying because of a sudden illness or event, such as a heart attack or an accident. Certain things about dying (and living) with advanced cancer can be predicted and discussed, including the cause of death, when death will finally occur, and how we know when a person is living the very last days of his or her life.

Many misconceptions exist about what can happen during the final days and weeks of a person's life. One stubborn myth about dying from cancer is that the person will finally die from only one cause. Someone might say, "It'll be the heart that goes last." When people have a chronic illness such as late-stage cancer, however, they usually do not die from one major event or for only one reason. Instead, they die because of many different factors that combine to slow down the body's important systems, such as the heart and lungs. In a sense, the physical body slowly gives up.

We cannot say exactly how long someone will live with a chronic illness. Many times, family members and friends want to know this information. They want to prepare themselves, make plans, or understand what will happen in the next few weeks or months. Doctors and nurses can give predictions of how long the person has to live, but these are only estimates or best guesses. Sometimes, the guesses are accurate; sometimes, the guesses are not. For example, some people have lived much longer than their predicted three or four months. In fact, some of these people have gotten better, returned to work, taken up their hobbies again, and enjoyed life for much longer than expected. It was not until months later that they finally slowed down, became weaker, and died.

Certain physical signs warn us that the end of life is growing close. Most people with an advanced, chronic illness such as cancer spend more time in bed or on a couch or chair. People with any type of advanced cancer eat much less food, and they drink fewer liquids. They also sleep more, lose weight, and become much weaker.

Not every warning sign is physical, however. People may talk about "leaving" or "having to go." Their dreams make them feel as if they want to "get going" or "go home." Although this is not common in every situation, this language and the emotion behind it are ways of talking about dying. The patient also may ask to see special friends or relatives, and some haziness or confusion can occur as one day blends into another. Keeping track of the day of the week becomes less important, as do other details.

The last days of life are unique for each person as well. They are very personal, and they are very private. People usually are less interested in the outside world, and they want the closeness of only a few people—or maybe just one other person—to comfort them. Exceptions do occur, of course. Some want many friends and family members around them, but this is rare.

So, this is the general picture of a patient in the final weeks of life: very weak; drowsy, with much sleeping; unable to eat any food and difficulty swallowing fluids; less able to talk and to concentrate; bodily comfort (as long as medicines are continued); and peace with dying.

Goals

- Know when to recognize situations that require professional help for the patient to reach a natural death.

- Keep the person comfortable.
- Give general nursing care.
- Welcome visitors and children.
- Tell others how they can help.

When to Get Professional Help

Health professionals can play an important role during the final days of life, but their advice and treatments (if any) will not be geared toward curing the person. At this point, it is hard to change the underlying physical problems, but the discomfort that results from those problems can be eased.

Call the doctor or nurse if any of the following situations exist:

The person you are caring for has difficulty becoming comfortable. You will know when people with advanced cancer are uncomfortable. They may tell you, or they may be tossing or moaning. If they are not conscious or awake, they may be frowning. Call the hospice or home care staff for help. If home care nurses or hospice staff are not available, call the doctor's office and ask that a visiting nurse or hospice nurse come to your home because the person is uncomfortable, and at this point, you do not know what to do.

The person you are caring for is confused or seeing things that are not there. Occasionally, being confused about the time of day, day of the week, or the date is normal, but severe confusion can upset people with cancer as well as you. Severe confusion might mean that they do not know where they are or who they are with. This can be a real problem if they are unhappy about where they think they are or afraid of what they see or hear. They may even see things that are not there. Sometimes, these visions are of people who have already died, such as a mother or a child. These are called hallucinations. If these visions comfort the person, they are not a problem. However, if they scare or upset the person, or if the hallucinations are affecting or upsetting the family, they are a problem. Call about severe confusion or upsetting hallucinations.

The person you are caring for is suffering from severe fear or anxiety. Try to understand what is frightening the person, but do not make assumptions. You could be wrong, and that would hinder your ability to help. It is okay to ask the person what worries them most. This allows you to focus on the real issue rather than guessing about what the person is afraid of. For example, you may assume the person is afraid of dying when, in reality, he or she is afraid of being left alone or running out of money.

Sometimes, anxiety is caused by medicine. If so, the medicine can be changed, and anti-anxiety medicines can be used. Visiting nurses can talk with the doctor and ask to have these medicines ordered.

You feel tired and overwhelmed. Needing help from other people is not a failure on your part. Your health is important if you are going to provide the best care for the patient. Eating and resting are crucial. Sometimes, it is hard to ask for help when you are caring for someone through the final days of their life—but you should. Call for help from a visiting nurse agency or a hospice. These groups will send out nurse's aides to give baths, do light laundry, change the bed, and give you both help and support. Registered nurses and other professionals will help you to manage medical problems that arise. Family and friends are important now as well. Ask them to help, and give them specific tasks that will help you as well as make them feel useful.

You do not think that you can handle keeping the person at home. Some caregivers are comfortable helping someone during the final days of life. Perhaps they have done this before; perhaps they have watched others do it. Giving nursing care and dealing with problems are not so upsetting to them.

Other caregivers have more difficulty. If they work outside the home, they may be overwhelmed by the strain of "two jobs." They also may have children. The task of caregiving may be new for them as well. They may have never been with someone during the final days of life or have helped with a natural death. They may have too much going on in their own lives to be able to handle the added demands of caring for a person with advanced cancer.

If you are not sure that you can handle caregiving near the end of a person's life, talk about your worries with someone. Social workers at the hospital or hospice are very helpful. Even if the person with cancer does not go to that hospital anymore or just goes to an outpatient clinic, call the hospital and ask for their department of social work. If you have visiting nurses, ask them to send a social worker to your home. They can help you to sort out which parts of caring for someone at home are most difficult, then you can discuss if you should move the person somewhere else, such as to a nursing home, or if someone else can take over some of your responsibilities at home. That decision, of course, is always up to you and the person being cared for. Include the patient in all of these decisions and discussions as much as possible.

The person with cancer is having trouble breathing. Report problems with breathing, especially if the person finds it hard to draw air into the lungs or release air. Labored or difficult breathing is very upsetting, but professional staff can help. They might order oxygen or other medicines to relieve anxiety. Sometimes, the patient is worried about running out of oxygen. If this is true, tell the supply company to bring you more than one tank, and set it up where the person with cancer can see it and feel reassured that a back-up tank is handy. Use a fan to keep air in the room moving, which can make breathing seem easier. Run the fan near their face or open windows.

Another way to ease breathing is giving anti-anxiety medicines and narcotics. Ask the nurses to arrange this with the physician. These medicines are available in several forms; pills, liquids, and suppositories are most frequently used. Shortness of breath can and should be relieved even up to the time of death.

What You Can Do to Help

Keep the Person Comfortable

Use an eggshell mattress and foam cushions. Many people with cancer lose weight; therefore, they may be less comfortable lying on their former mattress or sitting in chairs that used to suit them. Eggshell mattresses are made of foam and are softer than conventional types. Some people also cut up foam rubber to put on chairs or couches. The foam softens the seat and makes it more comfortable. Eggshell cushions and mattresses can be bought at large department stores or medical supply stores. Sometimes, visiting nurses will order a special mattress to prevent bedsores.

Use lip balm or salve to prevent chapped lips. Dry lips and mouth can be a serious problem when a person is not drinking much. Some of this discomfort can be prevented by using lip balms. Avoid using petroleum jelly if the person is on oxygen, however, as it can clog the line.

Use the end of a straw to give small sips of liquids. Some people have trouble drinking from a glass because of weakness. If so,

271

give fluids by dipping the straw into the glass and then holding your finger over the end of the straw. This holds liquid in the straw. Drip the liquid into the person's mouth by loosening the finger for short periods of time.

Use a special spoon to give liquid medicine. Pharmacies carry special spoons that help to avoid spilling liquid medicine. The spoon handle is enclosed and looks like a tube. You can pour the medicine into the scoop part, and it will flow down into the tube and into the person's mouth. It is much easier to take medicine such as Maalox® with this type of spoon, but you also can use a syringe. Have the nurse show you how to use it. If the person is having trouble swallowing, a few drops under the tongue will still be absorbed.

Easing discomfort caused by fever. Sometimes, fevers develop because not enough liquid is taken. If so, encourage the person you are caring for to drink more. Cool cloths applied to the brow can help as well, but do not give icy or cold baths. In some cases, the doctor may order antibiotics to fight the infection if, for example, an infection is causing pain or discomfort.

Manage and prevent problems with bleeding. Minor skin bleeding sometimes occurs because of bumping the arms or wrists on furniture. This is because the skin is not as tough as it once was. Medicines also can cause changes in the skin so that it is easily scraped open. Small gauze pads can be placed over any open spots and wrapped with 1- or 2-inch gauze to stay in place. Avoid using tape; however, as it might tear open the skin when removed.

If a nosebleed occurs, tilt the head back, but do not have the person lie flat. This could make the person choke on blood dripping from the nose into the throat. Put ice wrapped in a washcloth on the nose for short periods, such as two minutes.

Pressure on the skin and nose stops most bleeding. Bleeding inside the body or in the urine and stool, however, cannot be stopped in this way, because you cannot put pressure on these areas. If bleeding from the nose or other places continues, call the visiting nurse. The physician might order medication to slow down the bleeding as well.

Consider using an electric hospital bed. Electric beds are easy to operate. The person with cancer can control the positions, and so can you. Hospital beds also can be non-electric, using a crank at the bottom to raise it up or bring it down and to elevate the head or feet.

Cranking takes more work and bending, however. Many families set the bed in a living room or den on the first floor so that they will be near, and visitors will have more room to visit.

Let the patient plan the day. Letting the patient plan the day will show respect and support his or her dignity. Let the person plan what to do, what to eat or drink, when to sleep, and when to visit with others. Some people find watching television helpful.

Touch and talk. Even if the person is sleeping much of the time or slips into a coma, touching and talking remain important. Touch can include back rubs or holdings hands. Visitors can read scriptures or stories or review old times. Some people read poems, and background music can help. All of these decrease a person's sense of being alone and can be very comforting.

Invite ministers and church members to visit. Prayers and conversations with ministers and fellow church members can be very comforting for some people. Priests or deacons may want to bring sacraments, such as last rites or communion. Many home health agencies and hospice groups have a chaplain on staff who can visit as well. These visits should not be forced. It is up to the person with cancer to decide who would be comforting.

Understand that what you do is not wrong. Some caregivers worry they are not doing enough to keep the person comfortable or are not doing the right things. A few may even feel responsible for bringing on an early death. Nothing you can do (or not do) will change what is happening or lead to an early death. There really are no mistakes made at the end of life. The important point to remember now is that the goal is comfort.

Give General Nursing Care

Use a pan for bathing. If the person you are helping does not want to get in the tub or shower anymore, he or she can sit on top of the toilet seat or on a chair in front of the sink and bathe. If the person does not feel like getting out of bed, you can help with a bath in bed. Think back on how this was done in the hospital or the way you bathed small children. You need to set a pan of warm to hot water on a table or sturdy chair, then wring the washcloth well, soap it, and help the person to bathe. Be sure to keep him or her covered with a soft sheet or blanket to avoid a chill; this is important for privacy, too. It is wise to start with the face and then do the arms and legs, the chest and back, and finish with the private area. A nurse or nurse's aide can help you with bathing.

Soak the feet in warm water. Many people enjoy the feeling of warm water and miss bathing in a shower or tub. You can make up for this by helping the person to soak his or her feet in a pan of warm water. Do one foot at a time, and leave it soaking for about 10 minutes.

Change the sheets at least twice a week. If the person is spending a lot of time in bed, the sheets will get soiled more quickly. Fresh sheets usually are enjoyed. If the person is resting on couches or sleeping in a reclining chair, a fresh sheet cover is nice in these locations as well.

Help with mouth care twice a day. Keep up the same routines for dental and mouth care, including denture care if needed. A fresh mouth makes the person feel better.

Use lotions that do not contain alcohol. Skin dryness can become a problem as a person drinks less. Read the label on any lotion you are using and avoid lotions containing alcohol. Gently rub lotion on the elbows, heels, back, and spine. These places are very dry and can break down.

Prevent bedsores. When a person is in bed for a long time, some spots on the body can develop sores because of constant pressure. At first, they are pink, but then they turn red, the skin opens, and the size of the sore quickly increases. Bedsores start under the skin, and you may not even know they are there until they become severe. Bedsores often hurt, and the most likely places for them are where bones are sticking out, such as at the ankle bones, heels, end of the spinal column, hips, and elbows. Visiting nurses and hospice staff can help you to prevent bedsores. Call for their help if you notice very red areas or open sores.

Do not force food. Forcing food will distress the person with advanced cancer as well as the family. It is natural for a dying person to want less food. This is the body's natural way of approaching death—by shutting down.

It is hard to give up trying to feed someone you care about. Using intravenous (IV) fluids or special tube feedings for nutrition are not part of dying naturally, but if the person with cancer wants these treatments that is his or her right. Talk this over with the home care nurses, hospice staff, and physician. You can still offer sips of water. Cut a straw into a shorter length so that he or she can sip liquids. If the patient is too tired to sip, drop water into his or her mouth just to freshen it and give comfort. This will be very much appreciated.

Welcome Visitors

Not everyone is comfortable visiting a person in the final weeks of life. Some people want to stay away. Others want to come and help. The person who is sick should have control over who will visit. Here are some ideas to help manage visitors:

Set time aside for bathing and rest. Stay in control of the schedule; otherwise, visitors may come and go all day. Let people know if a visit is better in the afternoon or evening so that both you and the patient have time for rest and personal care.

Tell visitors if they are staying too long. At this point, it is okay to be honest. Visitors want to know what both of you want. If you or the person with cancer are tired, ask for shorter visits or telephone calls.

Ask the person with cancer who he or she would like to see, and invite those people. The person with cancer has a right to control the social scene. He or she may not want to see certain people; or if it is a bad day, may not want to see anyone.

Cope with Changes

Helping someone who is very ill brings on many challenges. You may have to take on new responsibilities. You also may face new physical, emotional, or mental strains. Here are some ways to help deal with these challenges:

Locate bills, checks, accounts, and important papers such as insurance policies. The person with cancer may have shared decision-making about finances with you previously. If not, it is time to locate important papers like these and talk about what they mean and what needs to be done.

Learn new household chores. If the person with cancer has done certain household chores in the past, such as shopping, preparing meals, or cleaning clothes, you will have to do them yourself now or ask someone else to do what needs to be done. Nurse's aides and home helpers can do some shopping and run errands, but they may not visit daily and do not always have the time for these chores. It often is better to depend on friends, neighbors, or relatives for these things (unless you want to do them yourself).

Ask the bank ahead of time how accounts are handled after someone dies. The bank will probably tell you that two names are needed on an account to be able to withdraw funds after someone has died. If you do not have two names on the account, put them on weeks before the person with cancer dies.

Talk with a friend about your feelings. Being with a close friend or someone you can talk to is an excellent way of sorting out your feelings. Knowing that others care and are there to listen gives many people support, strength, and confidence during this difficult experience.

Plan something nice for yourself once a day. Many caregivers do not take any time for themselves, and they sometimes feel guilty if they do. Going to lunch with someone or taking a nap are two examples of short activities that can help you to keep anxiety or stress from building to the breaking point.

Seek professional help for your emotional problems. Many people are reluctant to ask for help from counselors; they think that it means they are "crazy" or not strong enough. Professionals such as counselors, ministers, psychologists, psychiatrists, social workers, or nurses are experienced in listening and can help you deal with your stress. These people are there to help you with emotional, mental, or psychologic problems.

Physicians can evaluate if certain medicines will help you. For example, antidepressants may help. If your doctor does prescribe an antidepressant, he or she will follow you closely and watch for side effects such as blurred vision, feeling "out of it," or extreme fatigue. If any of these side effects happen, the doctor will change either the drug or its dose. Anti-anxiety drugs also can help, especially if you are having trouble sleeping.

Possible Obstacles

An obstacle other caregivers have faced: Different family members disagree about what to do.

Response: Tensions sometimes run high during the final days of life. People may have different opinions about a lot of issues, and it is not easy to resolve these, especially when people are upset. If a decision does not need to be made now, try to postpone any discussions of controversial issues. If a decision is needed immediately, imagine that you are looking back on it a year from now—and make the decision you think that people will feel best about at that time. Some decisions will not please everyone. Just make the best decision you can—and live with the consequences. Always be sure that the patient's comfort comes first.

Try holding to what you know the patient wants or would want, but if this cannot happen, accept your own limitations. For example, if he or she wanted to die at home but this is not possible, realize that you did all you could at home and that dying in the hospital or nursing home was the only way to ensure the person's comfort.

Think of Other Obstacles That Could Interfere with Carrying Out Your Plan

What additional roadblocks could get in the way of the recommendations in this plan? For example, will the person with advanced cancer cooperate? How will you explain what is needed to other people? Do you have the time and energy to carry out the plan?

You need to develop plans for getting around these roadblocks. Use the COPE ideas (creativity, optimism, planning, and expert information) in developing your plans.

Carrying Out and Adjusting Your Plan

Keep track of your own energy. Remember, you do not have to help the person at home alone, and you can say no to the responsibility for this task if you want. If you are worried about doing a good job or unsure that you want to be doing any of these things at all, ask for help. Doctors, nurses, and social workers can help you. Continue watching for signs that immediate professional help is needed.

Keeping someone who is very sick at home can be tiring and stressful. Be open to changing your plans about how to do this, and be honest about whether you want to do this at all. If you move the person to a nursing home, you can always move him or her back home, or to someone else's home, when you have more energy or help.

Chapter 35

The Dying Process

When a person enters the final steps of the dying process, two different dynamics are at work which are closely interrelated and interdependent. Therefore, as you seek to prepare yourself as this event approaches, the members of your hospice care team want you to know what to expect and how to respond in ways that will help your loved one accomplish this transition with support, understanding, and ease. This is the great gift of love you have to offer your loved one as this moment approaches.

Two Dynamics

On the physical plane the body begins the final process of shutting down, which will end when all the physical systems cease to function. Usually this is an orderly and undramatic progressive series of physical cues which are not medical emergencies requiring invasive interventions. These physical changes are a normal, natural way in which the body prepares itself to stop, and the most appropriate kinds of responses are comfort enhancing measures.

The other dynamic of the dying process is at work on the emotional/spiritual/mental plane and is a different kind of process. The spirit of the dying person begins the final process of release from the body, its immediate environment, and all attachments. This release also tends to follow its own priorities, which include the resolution of whatever is unfinished of a practical nature—reconciliation of close relationships and reception of permission to let go from family members. These events are the normal, natural way in which the spirit prepares to move from this materialistically-oriented realm of existence into the next dimension of life. The most appropriate kinds of responses to the emotional/spiritual/mental changes are those which support and encourage this release and transition.

When a person's body is ready and wanting to stop, but the person is still unresolved or not reconciled over some important issue or with some significant relationship, he or she will tend to linger even though very uncomfortable or debilitated in order to finish whatever needs finishing. On the other hand, when a person is emotionally/spiritually/mentally resolved and ready for this release, but his or her body has not completed its final physical process, the person will continue to live until the physical shut down is complete.

The experience we call death occurs when the body completes its natural process of shutting down and when the spirit completes its natural process of reconciling and finishing. These two processes need to happen in a way appropriate for the values, beliefs, and lifestyle of the dying person so that the death can occur as a peaceful release.

The physical, as well as the emotional/spiritual/mental signs and symptoms of impending death which follow are offered to help you understand the natural kinds of things which may happen and how you can respond appropriately. Not all these signs and symptoms will occur with every person, nor will they occur in this particular sequence. Each person is unique, and what has been most characteristic of the way your loved one has lived consistently will affect the way this final shut down and release occurs. This is not the time to try to change your loved one, but the time to give full acceptance, support, and comfort.

Normal Physical Signs and Symptoms of the Dying Process and Appropriate Responses

Coolness—The person's hands, arms, feet, and legs may become increasingly cool to the touch, and at the same time the color of the skin may change. This is a normal indication that the circulation of blood is decreasing to the body's extremities and being reserved for the most vital organs. Keep the person warm with a blanket, but do not use an electric blanket.

Sleeping—The person may spend an increasing amount of time sleeping and appear to be uncommunicative and unresponsive. This normal change is due in part to changes in the metabolism of the body. Sit with your loved one, hold his or her hand, do not shake or speak loudly, but speak softly and naturally. Do not talk about the person in the person's presence. Speak to him or her directly as you normally would, even though there may be no response.

Disorientation—The person may seem to be confused about the time, place, and identity of people surrounding him or her. This is also due in part to the metabolism changes. Identify yourself by name before you speak rather than to ask the person to guess who you are. Speak softly, clearly, and truthfully when you need to communicate something important for the patient's comfort, such as, "It is time to take your medication," and explain the reason for the communication, such as, "so you won't begin to hurt." Do not use this method to try to manipulate the patient to meet your needs.

Incontinence—The person may lose control of urine and/or bowel function as the muscles in that area begin to relax. Discuss with your hospice nurse what can be done to protect the bed and keep your loved one clean and comfortable.

Restlessness—The person may make restless and repetitive motions. This often happens and is due in part to the decrease in oxygen circulation to the brain and to metabolic changes. These changes may also temporarily alter personalities. Do not interfere with or try to restrain such motions. To have a calming effect, speak in a quiet natural way, lightly massage the forehead, read to the person, or play some soothing music.

Fluid and food decreases—The person may begin to want little or no food or fluid. This means the body is conserving for other functions the energy which would be expended in processing these items. Do not try to force food or drink into the person, or try to use guilt to manipulate them into eating or drinking something. To do this only makes the person much more uncomfortable. Small chips of ice, frozen Gatorade®, or juice may be refreshing in the mouth. Glycerin swabs may help keep the mouth and lips moist and comfortable. A cool, moist washcloth on the forehead may also increase physical comfort.

Urine decrease—The person's urine output normally decreases due to the reduced fluid intake, as well as a decrease in circulation through the kidneys. Consult with your hospice nurse to determine whether there may be a need to insert or irrigate a catheter.

Breathing pattern change—The person's regular characteristic breathing pattern may change with the onset of a different breathing pace which alternates with periods of no breathing. This is called Cheyne-Stokes respiration and is very common. It indicates a decrease in circulation in the internal organs. Elevating the head may help bring comfort. Hold his or her hand. Speak gently.

Normal Emotional/Spiritual/Mental Signs and Symptoms with Appropriate Responses

Withdrawal—The person may seem unresponsive, withdrawn, or in a comatose state. This indicates preparation for release, a detaching from surroundings and relationships, and a beginning of letting go. Since hearing remains until the end, speak to your loved one in your normal tone of voice, identify yourself by your name when you speak, hold his or her hand, and say whatever you need to say that will help the person let go.

Vision experiences—The person may speak or claim to have spoken to individuals who may have already died. They may say they see or have seen places not presently accessible or visible to you. This does not indicate a hallucination or a drug reaction. The person is beginning to detach from this life and is being prepared for the transition so it will not be frightening. Do not contradict, explain away, belittle, or argue about what the person claims to have seen or heard. Just because you cannot see or hear it does not mean it is not real to your loved one. Affirm his or her experiences. They are normal and common. If the experience frightened your loved one, explain to him or her that it is normal.

Restlessness—The person may perform repetitive and restless tasks. This may indicate that something is still unresolved or unfinished thus disturbing him or her, and preventing him or her from letting go. Your hospice team members will assist you in identifying what may be happening, and help you find ways to help the person find release from the tension or fear. Other things which may be helpful in calming the person are to recall a favorite place your loved one enjoyed, a favorite experience, read something comforting, play music, and give assurance it is okay to let go.

Fluids and food decrease—When the person wants little or no fluid or food, this may indicate that the person is ready for the final shut down. You may help your loved one by giving him or her permission to let go whenever he or she is ready. At the same time, affirm your loved one's ongoing value to you and the good you will carry forward into your life that you received from him or her.

Decreased socialization—The person may only want to be with a very few people, or even just one person. This is a sign of preparation for release, and an affirming of whom the support is most needed from, in order to make the approaching transition. If you are not part of this inner circle at the end, it does not mean you are not loved or are unimportant. It means you have already fulfilled you task with him or her and it is time for you to say, "Goodbye." If you are part of the final inner circle, the loved one needs your affirmation, support, and permission.

Unusual communication—The person may make a seemingly out of character or non sequitur statement, gesture, or request. This indicates that he or she is ready to say good-bye and is testing to see if you are ready to let him or her go. Accept the moment as a beautiful gift when it is offered. Kiss, hug, hold, cry, and say whatever you most need to say.

Giving permission—Giving permission to your loved one to let go without making him or her feel guilty for leaving, or trying to keep him or her with you to meet your own needs can be difficult. A dying person will normally try to hold on, even though it brings prolonged discomfort, in order to be sure that those who are going to be left behind will be all right. Therefore, your ability to release the dying person from this concern and give him or her assurance that it is all right to let go whenever he or she is ready is one of the greatest gifts you have to give your loved one at this time.

Saying good-bye—When the person is ready to die and you are able to let go, then is the time to say, "Good-bye." Saying good-bye is your final gift of love to the loved one, for it achieves closure and makes the final release possible. It may be helpful to lie in bed with the person and hold him or her, or to take their hand and say everything you need to say so afterward you need never to say to yourself, "Why didn't I say this or that," to him or her.

It may be as simple as saying, "I love you." It may include recounting your favorite memories, places, and activities you shared. It may include saying, "I'm sorry for whatever contributed to any tensions or difficulties in our relationship." It may also include saying, "Thank you for...." Tears are a normal and natural part of saying good-bye. Tears do not need to be hidden from your loved one or apologized for. Tears express your love and help you to let go.

How Will You Know when Death Has Occurred?

The signs of death include such things as: no breathing, no heart-beat, release of bowel and bladder, no response, eyelids slightly open, eyes fixed on a certain spot, no blinking, jaw relaxed, and mouth slightly opened. If you are using hospice, call the hospice office number at the time of death. There are telephone calls which must be made at that time by the hospice staff. A hospice nurse will come to assist you if needed or desired. If not, phone support is available.

The body does not have to be moved until you are ready. If the family wants to assist in preparing the body by bathing or dressing, that may be done.

Chapter 36

What to Do when Death Occurs

When Death Occurs

When a loved one dies, you may experience a wide range of emotions. You may experience sadness, confusion, loneliness, anger, anxiety, and perhaps even guilt or relief. This is a time to honor family and cultural rituals. These rituals allow you to acknowledge the reality of the death and to begin the healing journey. At the same time, you must complete a variety of tasks. You need to call family and friends. You need to arrange for the care of the body. You need to hold a funeral or memorial service. You need to alert various government agencies and businesses about the death, and settle the estate. This chapter will help you get through the hours, days, and weeks immediately following the death of a loved one.

Signs That Death Has Occurred

Even when death is expected, it is often difficult to accept. These signs indicate that a person has died.

- no breathing
- no heartbeat or pulse
- loss of control of bowel and bladder (the sheets or undergarments may be soiled)

From "When Death Occurs: What to Do When a Loved One Dies," © 2004 Center on Aging, University of Hawaii at Manoa. Reprinted with permission.

- no response to touch or words

- eyes remain fixed on a certain spot, eyelids may be opened or closed

- jaw is relaxed, the mouth slightly open, fluid or drainage from the nose or mouth

Many people wonder when the body will become stiff or worry that it will begin to smell. The stiffening is called rigor mortis. This is a temporary condition that begins three to four hours after death and ends twenty-four to thirty-six hours after death. As far as odor is concerned, generally, after the body has been bathed, there should be minimal or no offensive odor. If the eyes remain open at death, it is all right to close them; however, know that they may open again. It is okay to leave them open. Families who want to keep an unembalmed body at home for a viewing or service may use dry ice to preserve it temporarily.

Who to Call First

If death occurs in a hospital or nursing home and you are the first to be aware of the death, alert the nursing staff. The doctor will certify the death. The institution will need to know which mortuary or funeral home to call, and will perform that task for you.

If death occurs at home and is expected, call your doctor. This does not have to be done immediately, particularly if death occurs in the middle of the night. If you call 911, inform the operator that the death was expected. Unless the deceased is wearing a *comfort care only* bracelet or necklace, emergency medical personnel will most likely attempt resuscitation. If hospice is involved, the on-call nurse should be notified.

If the death was unattended and unexpected at home or elsewhere, call 911. The police and emergency medical personnel will determine the next appropriate steps. Under certain circumstances, the coroner will be contacted.

If the death occurs out of state and there is a pre-paid funeral plan, check the policy for travel protection benefits. If none exist, call the mortuary in the town where you want the deceased to be buried or cremated. They will help you to arrange transport of the body.

The First Few Hours

The mortuary does not need to be contacted immediately. This is a time to call your family members, friends, and clergy to be with the deceased. Give yourself adequate time to experience what has just happened. You may want to hold or touch a loved one who has died and say your good-byes. Sharing stories with friends and family also can help to begin the grieving process.

This is the time to honor any family or cultural rituals. Some cultures have customs about bathing and clothing the body after death. Some cultures believe that the dead can carry messages to loved ones that have already died. Some cultures expect the dead to be buried with possessions that have meaning or would be useful in the next life.

Death rituals can help us:

- deal with our loss at a time of grief

- release the person who has died

- reflect on the past, deal with the present, and look to the future

- bind together with other mourners, allowing for a possibility to share common thoughts, memories, and feelings

When you have said your goodbyes, it is time to surrender the body of your loved one to the mortuary, funeral home, or medical school. Your chosen mortuary or funeral home will send a vehicle to pick up the body. If you have chosen body donation, the medical school will arrange transportation. If death occurs in a hospital or nursing home, the body may be moved temporarily to the morgue while transportation is arranged. You may even transport the body in your own vehicle.

There are a number of options for final disposition of the body. Burial, cremation, and body donation are most common. Some people, however, may prefer unusual alternatives, such as becoming part of an artificial reef to help the environment, or to have their ashes launched with others for perpetual orbit in space. Culture, religion, and personal preference all play a role in determining what the deceased and family want done.

Arranging the Service

Once the body has been moved, you need to begin planning the funeral or memorial service in accordance with the wishes of the deceased. Hopefully, plans have been made ahead of time. If not, find someone to assist you, for example your minister, a trusted friend, or a family member. If the funeral home or mortuary has not been selected ahead of time, a funeral or memorial society can help.

You need to tell family and friends about the death and the service. Ask for help with this task by calling three to five reliable contacts and asking them to each call three to five others. Your faith community can help spread the word among its membership, and announcements can be posted in the newspaper or sent through e-mail. If the deceased was working or volunteering at the time of the death, alert someone at their workplace.

If the death occurs in a distant community, you may be eligible for a discounted airline ticket. Travel agents and airline representatives may ask to see a copy of the death certificate. Most employers allow you to take funeral leave. Ask about your benefits, and don't hesitate to ask to take vacation or sick leave if you need more time off.

Practical Matters

After you have surrendered the body, there are many tasks to complete. Survivors are often at a loss for how to proceed. Here are the steps to follow:

Obtain Certified Copies of the Death Certificate

The family doctor or medical examiner will supply and sign the death certificate within twenty-four hours of death and state the cause of death. The remainder of the form usually is completed by the mortuary handling the final affairs and filed with the state registrar. You will need a certified copy of the death certificate every time you apply for benefits or need proof of the death. It is best to get ten to fifteen certified copies, depending on the complexity of the estate. Photocopies will not be accepted.

Obtain Certified Copies of the Marriage Certificate

If you are the spouse, you may need proof of marriage before you can inherit from the estate, existing policies, or investments. You will also need proof of marriage when applying for Social Security benefits. Death and marriage certificates are kept by the state where the death or marriage occurred. Visit http://www.cdc.gov/nchs on the Internet for state-by-state information on requesting certified copies of death and marriage certificates.

Notify the Lawyer or Executor of the Estate

Settling an estate can be a complicated affair. There may be a need for legal advice on matters such as:

- recording of property deeds
- disposition of stocks and bonds, investments, savings and checking accounts, and other assets
- disbursement of the deceased's estate

Life Insurance

Contact the local life insurance agent or the home office of the life insurance company. Locate insurance policies for death benefits. You usually need to show two documents: a death certificate and a statement of claim. Companies reserve the right to request further information. Claims should include the:

- full name and address of the deceased
- policy number(s) and face amount(s)
- the deceased's date and place of birth as well as the date, place, and cause of death
- the deceased's occupation and date last worked
- the claimant's name, age, address, and Social Security number

Social Security

You will need to contact the Social Security office to check eligibility for lump-sum benefits and to inquire about monthly benefits. Remember, you must apply for Social Security benefits. They are not automatic. Delays in applying may result in the loss of certain benefits.

When applying for Social Security benefits, you will need:

- a certified copy of the death certificate
- the deceased's Social Security number
- approximate earnings of the surviving spouse in the year of death
- record of deceased's earnings in the year prior to death (W-2 form or tax return)
- Social Security numbers of the surviving spouse and minor or disabled children (disabled before age twenty-two and who remain disabled)
- birth certificates of the surviving spouse and minor or disabled children (disabled before age twenty-two and who remain disabled)

- proof of marriage (certified copy of certificate)
- proof of citizenship
- picture identification
- checkbook or bank account number so that benefits can be deposited directly into your account.

Eligibility for Civil Service and Veteran's Benefits

Survivors of civil service or federal workers may be eligible for benefits if the deceased was the spouse and he or she died after eighteen months on the job. Visit the Office of Personnel Management at http://www.opm.gov or call 1-888-767-6738 for more information.

If the deceased was a veteran, he or she is entitled to burial benefits in a national or state Veteran's cemetery. For more information, visit the National Cemetery Administration website at http://www.cem .va.gov or call 1-800-827-1000.

Other Important Contacts

- If your loved one was employed at the time of death, contact the employer to check for death benefits.
- Notify the companies with which the deceased had regular service.
- Call any banks where the deceased had accounts. It is best to name a beneficiary on individual accounts before death occurs. However, if this has not been done, the surviving spouse or family member may complete an affidavit from the bank.
- Alert credit card companies. If you held a joint account with the deceased, the company may want to issue you a new card.
- If the deceased ordered medications by mail, you should cancel the service.
- Cancel or change the name on any automatic bill-paying services and magazine and newspaper subscriptions.
- Any mail addressed to the deceased should be marked "Deceased— Return to Sender," and given to the mail carrier or post office.

Handling Your Emotions

People react differently to a death. Even when death is expected, the emotional impact of losing a loved one can be overwhelming. In the midst of all the tasks, you may experience a range of emotions including sadness, confusion, loneliness, guilt, anger, and anxiety. You may feel like you are on an emotional roller coaster. One day you may feel completely lost, the next day you may feel normal and productive, and the next day you may feel down in the dumps. These changing feelings are a normal part of the grieving process.

Checklist Summary

- Call your minister, family members, or friends to be with you immediately after the death of your loved one.
- Call the funeral home, mortuary, or medical school about transporting the body.
- Contact the people who can help arrange the service.
- Notify the local newspaper of the death and include information in the obituary on location of service, donations, flowers, etc.
- Alert other family, friends, workplace, and faith and volunteer communities about the death.
- Obtain ten to fifteen certified copies of the death certificate, depending on the complexity of the estate.
- Contact the Social Security office.
- Contact the life insurance company of the deceased.
- Explore eligibility for Civil Service and Veteran's benefits.
- Notify the lawyer or executor of the estate.
- Alert credit card companies.
- Cancel prescription, newspaper, and other subscriptions.
- Cancel automatic bill payments.

Write down contact information for family, friends, funeral home or mortuary, employer, minister, lawyer, bank, credit card companies, and other service providers and use a notebook to keep track of your calls including the person called, purpose of the call, and the outcome of the call.

Part Six

Death and Children: Information for Parents

Chapter 37

Caring for a Terminally Ill Child

Despite the best efforts of your child's medical team, cancer treatment sometimes stops working and a cure is no longer possible. The focus of treatment switches to helping your child remain comfortable and pain-free as he or she approaches the end of life. Parents play a crucial role in helping prepare their child for a peaceful and dignified death.

Palliative Care and Hospice

When a cure is no longer possible, the focus of your child's treatment will shift to palliative care. Palliative care is aimed at comfort rather than a cure and focuses on relieving symptoms and pain. Hospice is a special type of palliative care with a broad range of services provided by a team of doctors, nurses, social workers, therapists, clergy, and others. Hospice focuses on the quality, not the length of life, and helps ensure that the child's last days are spent as peacefully as possible. Hospice caregivers also help family members learn how to care for their child so parents and others can be as involved as they want to be. Hospice caregivers support the entire family emotionally, socially, and spiritually, both before and after the child's death.

Hospice services can be provided at home, in a hospital, or in a private, long-term care facility. Many families want their child to die in the comfort of their own home surrounded by their family, pets, and special belongings. Some families find the reassurance of the hospital environment more comforting and many children develop close relationships with the nurses and the other children at the hospital. If possible, the child should be involved in making the decision to die at home versus in the hospital. In most cases, the decision can be revisited if home care becomes too difficult or if a child in the hospital wishes to be at home.

Talking to Your Child about Death

Taking to your child about his own death is probably the most difficult step in caring for a terminally ill child. Many parents think they can protect their child by not telling the truth. However, most children already know or suspect that they are dying. They sense the truth from listening to and watching the adults around them, as well as from experiencing the changes inside their body. It is important to be honest and open so your child feels free to discuss fears and questions. Your child will feel less anxious and alone if he or she knows what to expect and can count on you for support and love. If your child senses they cannot talk to you, he or she will feel isolated, lonely, and more afraid. Not talking about your child's death also prevents both you and your child from bringing closure to his life—by sharing memories, expressing love, and saying good-bye.

Some of the questions your child asks about death may seem inappropriate or upsetting. Knowing how your child views death will help you understand and respond to these questions. Your child's understanding of death is influenced by your family's beliefs, things viewed on television, read in books, and his or her age. Preschool-aged children are too young to understand the concept of death, but they do fear separation. They need extra reassurance with frequent touches and hugs. School-aged children are just beginning to understand death, but their understanding is not well developed. They may view death as a separation or as a person, such as a ghost or an angel. Teenagers have a more adult understanding of death, but this understanding directly challenges their feelings of immortality and growing need for independence.

The following are points to keep in mind when talking to your child about death:

- Use simple, direct language that your child can understand. Use the words death and dying rather than misleading or confusing terms such as passing away or going to sleep.

- Have many conversations with your child and let him or her know that you or someone else is always available to talk. Encourage your child to express emotions—positive and negative. Younger children may express their feelings through play or art.

- Reassure your child that he or she will not be alone. It is critical that children know their parents will be with them when they die and that parental love and support will continue until death and afterward.

- Reassure your child that death is not painful and that after death, any pain and suffering go away and never come back.

- Children need to know that they made a difference in the lives of others. Remind your child of the special things he or she has done and the teachers, friends, nurses, and others who will always remember him. Reassure that your special feelings and love will continue forever.

- Discuss your family's religious or spiritual beliefs about death and what happens after death.

- Many dying children feel guilty for leaving their parents and worry about what will happen to their family without them. You may need to give your child permission to die so he or she can do so peacefully and without guilt.

Meeting Your Child's Needs

Although parents often feel powerless, there are many things you can do to help meet your child's physical and psychosocial needs. As your child approaches death, his or her needs will change. Paying close attention to your child's behavior will help you adjust to these changing needs.

- Allow your child to be a child. Give time to play and engage in other age-appropriate activities such watching television, reading, or playing games.

- Allow your child to continue attending school, even if for only a few hours each week. If your child cannot go to school, ask the teacher to have the class write letters, draw pictures, or make videotapes.

- Encourage visits and contact with family and friends, as long as it is meaningful and not too stressful for your child.

- Give your child as much privacy and independence as possible in personal care, decision-making, and the desire to be alone.

- Encourage your child's end-of-life wishes such as giving away special belongings or writing letters to friends.

- Give your child time to say good-bye to family, friends, teachers, and other special people. This can be done in person, with letters, or through a parent.

- Stick to comfortable routines. If possible, try to keep the same caregivers.

- Make caregivers aware of your child's needs, especially the need for pain management.

- Without using graphic or frightening descriptions, talk about the physical symptoms and changes your child can expect. Knowing what to expect will make him or her less anxious and afraid.

- Continue to set limits on your child's behavior and practice normal parenting. Without limits, your child will feel overwhelmed and out of control.

- Encourage, but do not force, your child to talk with a counselor.

Help for Parents

Parents are not supposed to outlive their children; and nothing can erase the anguish and distress that parents experience. The following are suggestions to help parents cope as they help their child achieve a comfortable and peaceful death:

- It is normal to experience emotions such as anger, guilt, and frustration, as well as financial worries and marital conflict. Talk with your spouse or someone else about your feelings and fears.

- Seek support from a professional grief counselor or attend a support group with other parents. Your hospital or hospice caregivers can help you locate a counselor or support group.

- The dual role of parent and caregiver can be physically and emotionally exhausting. Take advantage of offers for help from family and friends. Use respite care services to allow yourself a break from caregiving.

- Ask the hospital or hospice staff to go over symptoms that occur close to death, such as skin and respiratory changes. Knowing what to expect will help you feel more prepared and enable you to be with your child when death occurs.

• Make funeral arrangements in advance, as well as other plans such as whether to have an autopsy or an advance directive. Making these plans in advance frees you to spend time with your child and avoids having to make decisions in a crisis.

• Take time to just be with your child and tell how much you love him or her. Some parents and children, as well as siblings, find it helpful to look through photo albums and share stories and memories of times spent together.

Chapter 38

Making Decisions when Your Child Is Very Sick

When Your Child Is Admitted to the Intensive Care Unit

The first sight of your child in the intensive care unit (ICU) can be upsetting and confusing. Your child may not recognize you and will be lying in bed, connected to machines with lines and tubes, and may be given medications to stay still. This is a difficult and stressful period for you and your family. You may find this chapter helpful in understanding what is happening in the ICU and what you may be able to do to help your child.

Why does my child look like that?

Each of the wires and tubes you see is to help the doctors and nurses care for your child. Some of the wires and tubes that your child may have include:

Head

- Brain: brain pressure monitor, brain fluid drain
- Mouth: breathing tube, feeding tube
- Nose: feeding, breathing (nasotracheal tube), suction tubes

- Face: oxygen mask, oxygen tubes in the nose (nasal cannula or nasal prongs), pressure mask

Chest

- Sides: lung drain of fluid or air (chest tube, pigtail catheter)
- Front: heart pressure monitors, heart fluid drain (pericardial catheter), electrical wires to the heart (pacemaker wires)

Abdomen / Groin

- Side: feeding tube or button
- Side: fluid drains
- Groin: urine tube (Foley catheter)

Body

- Entire body: heart and breathing monitor wires (cardiorespiratory [CR] monitor)
- Head, hands, arms, feet: fluids and medication tubes (intravenous or IV)
- Neck, collarbone, groin: deep IV (central line)
- Arm, leg: blood pressure cuff
- Wrist side-arm, ankle, foot, groin: constant blood pressure monitor
- Finger, toe, ear, nose, forehead: blood oxygen monitor

You may see a nurse or technician draw small amounts of blood from your child either by using a needle (as a result, there may be some bruising that will heal over time) or from a central line or a-line. These blood samples provide important information that helps keep a close watch on your child's condition. As your child improves, less blood will be taken and many of the wires and tubes will be removed.

Your child may appear to be asleep or may not move when you touch him or her. Some children may not move because of an overwhelming illness of the brain. Your doctor may have given your child one or more of the following medicines:

- Sedative: to help your child relax, sleep, and not remember what is happening
- Analgesic: to decrease or eliminate pain

- Muscle relaxants: to keep your child from moving

You should continue to touch, caress, speak, sing, and read to your child when he or she is sedated and appears to be asleep. It is often comforting and reassuring for your child. Occasionally, the nurses or doctors may ask you not to stimulate your child if this leads to high brain pressure.

What medical problems may happen to children in the ICU?

Often, children are admitted to the ICU because of a single problem, such as a severe case of pneumonia or an injury to the head. However, the function of other organs in the body may be affected because of the body's response to your child's illness or injury. Here are some of the changes that may occur in your child:

- Shock: low blood pressure, cool or flushed skin
- Kidney injury: little to no urine production
- Liver injury: yellow skin (jaundice), tremors, strange behaviors, unconsciousness (coma), or bleeding
- Lung injury: not getting enough oxygen in, or carbon dioxide out, and may need a breathing tube or ventilator to help your child breathe
- Brain injury: swollen brain, which may cause your child to act strangely, to be unconscious (coma), or to have seizures

What are all these machines hooked up to my child?

As a result of certain illnesses, your child may be connected to some of the various machines listed to support his or her organs until he or she is sufficiently healed:

- Kidney: dialysis to purify the blood and balance blood salts
- Lungs: pressure mask, breathing machine (ventilator), lung by-pass
- Heart, heart-lung: bypass

Who are the people taking care of my child?

A health care team will be taking care of your child around the clock. This team includes any or all of the following:

303

- Doctors: Several teams of doctors may be caring for your child. An attending physician heads each team of physicians. These teams include an ICU doctor (pediatric intensivist) who is a specialist in treatment of critically ill children, a surgeon who may need to perform an operation for your child and works closely with the ICU doctor, and other specialists. In many ICUs, there are also doctors in training. These include medical students, residents, and fellows. Each team will have an attending physician and may have many doctors in training who work closely with the attending physician in caring for you child.

- Nurses: Specially trained to closely monitor and provide clinical care for your child.

- Pharmacists: Specialists who monitor your child's medications and dosages during the course of the illness.

- Dietitians: Nutrition specialists who help manage your child's nutrition, including tube feedings or IV feedings.

- Respiratory therapists: Specialists who help your child with breathing treatments, measure lung function, and provide oxygen and ventilator care.

- Physical therapists: Specialists who help tone and strengthen weak muscles and loosen stiff joints that your child may develop during his or her ICU stay.

- Occupational therapists: Specialists who access and teach your child to regain skills such as eating and dressing.

- Child-life specialists: Specialists who help your child cope with being in the ICU. These experts in child development can also help prepare siblings for a visit to the ICU.

- Social workers: Specialists who support you and your family and who guide you to resources as needed during your child's stay in the ICU.

- Psychologists: Specialists who provide counseling to you and your child during your child's illness.

- Chaplains: Clergy who provide spiritual support to you and your child; usually nondenominational, but denominational upon request.

- Unit clerks: Desk clerks who order tests, coordinate patient transfers, and keep the administrative aspects of the ICU running smoothly.

- Discharge planners: Staff who help coordinate the transfer of your child to other hospitals or care facilities and arrange for equipment that you may need at home to help care for your child.

- Parents/Guardians: The most important member of the team is you.

What can I do?

You know your child better than anyone else and can provide helpful observations about him or her. Here is what you can do:

Participate in the care of your child: When appropriate, wash, feed, or hold your child (always ask your child's nurse first if this is okay). Be aware of daily and long-term goals to help your child get better. Understand what the core goals are as well as the big picture in order for your child to leave the ICU. Recovery is a process that may be unpredictable and is based on your child's progress. Every child recovers differently even from similar illnesses.

Ask questions to stay informed: Feel free to ask questions as many times as you need. Your care providers realize that you are under a great deal of stress and may not remember everything the first time you hear it. Write down the names of your care team members and what their roles are. If you think of questions when the doctors are not around, ask your nurse or write them down to ask later.

Bring in pictures of your child or family: This helps your care team see your child the way you do and personalizes your child's care.

Bring in favorite toys, blankets, books, movies, and music: Familiar objects are comforting for children. Distraction with familiar toys and objects can help your child stay calm and recover more quickly.

Learn more about your child's illness: Your doctor or nurse can provide you with written material, helpful websites, and can explain to you what is going on.

Mail: Your child may enjoy receiving mail from family and friends. Your child's nurse can give you the address of the ICU.

How can I take care of myself?

The people taking care of your child all need to take breaks from the tiring and emotionally challenging work of caring for your child. You need to take breaks too. Here are some suggestions:

- eat healthy
- get enough sleep
- exercise or stretch your limbs periodically
- accept the help and support of family and friends
- keep a positive attitude
- use faith and spiritual support and activities, such as meditation
- keep a journal of thoughts, feelings, or your child's progress
- read inspirational material
- appoint a family member or close friend to take messages or to be a spokesperson for you
- make sure someone looks after your house, pets, and checks your mail and phone messages

How will this affect my other children?

The illness or death of a sibling can affect other children in your family. Here are some things to look for:

- Children feel responsible for sibling's illness because they wished him or her ill in the past.
- Children feel ignored or that you are favoring the sick child by spending so much time at the hospital.
- Children act out or may regress (for example, loses bladder control).
- Children do poorly in school due to prolonged disruption in family life.

Often it is helpful to address these issues yourself or with the help of a specially trained psychologist or child-life therapist. Many families find family therapy helpful in resolving these issues. Take some time to be with the rest of your family and to restore balance to your own life.

End-of-Life Care

A child in the ICU will have every reasonable treatment during his or her critical illness. Occasionally, a child's illness is too overwhelming for current medical care to support the body, or there may be no cure available, in which case your child may not survive their illness.

Your doctors may approach you (or you may wish to approach your doctors or nurses) to discuss the discontinuation of mechanical treatments such as breathing or dialysis machines or to discontinue blood pressure medications that may only be prolonging your child's dying process. The doctor may discuss limiting some of these care options with you. Here are some basic terms to know:

CPR (cardio-pulmonary resuscitation): Heart and breathing support using chest compressions, medications, and/or a breathing tube. Various combinations of these treatments are also possible.

Defibrillator: A machine that sends an electrical stimulus to restart the heart.

Brain death: Irreversible death of the entire brain; breathing stops in the absence of a ventilator. The kidneys may not work properly. Some spinal reflexes may remain. This is death by legal and medical standards. A brain dead child may be eligible to become an organ donor.

Making Decisions when Your Child Is Very Sick

Having a child in the intensive care unit is never easy. It is particularly difficult when your child is very sick or has suffered a severe injury and the physicians are not sure if he or she will survive. There are also times when providing medical support to your child may actually cause him or her pain and suffering. When that happens, continuing with painful or uncomfortable procedures may not be what is best for your child. Because the health care providers deeply care about your child, they will always try to do what is in his or her best interest, even if it means making difficult or heart-wrenching decisions. This section will help you understand some of the decisions you may face surrounding these issues. Hopefully, it will help you make choices that you feel are best for your child.

Intensive Care Vocabulary

Your physician may talk to you about different types of treatment. Some treatments are aggressive. This means that the health care provider will try to treat your child with strong medicines or medical machinery. Other treatments focus on keeping children comfortable and eliminating any pain. Some words and phrases that your physician may use might be new to you. The following list may help you understand your child's options.

Palliative care or end-of-life care: In general, this is care given to a very sick or injured child when medical technology cannot make him or her better. Often, the focus of the care is to keep the child comfortable and to ensure that he or she does not feel any pain, discomfort, or anxiety.

Intubation: The physician places a breathing tube through a child's nose or mouth directly into the child's lungs. This is done to help the child breathe. The tube may be attached to a ventilator (also known as a respirator or mechanical ventilation), which can breathe for the child or help the child to breathe.

Electrocardioversion or defibrillation: When the physician uses an electrical current or electrical pulse, to change the heart's rhythm. People sometimes refer to this as jump-starting the heart, but this is not accurate. The electricity does not cause the heart to start if it has stopped; it actually temporarily quiets the heart so that it can restart in a more organized way.

Cardio-pulmonary resuscitation (CPR): During CPR the physician or nurse pushes on the child's chest to squeeze the heart so that the blood will be pumped around the body. This action is known as a chest compression. CPR may also include intubation. Additionally, children are often given medicines to help make their heart beats stronger or faster (these medications are called cardiotonic drugs, vasoactive drugs, inotropes, or pressors). CPR may also include electrocardioversion or defibrillation.

Do-not-resuscitate (DNR): Resuscitation includes different medical procedures including, but not limited to, those listed. Your child's physician may talk to you about limiting aggressive treatment if it is not beneficial. Chest compressions and electrical shocks may be painful, and occasionally it is better for a child not to undergo these procedures.

Limitation of care: This is a term sometimes used to include any limitations on aggressive procedures. Limitations may include DNR or DNI (do-not-intubate) orders. Other limitations may be set on the use of antibiotics, the administration of tube feeds (which is when a feeding tube is placed into a child's stomach through the nose or mouth for the purpose of giving liquid nutrition), the use of IV fluids, or any other medical procedure.

Withdrawal of support: When health care providers withdraw support, they remove machines, medications, or fluids that are prolonging a child's life, but not making him or her better. The health care provider will always continue to provide pain medication and ensure that a child is comfortable. When there is no chance that a child's health will improve, or the treatment is painful or uncomfortable, the parents and physicians may feel it is best to allow the child to die peacefully and comfortably rather than prolong the dying process.

Brain death: There are two different kinds of death recognized by law. The most common way of death is the cessation of the heart beat. Death also occurs when the brain completely stops working. This is called brain death. If a person is declared brain dead, the heart may continue to beat, but the person cannot breathe without machines, feel pain, or have any thoughts or feelings. When this happens, the machines will be turned off. This is not withdrawal of support because the child has already died.

Discussing Your Child's Care

It is important to discuss your child's care with the physician, even when it may be difficult. This does not mean that you have to make a decision about how to treat your child or that your child's physician will make a decision. But it is important to keep the lines of communication open at all times. If the physician feels that your child's illness or injuries are so serious that he or she may not survive, or if the treatment for your child may be painful or uncomfortable and will not cure him or her, your physician may wish to discuss end-of-life care for your child. These conversations are difficult; however, the child's best interest is always the priority. Sometimes parents will initiate these conversations because they do not want to see the child uncomfortable or in pain. A parent should always feel comfortable discussing this topic with the child's physician.

When talking about end-of-life care it is important to have good support such as a relative or friend with you. Some families choose to have a member of their religious affiliation with them. A social worker or your child's nurse can give you support as well. They have helped many families in similar situations and can help you think of questions to ask the physician.

Something to consider is whether or not your child's brothers and sisters should be involved with end-of-life discussions. This is different for every family. Young children may not understand what is being discussed or may be frightened by the conversations. Additionally, siblings sometimes feel guilty or even jealous when a child is in the ICU. The social worker or child life specialist may be able to help you decide how to involve your other children.

Remembering a Child Who Has Died

The loss of a child is one of the most profound and life-altering experiences that a person will ever face. It is important for you to know that you are not alone. Together with your family and friends, your team of physicians, nurses, social workers, and child-life experts are available to you at any time—day or night. All of your questions need to be answered, and you should feel secure with your decisions.

After a child dies, encourage families to spend as much time at the bedside as needed before leaving the hospital. Everyone should have a chance to say good-bye. Parents are welcome to help the nurse clean and bathe their child, or dress him or her in a favorite outfit. Holding and rocking your child may also provide comfort. Some families wish to leave before their child dies. This is a personal decision that should be made based upon what is best for the family.

Many parents find that having pictures taken of their child in their last hours is reassuring. Handprints and footprints can be made for you, and many parents find these keepsakes reassuring. A lock of hair, your child's favorite stuffed animal, a picture he or she painted, or writing a letter to your child may all be reassuring to you.

The social worker can discuss funeral arrangements. A funeral home will need to be selected and the parent or guardian will be asked to sign a Release of Remains either at the hospital or at the mortuary. A social worker, your pastor, relatives, and friends may be helpful to you. The mortuary will discuss the many options and your family's wishes.

Throughout the hospitalization, most of your energy is focused on your child. Parents sometimes forget to eat, and may get little or no sleep. Emotions run high and there may be conflicts between family members. When a child dies, the focus is lost. Your role as a parent is altered forever, and nothing can take that pain away. Making decisions, walking, talking, eating—things that we take for granted—suddenly become difficult. While there may be others that need taking care of, you must remember to take care of yourself. Communication with your loved ones is essential.

Getting back into life's routines may seem impossible, but there are many resources to help. Some parents find certain books helpful in their grief. Others find support groups or web-based bulletin boards helpful. You are not alone.

The Gift of Life

The death of a child is devastating. Some parents, however, find that helping other families with ill children is comforting. Often organs and tissues from children who die can be donated to other children, or sometimes to adults, who suffer from certain illnesses that can be cured by organ transplantation. The gift of a kidney, liver, or heart may save the life of someone else. All vital organs may be donated. Many tissues, like corneas, bone, and skin can also be donated to help others.

The decision to donate is completely up to you. Some families choose to donate, while others prefer not to donate. There are many options with organ donation and you may discuss them all with you child's physician or a representative from your local organ donation service.

Additional Information

Compassionate Friends
P.O. Box 3696
Oak Brook, IL 60522-3696
Toll-Free: 877-969-0010
Fax: 630-990-0246
Website: http://www.compassionatefriends.org
E-mail: nationaloffice@compassionatefriends.org

Leukemia & Lymphoma Society
1311 Mamaroneck Ave.
White Plains, NY 10605
Toll-Free: 800-955-44572
Phone: 914-949-5213
Fax: 914-9494-6691
Website: http://www.leukemia-lymphoma.org

Society of Critical Care Medicine
701 Lee St., Suite 200
Des Plaines, IL 60016
Phone: 847-827-6888
Fax: 847-827-6886
Website: http://www.sccm.org
E-mail: info@sccm.org

Chapter 39

Children's Hospice, Palliative, and End-of-Life Care

An Unmet Need

Children are not supposed to get sick or to die, but they do.

- Over 50,000 children die each year in the United States alone.

- Worldwide, an estimated seven million children and their families could benefit from children's hospice support or palliative care.

- Today, less than one percent of children needing hospice care in the United States receive it.

The number of children receiving hospice and palliative care is on the rise thanks in large part to those programs of Children's Hospice International, which raise the awareness of special needs of children.

Children are not immune to serious illness and death. The devastating impact this can have on their families often leads to increased incidence of job loss, alcoholism, and drug abuse by the survivors. Most parents want and need to have some involvement and control over their children's care. Children's hospice care encourages their participation and thus eases their emotional strain and grief.

Making a Difference

Children's hospice care prepares parents to assume the role of primary caregiver. It supports the inclusion of the patient and the family in the decision-making process to the best of the family's ability and commensurate with their desires. It is an interdisciplinary concept of bringing together physicians, nurses, social workers, therapists, teachers, clergy, administrators, and volunteers as a team to provide the care and support needed. The child and family are the leaders of the team. The focus of hospice care is on life and living, improving the quality of life or the patient and the ongoing lives of the family.

Differences between Hospice Care for Children and Adults

Why the Adult Hospice Model Fails Children

- Parents are not prepared to make an either/or choice between treatments aimed at achieving comfort and treatments aimed at disease management/elimination.

- Pediatricians are strongly involved with and committed to their children and resist turning over control of the care plan to others at the end of life.

- Childhood diseases are treated as aggressively as possible, with the overall goal of extending the life of the child as much as possible at any cost.

- Parents identify the point of diagnosis as the most devastating time of emotional/spiritual adjustment.

- The expertise and skills involved with children (development issues/needs) are not inherent in the skills base of hospice workers who care for a predominantly elderly population.

- Entrance into hospice (requiring a six-month prognosis) assumes a cancer trajectory, not other diseases with different trajectories, although there is no scientific basis for the six-month rule.

- Scope of services of the typical adult hospice does not include pediatric/adolescent specific services.

- Small number of pediatric cases affects economies of scale within hospice resources.

- Entrance into hospice care is based on a patient informed consent model, and children are dependent on the informed consent of their legal guardians.
- Reimbursement, not best clinical practice, nor what is often in the best interest of the child, drives choices made available to parents/guardians.

Patient Issues

- Patient is not legally competent.
- Patient is in a developmental process which affects understanding of life and death, sickness and health, God, etc.
- Patient has not achieved a full and complete life.
- Patient lacks verbal skills to describe needs, feelings, etc.
- Patient will protect parents and significant others at own expense.
- Patient is often in a highly technical medical environment.

Family Issues

- Family needs to protect the child from information about his/her health.
- Family needs to do everything possible to save the child.
- Family may have difficulty dealing with siblings.
- Family stress on finances.
- Family fears that care at home is not as good as at the hospital.
- Grandparents feel helpless in dealing with their children and grandchildren.
- Family needs relief from burden of care.

Caregiver Issues

- Caregivers need to protect children, parents, siblings.
- Caregivers feel a sense of failure in not saving the child.
- Caregivers lack understanding children's cognitive level.
- Caregivers feel a sense of ownership of children, even at expense of parents.

- Caregivers have out-of-date ideas about pain in children, especially infants.
- Caregivers lack knowledge about children's disease processes.
- Influence of unfinished business on style of care.

Institutional/Agency Issues

- Less reimbursement or none for children's hospice/home care.
- High staff intensity caring for children at home.
- Ongoing staff support necessary.
- Children's services have immediate appeal to public.
- Special competencies are needed in pediatric care.
- Assess how admission criteria may screen out children.
- Address unusual bereavement needs of family members.

Chapter 40

Sudden Infant Death Syndrome (SIDS)

SIDS stands for sudden infant death syndrome. This term describes the sudden, unexplained death of an infant younger than one year of age. Some people call SIDS crib death because many babies who die of SIDS are found in their cribs. But, cribs do not cause SIDS.

Fast Facts about SIDS

- SIDS is the leading cause of death in infants between one month and one year of age.

- Most SIDS deaths happen when babies are between two months and four months of age.

- African American babies are more than two times as likely to die of SIDS as white babies.

- American Indian/Alaskan Native babies are nearly three times as likely to die of SIDS as white babies.

What should I know about SIDS?

Health care providers do not know exactly what causes SIDS, but they do know:

"Safe Sleep for Your Baby: Ten Ways to Reduce the Risk of Sudden Infant Death Syndrome (SIDS)," National Institute of Child Health and Human Development, NIH Pub No. 05-7040, updated December 2005.

- Babies sleep safer on their backs. Babies who sleep on their stomachs are much more likely to die of SIDS than babies who sleep on their backs.

- Sleep surface matters. Babies who sleep on or under soft bedding are more likely to die of SIDS.

- Every sleep time counts. Babies who usually sleep on their backs but who are then placed on their stomachs, like for a nap, are at very high risk for SIDS. So it is important for everyone who cares for your baby to use the back sleep position for naps and at night.

What can I do to lower my baby's risk of SIDS?

Here are ten ways that you and others who care for your baby can reduce the risk of SIDS.

Safe Sleep Top 10

1. Always place your baby on his or her back to sleep, for naps and at night. The back sleep position is the safest, and every sleep time counts.

2. Place your baby on a firm sleep surface, such as on a safety-approved crib mattress, covered by a fitted sheet. Never place your baby to sleep on pillows, quilts, sheepskins, or other soft surfaces.

3. Keep soft objects, toys, and loose bedding out of your baby's sleep area. Do not use pillows, blankets, quilts, sheepskins, and pillow-like crib bumpers in your baby's sleep area, and keep any other items away from your baby's face.

4. Do not allow smoking around your baby. Do not smoke before or after the birth of your baby, and do not let others smoke around your baby.

5. Keep your baby's sleep area close to, but separate from, where you and others sleep. Your baby should not sleep in a bed or on a couch or armchair with adults or other children, but he or she can sleep in the same room as you. If you bring the baby into bed with you to breast feed, put him or her back in a separate sleep area, such as a bassinet, crib, cradle, or a bedside co-sleeper (infant bed that attaches to an adult bed) when finished.

6. Think about using a clean, dry pacifier when placing the infant down to sleep, but do not force the baby to take it. (If you are breast feeding your baby, wait until your child is one month old or is used to breast feeding before using a pacifier.)

7. Do not let your baby overheat during sleep. Dress your baby in light sleep clothing, and keep the room at a temperature that is comfortable for an adult.

8. Avoid products that claim to reduce the risk of SIDS because most have not been tested for effectiveness or safety.

9. Do not use home monitors to reduce the risk of SIDS. If you have questions about using monitors for other conditions talk to your health care provider.

10. Reduce the chance that flat spots will develop on your baby's head: provide tummy time when your baby is awake and someone is watching; change the direction that your baby lies in the crib from one week to the next; and avoid too much time in car seats, carriers, and bouncers.

Babies Sleep Safest on Their Backs

One of the easiest ways to lower your baby's risk of SIDS is to put him or her on the back to sleep, for naps and at night. Health care providers used to think that babies should sleep on their stomachs, but research now shows that babies are less likely to die of SIDS when they sleep on their backs. Placing your baby on his or her back to sleep is the number one way to reduce the risk of SIDS.

Won't my baby choke if he or she sleeps on his or her back?

No. Healthy babies automatically swallow or cough-up fluids. There has been no increase in choking or other problems for babies who sleep on their backs.

Spread the Word

Make sure everyone who cares for your baby knows the Safe Sleep Top 10. Tell grandparents, baby sitters, childcare providers, and other caregivers to always place your baby on his or her back to sleep to reduce the risk of SIDS. Babies who usually sleep on their backs, but who are then placed on their stomachs, even for a nap, are at very high risk for SIDS—so every sleep time counts.

Additional Information

Back to Sleep Campaign
31 Center Drive, Room 2A32
Bethesda, MD 20892
Toll-Free: 800-505-CRIB (2742)
Fax: 301-496-7101
Website: http://www.nichd.nih.gov/SIDS

Chapter 41

Stillbirth, Miscarriage, and Infant Death

Coping with Grief

Most parents who experience the death of a child describe the pain that follows as the most intense they have ever experienced. Many parents wonder if they will be able to tolerate the pain, to survive it, and to be able to feel that life has meaning again. The intense pain that grieving parents experience may be eased somewhat if they know what has helped other families overcome a similar grief.

Emotions that may be experienced include sadness, guilt, anger, and fear. Sadness is a normal emotion felt as a result of your loss. Parents may blame themselves for something they did or neglected to do. "If only" becomes a familiar phrase. Parents may feel angry with themselves, their spouse, the childcare provider, the physician, or their baby for having died. Parents might find themselves angry with God, and religious beliefs may be questioned. Many parents experience an overall sense of fear that something else horrible is going to happen. Grieving parents often fear that they are going crazy. These are all normal reactions.

After the initial shock and numbness of the first few days begin to wear off, parents find that they are left with prolonged depression.

This chapter includes: "Coping with Grief: Parents," © 2004 First Candles/ SIDS Alliance. Reprinted with permission. For additional information, visit http://www.sidsalliance.org. Also, "Ways to Support a Parent Whose Baby Has Died," "When a Baby Is Born Still," and excerpts from "Early Pregnancy Loss," © 2004 National SHARE Office. All rights reserved. Reprinted with permission.

There are ups-and-downs that can be brought on by unsolicited mail giveaways of baby products; thoughtless or innocent remarks from others; or by the parents remembering that it is the same day of the week or date that the baby died. At these low points, it is often very helpful for them to talk to another bereaved parent. For some families, support may be obtained from friends and relatives, the clergy, physicians, counselors, or other health professionals who have helped others in similar situations.

Bereaved parents find it difficult to concentrate for any length of time, making it hard to read, write, or make decisions. Some people experience sensations of dizziness or pressure in the head. These feelings are common in grief and do not indicate that the person is losing mental balance.

Sleep may be difficult, leaving parents fatigued. If they have a family to care for or a job to get back to, they may need temporary assistance from their doctor in the form of mild medication to help them rest. Even with sleep, the feeling of exhaustion may persist.

Those in grief often experience muscular problems or other physical symptoms centering on the heart or stomach. Often they have no appetite, and they eat only because they know they must. They feel tied in knots inside. Mothers nearly always say that their arms ache to hold the baby.

Grieving parents may have an irresistible urge to get away, a fear or dread of being alone, or unreasonable fears of danger. If they have other children, parents fear for their safety, yet at the same time they may be afraid of or shun the responsibility of caring for them. Even with this extreme concern about their children, parents may be irritated or impatient with the child's behavior.

Many parents rely heavily on family and friends, but at the same time they may resent help and even feel guilty about their feelings. The situation is made even more difficult when the community around them does not seem to understand a sudden, unexpected, infant death. Friends and relatives are trying to help, but seem to say the wrong things or appear not to understand.

Grief Reactions of Parents May Be Different

Mothers and fathers express their grief in different ways. This fact is not always understood. For instance, mothers generally need to talk out their grief, while fathers tend to suffer in silence. Parents working outside the home are diverted by their work, while parents working at home are surrounded by constant reminders of the baby. Fathers may find it more difficult to ask for help and support from others and may seek diversions through their work; they may even take on extra work to escape thinking about it all the time.

Often the loss of the baby is the first grief situation either parent has experienced. Grief is so intense that they find themselves struggling for ways to relate to each other as well as to their friends and relatives. In order to prevent misunderstanding, most families find it helpful to maintain an atmosphere in which their feelings can be discussed openly even though that is difficult.

Another Baby—Maybe

Maybe you are one of the many people trying for another baby soon after a SIDS or stillbirth death. It is natural—you want to fill your empty arms. Yet you may feel frightened that it will happen again. You will need to figure out how long to wait and what seems right for you. For many parents, the thought of having another baby brings comfort. Others comment that they feel they are betraying their baby who has died. The right time to embark on this will vary depending on your individual circumstances. Trust yourself about the timing.

When a baby dies, well-intentioned people generally try to persuade parents that having another baby as soon as possible is the only answer to accepting that death. If you had infertility problems or other losses, it may seem especially cruel. Rather strong attempts may sometimes be made to convince you that healing can only be accomplished this way. But healing is actually nothing more than incorporating an event into your life in a way that enables you to live with it in an appropriate fashion. Doing that takes time. You cannot necessarily speed up the process of healing by having or not having another baby.

If you decide not to have another baby and that decision is based upon your own reasons, be secure with the fact that this decision is right for you. If you decide not to have another baby, but you think this decision is based more on fear than on practical considerations, do not hesitate to seek some counseling. You will not be the first or the last person to experience this feeling.

If you are expecting a baby, you will probably be a little nervous and excited as well as afraid. It is hard to be patient. It may seem unfair to have to wait and go through this all again. The pregnancy can seem to last forever, and it may be hard not to believe that it won't happen again. Building a good support system can really help. Talk with your doctor or another health professional; you can also contact First Candle/SIDS Alliance. Speaking with other bereaved parents who have had subsequent children may help. Search within your group of relatives and friends for people who will listen to your fears—not give you lots of unsolicited advice. Reviewing the facts about SIDS, stillbirth deaths, and reducing the risks may also be reassuring.

For lack of a better term, your next child has been called the subsequent child. This new child is indeed a very special one, to you and to everyone else. The birth of a subsequent child can be an overwhelming emotional experience. When you see and hold your new baby for the first time, you may find that difficult memories come flooding back and intermingle with the pleasure you are feeling. The moment can be a mixture of great joy and intense pain.

The most uncomfortable period will be the point when your subsequent baby nears the age or the time of the pregnancy of the baby who died. It is one of those milestones that must be reached and passed. Once it is, most parents report that their moments of uneasiness start to decrease. Be assured that you are not the only person to experience discomfort or panic—nearly everyone does. You can only do your best in finding ways to handle it. If you find that you are feeling uneasy most of the time, be sure to consult your doctor, other health professional, or First Candle/SIDS Alliance for additional help.

The birth of your newborn represents hope and a promise of the continuity of life. Joy and sorrow are memories in your life that enable you to know the importance of hope. Many parents have weathered the crisis, panic, and great joy of their subsequent child's infancy. They acknowledge that while it was not always easy, and they had to work at handling their emotions, their effort was rewarded by one of the most wonderful periods in their lives.

Early Pregnancy Loss

The feelings you experience after an early pregnancy loss are often more intense than most people, including you, might expect. The death of a baby at any stage is a very real loss. Although your physical healing may be a short process, the emotional healing might take much longer.

What is an early pregnancy loss?

An early pregnancy loss is defined as any loss before 20 weeks gestation. Most pregnancy losses occur before the thirteenth week, called a first trimester loss. Loss during this time most commonly occurs because of a problem with the development of the baby or the placenta.

If a loss occurs before 20 weeks, you may not be able to determine the gender of the baby without chromosomal testing.

How can I expect to feel?

After an early pregnancy loss, you may feel anything from relief, to disappointment, to profound grief. These feelings may constantly change. You might experience a range of emotions at different times, or re-experience an emotion you have already felt. There is no right or wrong way to move through your emotions. You and your partner may grieve differently, and the community around you may grieve yet another way. And even though there are people who may share the common thread of having a loss, each individual's experience is always different. The following array of emotions makes up a normal process of grief. It is unlikely that you will experience these in an order or as stages. The intense feelings of your grief will not last forever; there will come a time when the heartache will be less painful. Incorporating your loss into your daily life takes patience and time. Not all of this time is spent in acute or deep grief. The degree that the varying emotions are felt lessens with time, and healing takes place. You may feel:

- shock
- confusion
- low self esteem
- denial
- anger
- guilt and/or self-blame
- frustration
- relief
- sadness and/or depression
- physical symptoms related to hormonal changes

When a Baby Is Born Still

For many families, the instant you knew you were pregnant your life changed forever. Throughout your pregnancy you may have felt excited. Maybe you already picked names or the perfect outfit for the baby, or even prepared the nursery. You may have also felt reluctant or worried about how this baby was going to affect the rest of your life. Whether you were feeling joy or apprehension, this new baby was an important part of your future.

The feelings you experience after a late pregnancy loss are often overwhelming and intense. The death of a baby at any stage is a very real loss. You will not only have to recover physically, but emotionally and spiritually.

The following information has been gathered by bereaved parents, friends, and professionals to help you realize the normalcy of all the emotions and fears you may experience during your grief journey.

What is a stillbirth?

A stillbirth is the delivery of a baby who has died, and is greater than 20 weeks gestation. In about half of all stillbirths, a cause for the baby's death can be discovered after evaluating the baby. It is possible for the baby to have birth defects or problems with the placenta or umbilical cord. Other causes may be found in maternal circumstances. Unfortunately, for many stillbirths, the cause of the baby's death remains undetermined. Stillbirth cannot be predicted, nor can we predict whom it will affect.

How can I expect to feel?

The discovery that your baby has died is a complete shock, and the emotions you have may be overwhelming. You may be asking, "Why did this have to happen?" This news and process can be devastating to families. You now have to go from the highs of awaiting a beautiful, healthy baby, to the lows of deep grief. You have not only lost a baby, but also the hopes and dreams you had planned for your future together. Your emotions and feelings will be constantly changing. You might experience a range of emotions at different times, or re-experience an emotion you have already felt. There is no right or wrong way to move through your feelings. Everyone's experience and way of grieving is different. While grieving, you may experience any or all of the emotions listed. It is very unlikely that you will experience these in any order or as stages. The intense feelings of your grief will not last forever; there will come a time when the heartache is less painful. Incorporating your loss into your daily life takes patience and time. Not all of this time is spent in acute or deep grief. The degree that the varying emotions are felt lessens with time and healing takes place. It is important for you to know what you are feeling is normal for you. You may feel:

- overwhelming shock
- confusion
- low self-esteem
- loss of control
- disappointment
- jealousy
- anger
- guilt and/or self-blame
- frustration
- sadness and/or depression
- physical symptoms related to hormonal changes

How are fathers or partners feeling?

This is likely a difficult time for fathers too. As a father or partner, you may be experiencing many of the same emotions as your wife or partner. Sometimes your feelings may be equally as strong. Even though you may have similar feelings, you may feel very detached from your partner right now, and you may have difficulty understanding how she is feeling. You may feel a sense of helplessness, as you cannot control what has happened or how you feel emotionally. Or, perhaps you have put your feelings aside so you can be there to support her. It is important to remember that you also need support at this time. Even if you have suppressed your grief, it is still there and will resurface again at some point. Another difficult issue you may face is other people downplaying the grief you are experiencing. Partners are not usually given much time off for a pregnancy loss and may feel torn about returning to work. You may not receive the support you need. It is normal to feel frustrated if you are constantly being asked how your partner is doing while it seems no one cares or asks about you.

It is important to know that the feelings and reactions you have are normal. It may be confusing or frustrating to experience this wide range of emotions. You and your partner will likely grieve in different ways and at different times. You can be supportive to one another, but know it is all right to take the time to grieve without being the strong one. You may find that you get help from someone you were not expecting it from. Try to be open to receiving that support. Also, be willing to seek out people or groups for support if it is not readily available to you.

How do I deal with the reaction of others?

It is difficult for someone who has never lost a baby to comprehend what you are going through. Often, people do not know what to say to you, and in their attempts to make you feel better they may say things that upset you or make you angry. Most people do not purposely try to be insensitive; they simply do not understand the impact the death of your baby has had on you. Some people do not understand the intimate relationship you and your baby already had since they were not able to experience the same close, tangible bond while you were pregnant.

The best way to deal with people when you are grieving is to be honest and tell them what you need. Instead of saying, "You just don't understand how I feel," say "I'm having a bad day; it really hurts my feelings when you say things like that." Some women have found it helpful to write notes or letters to their family, friends, and/or co-workers explaining the circumstances surrounding their loss, and what they need from them. Sometimes people are surprised at the depth of your feelings.

How can I best care for myself?

Take care of your body. Your doctor should give you specific directions for your care after delivery. Taking care of your physical health is just as important as taking care of your emotional health. Even though you will not be caring for a newborn at home, the grief you will carry can be exhausting. Because grieving has a physical component, it is very important to eat a balanced diet, exercise (even if it is just a walk around the block), drink plenty of water, and maintain a regular rest routine. Besides your emotional reactions, you will also be dealing with hormonal responses. Your body will go through the same hormonal and physical changes as you would if you had delivered a healthy baby. You can expect to experience mood swings, fatigue, insomnia, inability to concentrate, or irritability. Your energy levels can be erratic as well as your appetite.

Find support. There are many sources for support. Many people find it helpful to attend a pregnancy loss support group. You can also find on-line organizations designed to help grieving parents. For some, a close friend or relative can be of great comfort. If your sadness significantly interrupts your ability to function daily, it is important to contact your doctor or see a professional counselor.

Communicate. Tell others what you need and be specific. Other than verbally expressing your needs, you can write notes or letters to friends, family, and/or co-workers. Tell people what you need from them, especially when you want to talk about your baby, or even when you do not.

Take care of your mind and spirit. You may find a need for more spiritual bonds during this time. Contact clergy or simply set aside time for reflection or relaxation. Some people enjoy reading and writing. Journaling your experience may be an important part of your healing process.

How can I memorialize my baby?

You can start by collecting anything that reminds you of your baby to create a memory box, keepsake book, and/or shadow box. Examples of items to include are:

- sonogram pictures
- pictures of yourself pregnant, even if you didn't know you were pregnant or look pregnant
- pictures of your baby
- hospital birth certificate
- hospital bracelet
- cards of congratulations before your loss
- cards, flowers, and gifts after your loss
- footprint and handprint certificates
- permanent hand and foot prints
- crib card, comb, or measuring tape
- baby clothes and/or blanket
- naming ceremony/baptism booklet
- memory book

In the future you can:

- arrange a special service or funeral
- plant a special bush, tree, or garden
- create a bracelet or another piece of jewelry

- keep a journal
- make donations to charities in memory of your baby

Ways to Support a Parent Whose Baby Has Died

For many families who are pregnant with or have recently delivered a very loved and wanted baby, hopes and dreams are torn apart with the news that the baby has died. For the rest of the world around them, not much seems changed. Unfortunately, something very sad and life altering has happened that needs to be acknowledged. A baby has died.

The following information has been gathered by bereaved parents, friends, and professionals. Here are some ways to better acknowledge the death of a baby and communicate with parents experiencing grief.

The First Encounter

Say I'm sorry. If you can't find the right words, it is better to say, "I'm sorry," than nothing at all.

Avoid cliches such as:

- Everything happens for a reason.
- Thank goodness you are young; you can still have more children.
- There must have been something wrong with the baby.
- I understand how you feel (unless you have an experience to share).
- It was meant to be.
- You have an angel in heaven.
- At least you didn't get to know the baby.
- You are so strong, I could never handle this.
- I guess it's good it happened now.
- At least you have children at home.
- God would never give you more than you could handle.

What may seem comforting to you may be very hurtful to others. Clichés tend to minimize the loss and the emotions a parent has toward their baby.

I don't know what to say. If you are unaware of what to say, simply say, "I don't know what to say." Honesty can be more comforting than words with less meaning.

Silence can be okay. Sometimes there is just nothing to say. Just be quiet, be with them, hold their hand, touch their shoulder, or give them a hug.

Apologize for hurtful comments. If you do say something insensitive, acknowledge it and apologize. These comments can cause hurt and future resentment.

Responses to death. Do the same things for the death of a baby as you would if another family member died. Send flowers and/or sympathy cards, share special remembrances, make phone calls, or make/bring dinner. If you are a close family member or friend, it may be helpful if you ask to help maintain laundry, basic housecleaning, cooking, or watch other children at home (if applicable). Be sure to obtain permission from the bereaved family before disassembling the baby's room or removing baby items.

In the First Few Weeks

Ask and listen. Ask sincerely, "How are you?" and be ready to listen. They may have a lot to say and may repeat their story many times. In order to be helpful to their grieving process, you must be willing to listen. Sometimes parents can verbalize what they need, so you know what you can do or say to comfort them. You can also add, "I've been thinking of you," or "I've been praying for you," if either is appropriate to the situation.

Don't forget dad. Fathers and mothers grieve differently. Dads may not talk about the baby as much. Men tend to go back to work sooner and seem to reclaim their lives faster, but that does not mean that they are not grieving. Let them open up to you if they need to talk.

Be specific in your offer to help. "Call me if you need anything," or "Let me know how I can help," are generic statements for grieving families. Not all people are willing to ask for help. Offer to bring dinner Tuesday at 6:00, ask to take a newly bereaved mom to breakfast Thursday morning at 9:00, or ask dad if he wants to play nine holes

331

of golf Friday at 8:00. If their response is no, it is okay to offer again in a week or two.

Acknowledge the baby. One misconception is that the shorter the baby's life, the easier the grief process. The opposite is true. Whether the baby died during the pregnancy or lived a short time, the family lost future hopes and dreams. It is important when talking with parents to use the baby's name if one was given. By doing this you are showing the parents you value the short life of their baby. You will honor the family and baby, showing he/she is not forgotten.

Avoid giving advice. Everyone is an individual and grieves differently. There are no rules that define how a bereaved parent should feel or how soon he or she will return to the norms of daily life. Giving parents permission to grieve their own way can be healing.

In the Following Months and Years

Parents need time. The parents of a baby who has died will need more time to grieve than society allows. The average intense grief period is 18 to 24 months. Parents will go through ups and downs during that time. The future holds many milestones that will be missed, such as first steps, the first day of kindergarten, toothless grins, or a sweet sixteen. These milestones may bring tears to the parents, yet may have disappeared to others. Acknowledge a parent's grief and remember with them.

Open communication. Bereaved parents need a safe person and/or place to talk about their baby and the feelings they are experiencing. They need to be heard without being judged or receiving unwanted advice. Allow the parents to talk openly about the pregnancy, the birth, and any future plans or dreams they may be missing.

Remember special dates. Grieving parents may be saddened by special events or dates (birthdays, due date, delivery date, Mother's and Father's Day, holidays) because they are a reminder their baby is not here. These days may be difficult without their baby, and parents need your support at these times.

Make contact. After a few weeks, people generally stop coming by. Continue to call and check in on the family. Make a call, leave a message, or write a note to let them know you care. Most bereaved parents appreciate acknowledgment of their grief and the life of their baby.

Showing You Care in the Workplace

During and after the loss of a baby, the workplace can be a confusing and difficult place to grieve. The key to maintaining good working relations is to have open communication.

- Parents of a baby who died need adequate time off (refer to bereavement policies) and need a plan of action for returning. Mothers, especially, need appropriate time to recover and heal. Some parents need to return part-time and some can return full-time.

- Try to help parents maintain a normalcy at work. Ask them to lunch, or sincerely ask how they are doing.

- Grief can make a normal day of work unbearable. Employees and employers can try to alleviate feelings of being overwhelmed by either delegating or sharing job responsibilities.

- It may or may not be appropriate to share emotional issues publicly at work. Discuss what is appropriate, and understand that grief is a normal process that takes time to work through.

- Crying, having difficult days, feeling confused, or having trouble concentrating is normal for grieving parents. Providing a safe place for bereaved parents to express their feelings will aid in their healing process.

Additional Information

National SHARE Office
St. Joseph Health Center
300 First Capitol Dr.
St. Charles, MO 63301-2893
Toll-Free: 800-821-6819
Phone: 636-947-6164
Fax: 636-947-7486
Website: http://www.nationalshareoffice.com
E-mail: share@nationalshareoffice.com

First Candle/SIDS Alliance
1314 Bedford Ave., Suite 210
Baltimore, MD 21208
Toll-Free: 800-221-7437
Phone: 410-653-8226
Website: http://www.sidsalliance.org
E-mail: info@firstcandle.org

Mail Preference Service
Direct Marketing Association
P.O. Box 9008
Farmingdale, NY 11735-9008

You can write to Mail Preference Service to stop many unwanted junk mailings from coming to your house which may help decrease the amount of baby-related mail parents get the first year after their loss. Writing to the address will take you off many national mailing lists for awhile; however, if you would still want to receive certain catalogs (not baby-related), it might work best to just write to the specific companies sending the baby-related mailings.

Chapter 42

Grieving the Death of a Child

For the Newly Bereaved

The death of our children at any age from any circumstance is indeed one of the cruelest blows that life has to offer. The journey through this grief is a very long, dark, difficult, and painful one for bereaved parents.

In the early minutes, days, weeks, months, and even years of grief, we find ourselves in an all consuming grief and pain beyond description. We find it difficult to carry on our everyday lives or to think of little else except our child's death. Even our once wonderfully happy memories shared with our children while they lived now bring us pain for a time.

Bereaved parents do not get over the death of children, nor snap out of it as the outside world seems to think can and should be done. The death of our children is not an illness or a disease from which we recover. It is a life altering change that we must learn to live with.

With the death of our children, we are forced to do the impossible: build a new life and discover a new normal for ourselves and our families in a world that no longer includes our beloved children. It is very important for newly bereaved parents to know that they will experience a wide and often frightening variety of intense feelings after the death of a child. It is also very important for newly bereaved parents

"For the Newly Bereaved," by Mary Cleckley, in loving memory of her son. Reprinted with permission from Bereaved Parents of the USA. For additional information, visit http://www.bereavedparentsusa.org.

to understand and know that all of these feelings that you experience are all very natural and normal under the circumstances

Equally important for you to know and to believe is that as much as you cannot possibly believe it now, you will not always feel this powerful and all consuming grief. But right now you must follow the instincts of your soul and allow your bodies and hearts to grieve. The grief resulting from your child's death cannot be skirted over, around, or under. You must go through it in order to come out on the other side.

Be gentle and patient with yourself and your family. Allow yourself to cry, to grieve, and to retell your child's story as often as needed and for as long as you need. Eventually, you will smile and find joy again. You will never forget your child; he or she will be with you in your heart and memories for as long as you live.

Some of the things you may experience or feel are:

- depression

- a profound longing and emptiness

- wanting to die—this feeling usually passes in time; for eventually you will realize that you must go on for the sake of remaining family members, yourself, and your child who died

- profound sadness

- crying all the time or at unexpected times

- inability to concentrate on anything

- misplacing items constantly

- wondering why

- forgetfulness

- questioning yourself over and over: "If only I had....?" "Why didn't I...?"

- placing unnecessary guilt on yourself or others

- anger with yourself, family members, God, the doctor, and even your child for dying

- fearing that you are going crazy (very normal)

- great physical exhaustion—grief is hard work and consumes much energy

- difficulty sleeping or sleeping all the time to avoid the pain

- physical symptoms such as heaviness in your chest or having difficulty breathing (if these feelings persist see your physician), tightness in your throat, yawning, sighing, gasping, or even hyperventilating

- lack of appetite or over eating

- weight gain or weight loss

- anxiety (often associated with overprotective behavior toward surviving children and other family members)

- denial of your loss, thinking that your child will return (denial can be effectively treated by spiritual leaders as well as psychologists—seek help if your denial phase persists beyond a month)

- needing to tell and retell the story of your child's death

- inability to function in your job

- sensing your child's presence or an odor or touch associated with your child

- having difficulty grocery shopping because of seeing your child's favorite food(s) on the shelves

- irrationally upset with yourself if you smile or laugh, thinking how can I smile, my child is dead—your child will want you life to be as good and as happy as possible in spite of death's intervention

- feeling as if your spouse or other family members don't understand your grief or are not grieving as you think they should—remember everyone grieves differently

- losing old friends who don't seem to understand your pain and grief

- making new friends through support groups with members who have also experienced the death of a child and therefore understand your feelings

- feeling like you are making progress in your grief work, then slipping back into the old feelings—grief work usually is a succession of two steps forward and one step back over a long period of time

- becoming very frustrated with others who expect you to be over this in a month, six months, or a year, and who say so—or even being frustrated with yourself for expecting to be over this too soon

Grief work from the death of your child is a slow process. Be patient with yourself. Keep remembering that you are not the only one who has had these experiences. These experiences are all typical, natural, and normal feelings for bereaved parents. You cannot ignore them. You must work through them. It will require even more time to feel better if you try to deny your feelings. There are no timetables for grief; each person must take as long as it takes for him or her to work through their feelings.

Additional Information

Bereaved Parents of the USA
National Office
P.O. Box 95
Park Forest, IL 60466
Phone: 708-748-7866
Website: http://www.bereavedparentsusa.org

Chapter 43

Helping Children Cope with Death and Funerals

Understanding the Problem

People have different ideas about whether to include children—no matter what their age—at the bedside during someone's final days of life, at the time of death itself, and at the funeral. Opinions about this differ depending on the family's manner of handling such matters and also on the type of death involved. For example, was the death sudden, or did the illness last a long time? Some adults do not want children seeing someone they know growing weaker or hooked to tubing. Opinions also depend on what the child's relationship is with the person who has cancer. Is it a parent, brother, sister, close relative, or friend? If it is someone the child does not know very well, maybe it is less important for the young person to visit. Also, consider whether other helpful adults or older children can pay attention to the child and help with any questions and feelings.

Along with these practical questions, people's ideas about whether children should be involved also are shaped by what they were told when they were little and someone died. Our opinions are shaped by what we learn from our own families about what is right. Your opinions about including children are shaped by how you cope with sadness and death yourself. Everyone copes differently.

When to Get Professional Help

Normally, professional help is not needed to make decisions about including children in events. Most questions and concerns can be worked out by family members or friends. However, a few clues might tell you that children or teenagers are having unusual problems whether it is dealing with watching the person who has cancer grow more ill, with the idea of the funeral, or even with death itself. This is when professional help can make a difference.

Call on professionals such as teachers, school psychologists, ministers, youth group leaders, social workers, or hospice staff who have helped you if you do not know how to handle certain situations and want to talk with someone other than family members. Also, call if young people do any of the following:

- have trouble sleeping
- show disruptive behavior at school
- do poorly in school, if this is a change
- act differently, such as being quiet and sad when before they were happy and talkative

What You Can Do to Help

Usually, caregivers are busy making decisions near the time of death and before any funeral or memorial service. While you may want to pay more attention to how children or teenagers are feeling and their questions, you may not have time. You also may not have the energy. Do not attempt to take care of everyone else's needs at this point. Instead, think about asking someone special in your circle of family or friends to help.

Plan Ahead for Any Visits by Children

Usually, fewer and fewer people visit during the final days of life, regardless of whether the sick person is at home, in a nursing home, or in a hospital. If visitors or family have children, a common question that arises is whether to bring them. Here are several ways to handle this question:

Learn what the child knows about what is happening. If the child knows that Grandma is very sick, ask the parent or guardian to paint a more complete picture so that the child is prepared. For example, grandchildren may not have seen Grandma recently, but they know what a person looks like in bed. If Grandma has lost weight, say that she shrank a little but is all there, the same height but just smaller. Also, prepare the child by mentioning any other visible differences, such as hair or skin changes. Use simple words. Most important, reassure the child that Grandma knows the child is there even if she is sleeping. If she is awake but not talking, tell the child that Grandma will look but not talk because she is resting.

Ask the child what he or she thinks is happening, and invite questions. Children have their own ideas and questions about what is happening, and they can be very open about what concerns them. For example, their understanding of dying and death is not the same as ours. It is not formed until 8 or 9 years of age, and even then, children do not fully understand the permanence or finality of death. Teenagers have a much fuller understanding, but their questions may be harder to answer (for example, Why is life unfair to good people?) Different ages have different types of questions. Answer them simply, and if you do not have the answers, be honest and say so.

Suggest that two people come with young children to visit. If young children want to visit with the dying person, remember that their attention span for the visit may be short. After they greet and see the person, they may quickly lose interest in the visit. Other parts of the home or the hospital may become more interesting. Another adult or teenager can take them out and entertain them so that the child is not fidgeting or feeling forced to stay in one place.

Be prepared for different expressions of feelings from children and from teenagers. Even if you think young people are handling this well, they may have many new and unspoken feelings. Teenagers need time to think about their feelings. If they are close to the person who is dying, they may feel angry, sad, confused, disappointed, or abandoned. Some teens will talk about this; many will not. Young children can feel the same way, but they are unable to talk about it. Therefore, these feelings sometimes come out through sudden changes in behavior, such as acting like a younger child, toddler, or baby. In many cases, this is a safe way for them to let out their feelings.

Ask adults you trust to pay attention to young people who visit and listen to their feelings and questions. As a caregiver, you have a lot going on, and taking care of children or teenagers can seem overwhelming. This is a task you can share with adults you trust. When you think things are not quite right with younger relatives or children, ask others to check in with them. Friends of the family are good to ask; they can help by paying attention to young children and listening to teenagers.

Answer Concerns about Dying and Death

Children have different questions about death at different ages. They are able to understand death better as they grow older and gain more experience. For example, they may have seen a pet die, or a friend may have lost a parent. They may have read books or watched television and come to know that death is forever.

Young people's questions about death can be surprising, and they may challenge you at a time when you are tired and trying to make many decisions. The following suggestions may help you to handle questions during the days immediately surrounding the death:

Find someone who will listen to the children's concerns about dying and what happens after death. You probably know who your children trust, and if you do not, ask them. Children are honest. For example, if you are a mother with a young child, you might ask: "If you hurt your finger and couldn't find me, who would you want to help you?" Teenagers might want to know why you want them to talk with someone. In this case, say that you have found it helps to talk and sort things out aloud. (Of course, they may or may not take your advice.)

Use pictures, dolls, or books with young children. Young children may want to draw pictures illustrating how they feel or what they know. This way, questions can come up as you ask them what is in their pictures or why they used certain colors. Another way is for them to play with dolls. Ask them to play, and tell them that today, one doll is Grandma. Watch what they do. This also is a good way to get children ready to see Grandma if she looks different from the way that she looked the last time they saw her. Tell the child that Grandma sleeps a lot now and is in bed all the time. Ask the child to put Grandma in bed. Some children may take care of the doll in bed; others may get mad and throw the doll across the room. Young children experience many feelings when there is a sickness in the family. This is normal, and you can help them by accepting how they feel.

The hospice may have books to help you reach young children and their feelings. They also may have a list of books available at your local library. Storybooks can help young children to recognize their feelings even when they cannot express them. There are picture books for very young children and books for older children that deal with the serious illness and death of a loved one.

Suggest that an older child talk with someone outside the family. Older children or teenagers might confide in a school counselor, teacher, school nurse, minister, church leader, Sunday school teacher, youth leader, or neighbor. They may be open with friends, or they may say nothing at all. Tell them you want to know how they are doing, but add that you know it sometimes helps to talk with someone who is not related or close to the family. Then drop it. Do not push.

Be prepared for tough questions about life after death. Answers about where people go after death or why people suffer and die vary from family to family, from one religion to the next and even from one society to another. A Spanish family might believe things about heaven that differ greatly from the beliefs of a Chinese family. Some adults have very set ideas that life after death exists. They can describe heaven very clearly, and they know the way to get there. Believing in life after death—no matter what the religious viewpoint, faith, or path to get there—brings comfort and hope to many people. Other adults may say that the answers to these questions are a mystery. The best answer to say is what you honestly think in simple, short explanations.

It is important that young people be able to talk with someone who will listen to their concerns. During their lives, they will hear different answers to these types of tough questions: What happens after death? Why do good people suffer? The important thing is that the young person is thinking about these issues, which is a vital part of growing up.

Be prepared for tough questions about what happens to the body. Teenagers can understand the difference between being buried and being cremated, and children of all ages may be curious about what happens to the body after death. If you or others are uncomfortable talking about this, refer them to people you know and trust. These could be members of the clergy, relatives, or friends. Hospice staff can speak with them as well. Young people should talk about their concerns with someone who will listen. These questions often lead to matters of a more spiritual or religious nature, such as where does the spirit go?

Answer all questions. Answering questions is important, because what children might imagine can be far worse than what actually happens. Young children have simple questions that deserve simple answers. For example: "When they put that tube in Daddy? Is that what killed him?" Without the opportunity to talk about this, a child can grow up being afraid of needles or tubes. Others might say: "I heard Aunt Mary say that Grandma starved to death. Did she?" If children hear this—and with cancer, they often do—and believe it, they can feel guilty that they did not feed Grandma. They also can become angry that others did not feed her. Young children may ask the same questions many times. This is perfectly normal.

Remind children that it is no one's fault when someone dies. Children usually will not ask directly if it is their fault that a close relative has died. Guilt is a very common reaction even though it is not reasonable. With young children, say something like: "Just because you got angry at Mommy sometimes, that doesn't mean it's your fault that she got sick and died." It also is helpful to give children permission to be angry, because anger is a normal part of losing someone you love. You can say something like: "Sometimes I get so mad that Daddy isn't here anymore." Children need to know that these feelings are normal and acceptable.

Share Decisions about Who Should Go to Funerals or Memorial Services

Ask for help making decisions about children attending services or for help looking after them, either at services, at home, or at someone else's house.

Ask young people if they want to go to the service. Asking young people this question depends, of course, on their age. Very young children cannot help you to make a decision, but older ones can. Making decisions for these children leaves them out. Young children and teenagers should not be protected from the reality of death, nor should they be shut out of the meals or talks after the funeral or memorial service and burial, if there is one. Shutting them out makes them feel alone. It also gives them the idea that death is so horrible that it cannot be coped with.

Funerals can help young people face their grief. Letting them listen to the planning for the funeral and including their ideas makes them feel that they belong to something that will live on. It also gives them a chance to talk about what has happened. Letting them be part of the rituals (the things a family normally does when a death occurs) is an important way to learn about this part of living.

Young children (younger than 8 or 9 years) do not understand that death is permanent. They will ask when Mommy or Grandma is coming back. If young children are not included in the funeral ritual, it will be harder for them to understand what has happened. If they have attended the funeral, however, you can say: "Remember when we all went to see Grandma in the casket, and then we went to the cemetery?" Without this memory, it will be harder for you to help these children understand.

Ask young people before the service how they are feeling about what is happening. Even after young people know they are going to a funeral, new feelings can surface. Relatives may be arriving. They may meet people who are unfamiliar to them but who claim to remember when they were little. It can be a busy and confusing time. If you are to help them, you need to be aware of what they are feeling.

Tell children what to expect at the funeral home, what they will see, and what will happen both before and after the service. This helps them to prepare for this new experience.

Let them change their minds. Young people may decide they want to attend services but then change their minds. Let them decide. They know what they want to do. If it is important for you to have them there, such as with teenagers, ask them to attend for your sake.

Remind yourself as well as them that it is the memory of the person's life, not the person's death that is important. It is okay if a young person does not want to go. However, if a child is very firm that he or she does not want to attend the funeral of a close relative, it usually signals that the child is very troubled or confused. Children typically are fascinated by funerals and, most of all, want to be included as part of the family. See if you can get the child to tell you what is worrying him or her about the funeral. Children can have many misconceptions and fears that should be cleared up so that they can feel okay about saying goodbye to the person who has died.

Remembering relatives or friends when they were alive is what is important; however, funeral services help to remind us that death really has happened. Children of any age usually will benefit (just as adults do).

Include them in meals or gatherings after services. Children want to feel that they belong, and leaving them out of special gatherings after services sends a message that they are unimportant. Many times, their feelings are hurt. If a child is struggling with sadness or fear, he or she will feel that much sadder and more abandoned.

Deal with the Possible Disapproval of Other Adults

Expect some adults to disagree with your decision to allow children to attend a memorial or funeral service. Some adults cannot bear to see a child suffer because they are so upset themselves about the death. They want to protect the young person from feeling what they are feeling. Some relatives and friends may say it is a bad idea to let young people attend a funeral. They will say things like: "Seeing grown-ups cry will be too upsetting for her" or, "Children do not belong at funerals." If you and other adults decide it is a good idea to include the younger child, some adults may go so far as to say that this is cruel or awful. Although this is rare, should these adults see the child cry, whether at the funeral or later, you may hear them tell others that you should have followed their advice and hint that you made a bad decision. This can be difficult, but the opposite decision would have been difficult as well. This is a situation in which someone must make a decision, and you know your children best and will be the one dealing with their feelings later. The job of a parent is to help children deal with life and its sadness. Dealing with death is just one more part of learning about life.

Help Young People at the Memorial or Funeral Service

Assign someone to supervise young children. Very young children probably will lose interest in the service after a short time. Try to find an adult who can be with them and can leave the service if they are restless.

Let the child visit the church or place where the service will be held. Very young children like to know that they can get basic needs met in new places. Visit the church or place where the service will be held ahead of time. Show them where the restroom is, where the water fountain is, and any play areas. This helps them to feel more secure at the service, especially if the person who died was a parent. Remind them that they do not have to stay. They can go outside with an adult and play or take a walk.

Assign someone to supervise everyday tasks. Young people need supervision with everyday tasks such as bathing, dressing, eating, and sleeping. They need to keep playing or spending time with friends if they are home. They also need activities if they are traveling and staying somewhere else. If you, as the caregiver, are too busy to think about these things, ask someone who knows the child to make sure that his or her everyday routines are followed.

Expect Struggles with Grief Both Now and in the Future

Listen to what others tell children that can either help or confuse them. Other adults, and even relatives, may tell young people how to feel, such as "Be brave and strong." They also will have ideas about how they should behave, such as "Don't cry," or "Be extra nice to your mother this week—she just lost her father." They also might have ideas about what the person who died might want to see the young person doing, such as "Your father wouldn't want you to cry for him." Adults who say these things mean well; however, their advice comes from the messages they received from their own parents or relatives when they were young.

Young people and teenagers may be confused when one piece of advice differs greatly from another. One adult may say "Be strong and don't cry," while another may say, "It's okay to cry," or "Crying means we loved your father and will miss him very much." You should be aware of these conflicting messages so that you can help the child to understand why people feel differently and to be comfortable with how he or she acted.

Tell them it is okay if they do not know how they feel. Not everyone knows how he or she feels. If children or teenagers do not know, tell them it is okay. They should not feel guilty about feeling nothing while everyone around them is sad or upset. Their feelings may come months later, so it is important to continue to ask them how they are feeling after the funeral and burial.

Normal grief reactions. Many changes follow the death of a close family member or friend. It can help to make a list of everything that went away or changed to understand what the child is experiencing. If young people were close to the person who died, they will feel grief (just as adults do). Tears often come and go in the first weeks after a death. Young people might even feel relieved that the waiting is over and that the death has finally occurred. Children grieve differently than adults— they usually do not cry for long periods of time but are sad briefly and then carry on with their normal activities. This does not mean that they fail to understand what has happened. It means that they are not ca- pable of the same prolonged, intense reactions that adults experience.

Normal grief reactions include:

- Shock and disbelief. At the beginning of grief, death is hard to accept even if the person had been sick for a long time. This dis- belief can give some protection against intense feelings.

- Memory. Gradually, memories and pictures of the person be- come less clear in the mind. Some people may worry this means the person was not that special to them, and they may feel guilty that they cannot always remember what the person looked like.

- Dreams. People may have dreams about the person who has died. Some find these dreams very comforting, but others are upset by them and wake up feeling very sad.

- Tears. Months later, tears may unexpectedly flow, and this can surprise young people who thought they were getting over it. This may be because the child is accepting the heavy feelings that come with realizing that the person has died and will never return.

- Fears after a parent dies. Children can be fearful after the death of a parent, and they may wonder what will happen to them now. If one parent has died, they may fear losing the other. Familiar household routines can change. The remaining parent might be depressed and grieving, and he or she might have to go to work; therefore, leaving the younger person with more time alone. For whatever reason, young people can feel worried about themselves and what will happen in the future, and it is important to reassure them that you have thought about these things as well. You might say, "It would be very unusual for me to get sick, too. And there will always be other people to take care of you if something should happen to me. That isn't something you need to worry about."

- Anger and withdrawal. Teenagers may become especially angry after the death of someone close to them. They may feel that the world is unfair, and they may lash out at others or withdraw. Some feel panic about the future and are scared of getting close to others. They may wonder if they are going crazy. They can feel guilty about what they did or said to the person who is gone and be unable to forgive themselves. And just like adults, they also may regret what they did not do.

- Sadness. Feelings of sadness may come and go over a long period of time. If young people are allowed to talk with others who understand, healing is more likely. How well they knew the person who died and how much they depended on him or her will affect how long these feelings continue.

Expect special days to be emotional. Adults and children often feel grief most strongly when holidays are approaching, around the date of the death itself, and during other special times, such as anniversaries or birthdays. This can happen even when they are not looking at calendars or paying attention to the dates. Children may be upset at these times because they remember the person who died or they are responding to your feelings. Support groups for adults and children can help at these times. Group members can agree it is a harder time than usual, and they can tell similar stories about their reactions to special days that reassure the grieving person.

Consider a group for grieving children if you think the child could use support from other young friends or teenagers. Support groups can be found through local hospitals, churches, funeral homes, or the blue pages in many telephone books. They often can recommend reading materials to help you understand how to help children deal with death.

Possible Obstacles

Obstacle: Aunt Mary may never speak to us again, that's how strongly she feels about the children coming to the funeral.

Response: Forget Aunt Mary for now. You cannot please everyone, least of all at an emotional, chaotic time like this. Talk the decision over with the children and a trusted friend or other adult, and make the decision that you feel is best. Review this chapter for ideas about how to make the event easier for children and other adults.

Obstacle: Children are too young to know what's happening.

Response: Children know when something is wrong or different. Even young babies might be more demanding because their schedules have changed or they are getting less attention. If you do not deal with their feelings now, you will have to later—and it will be harder then.

Other Obstacles: What additional roadblocks could get in the way of the recommendations in this plan? For example, will the person with advanced cancer cooperate? How will you explain what is needed to other people? Do you have the time and energy to carry out the plan? You need to develop plans for getting around these roadblocks. Use the COPE ideas (creativity, optimism, planning, and expert information).

Carrying Out and Adjusting Your Plan

Get accurate information about how the child is feeling and reacting to the illness or death. Talk with him or her about what has happened and how he or she feels. Show understanding for what the child is experiencing and explain how you feel.

Talk with other adults who will be present about the child's feelings, and ask for their help. You probably will have many other problems to deal with during this period, so ask other adults to take over some of your responsibilities with the child.

Checking on Results

Be alert for problems the child may have in dealing with the situation, the loss, and the changes in his or her life. Encourage the child to tell you how he or she is feeling by showing that you want to understand. Try to notice problems early, before they become severe. Check with school personnel such as teachers and the school nurse to gauge how the child is doing.

If Your Plan Does Not Work

Be understanding. This may be a difficult period for the child, especially if he or she must deal with many life changes. Problems usually will decrease over time.

If the child remains very upset for many months or his or her behavior is destructive or very upsetting to others, get professional help. Some clergy are experienced and skilled in dealing with emotional problems related to death. Mental health professionals—especially those experienced with the child's age group—often can help by talking to you and the child about the problems.

Chapter 44

Guiding Children through Grief

In the past, children were thought to be miniature adults and were expected to behave as adults. It is now understood that there are differences in the ways in which children and adults mourn.

Unlike adults, bereaved children do not experience continual and intense emotional and behavioral grief reactions. Children may seem to show grief only occasionally and briefly, but in reality a child's grief usually lasts longer than that of an adult. This may be explained by the fact that a child's ability to experience intense emotions is limited. Mourning in children may need to be addressed again and again as the child gets older. Since bereavement is a process that continues over time, children will think about the loss repeatedly, especially during important times in their life, such as going to camp, graduating from school, getting married, or giving birth to their own children.

A child's grief may be influenced by his or her age, personality, developmental stage, earlier experiences with death, and his or her relationship with the deceased. The surroundings, cause of death, family members' ability to communicate with one another, and ability to continue as a family after the death can also affect grief. The child's ongoing need for care, the child's opportunity to share his or her feelings and memories, the parent's ability to cope with stress, and the child's steady relationships with other adults are other factors that may influence grief.

Excerpted from "Loss, Grief, and Bereavement (PDQ®): Supportive Care–Patient," PDQ® Cancer Information Summary. National Cancer Institute; Bethesda, MD. Updated September 2005, available at http://cancer.gov. Accessed March 1, 2006.

Children do not react to loss in the same ways as adults. Grieving children may not show their feelings as openly as adults. Grieving children may not withdraw and dwell on the person who died, but instead may throw themselves into activities (for example, they may be sad one minute and playful the next). Often families think the child doesn't really understand or has gotten over the death. Neither is true—children's minds protect them from what is too powerful for them to handle. Children's grieving periods are shortened because they cannot think through their thoughts and feelings like adults. Also, children have trouble putting their feelings about grief into words. Instead, his or her behavior speaks for the child. Strong feelings of anger and fears of abandonment or death may show up in the behavior of grieving children. Children often play death games as a way of working out their feelings and anxieties. These games are familiar to the children and provide safe opportunities to express their feelings.

Children's Grief and Developmental Stages

Children at different stages of development have different understandings of death and the events near death.

Infants

Infants do not recognize death, but feelings of loss and separation are part of developing an awareness of death. Children who have been separated from their mother may be sluggish, quiet, unresponsive to a smile or a coo, less active, undergo physical changes (for example, weight loss), and sleep less.

Age 2–3 Years

Children at this age often confuse death with sleep and may experience anxiety as early as age 3. They may stop talking and appear to feel overall distress.

Age 3–6 Years

At this age children see death as a kind of sleep; the person is alive, but only in a limited way. The child cannot fully separate death from life. Children may think that the person is still living, even though he or she might have been buried, and ask questions about the deceased (for example, how does the deceased eat, go to the toilet, breathe, or play?). Young children know that death occurs physically, but think it is temporary, reversible, and not final. The child's concept of death may involve magical thinking. For example, the child may think that his or her thoughts can cause another person to become sick or die. Grieving children under five years of age may have trouble eating, sleeping, and controlling bladder and bowel functions.

Age 6–9 Years

Children at this age are commonly very curious about death, and may ask questions about what happens to one's body when it dies. Death is thought of as a person or spirit separate from the person who was alive, such as a skeleton, ghost, angel of death, or bogeyman. They may see death as final and frightening but as something that happens mostly to old people (and not to themselves). Grieving children can become afraid of school, have learning problems, develop antisocial or aggressive behaviors, become overly concerned about their own health (for example, developing symptoms of imaginary illness), withdraw from others, or become too attached and clinging. Boys usually become more aggressive and destructive (for example, acting out in school) instead of openly showing their sadness. When a parent dies children may feel abandoned by both their deceased parent and their surviving parent because the surviving parent is grieving and is unable to emotionally support the child.

Ages 9 and Older

By the time a child is 9 years old, death is known to be unavoidable and is not seen as a punishment. By the time a child is 12 years old, death is seen as final and something that happens to everyone.

In American society, many grieving adults withdraw and do not talk to others. Children, however, often talk to the people around them (even strangers) to see the reactions of others and to get clues for their own responses. Children may ask confusing questions. For example, a child may ask, "I know grandpa died, but when will he come home?" This is a way of testing reality and making sure the story of the death has not changed.

Other Issues for Grieving Children

Children's grief expresses three issues:

1. Did I cause the death to happen?

2. Is it going to happen to me?

3. Who is going to take care of me?

Table 44.1. Grief and Developmental Stages

Age	Understanding of Death	Expressions of Grief
Infancy to 2 years	Is not yet able to understand death.	Quietness, crankiness, decreased activity, poor sleep, and weight loss
	Separation from mother causes changes.	
2–6 years	Death is like sleeping.	Asks many questions (How does she go to the bathroom? How does she eat?)
		Problems in eating, sleeping, and bladder and bowel control
		Fear of abandonment
		Tantrums
	Dead person continues to live and function in some ways.	Magical thinking (Did I think something or do something that caused the death? Like when I said I hate you and I wish you would die?)
	Death is temporary, not final.	
	Dead person can come back to life.	
6–9 years	Death is thought of as a person or spirit (skeleton, ghost, bogeyman).	Curious about death
		Asks specific questions
		May have exaggerated fears about school
	Death is final and frightening.	May have aggressive behaviors (especially boys)
		Some concerns about imaginary illnesses
	Death happens to others, it won't happen to me.	May feel abandoned
9 and older	Everyone will die.	Heightened emotions, guilt, anger, shame
		Increased anxiety over own death
		Mood swings
	Death is final and cannot be changed.	Fear of rejection; not wanting to be different from peers
	Even I will die.	Changes in eating habits
		Sleeping problems
		Regressive behaviors (loss of interest in outside activities)
		Impulsive behaviors
		Feels guilty about being alive (especially related to death of a brother, sister, or peer)

Did I cause the death to happen?

Children often think that they have magical powers. If a mother says in irritation, "You'll be the death of me" and later dies, her child may wonder if he or she actually caused the mother's death. Also, when children argue, one may say (or think), "I wish you were dead." Should that child die, the surviving child may think that his or her thoughts actually caused the death.

Is it going to happen to me?

The death of another child may be especially hard for a child. If the child thinks that the death may have been prevented (by either a parent or a doctor), the child may think that he or she could also die.

Who is going to take care of me?

Since children depend on parents and other adults to take care of them, a grieving child may wonder who will care for him or her after the death of an important person.

Grieving Children: Treatment

A child's grieving process may be made easier by being open and honest with the child about death, using direct language, and incorporating the child into memorial ceremonies for the person who died.

Explanation of Death

Not talking about death (which indicates that the subject is off-limits) does not help children learn to cope with loss. When discussing death with children, explanations should be simple and direct. Each child should be told the truth using as much detail as he or she is able to understand. The child's questions should be answered honestly and directly. Children need to be reassured about their own security (they often worry that they will also die or that their surviving parent will go away). Children's questions should be answered, making sure that the child understands the answers.

Correct Language

A discussion about death should include the proper words, such as cancer, died, and death. Substitute words or phrases (for example,

355

he passed away, he is sleeping, or we lost him) should never be used because they can confuse children and lead to misunderstandings.

Planning Memorial Ceremonies

When a death occurs, children can and should be included in the planning and participation of memorial ceremonies. These events help children (and adults) remember loved ones. Children should not be forced to be involved in these ceremonies, but they should be encouraged to take part in those portions of the events with which they feel most comfortable. If the child wants to attend the funeral, wake, or memorial service, he or she should be given in advance a full explanation of what to expect. The surviving parent may be too involved in his or her own grief to give their child full attention, therefore, it may be helpful to have a familiar adult or family member care for the grieving child.

Part Seven

Legal and Economic
Issues at the End of Life

Chapter 45

Getting Your Affairs in Order

Editor's Note: As you put your affairs in order, remember to record Internet business and banking information for the executor of the estate. Important information would include business e-mail account addresses and passwords, contracts for digital accounts, and how to pay fees and maintain business URLs for business websites. If you own an Internet business, detailed information about the business should also be recorded. For family members, knowing how to access personal files including digital photos and communications might also be appreciated.

Possible Situations at the End of Life

Ben has been married for 50 years. He always managed the family's money. But since his stroke Ben cannot walk or talk. Shirley, his wife, feels overwhelmed. Of course, she is worried about Ben's health. But, on top of that, she has no idea what bills should be paid or when they are due.

Eighty-year-old Louise lives alone. One night she fell in the kitchen and broke her hip. She spent one week in the hospital and two months in an assisted living facility. Even though her son lives across the country, he was able to pay her bills and handle her Medicare questions right away. That's because several years ago, Louise and her son talked about what to do in case of a medical emergency.

National Institute on Aging (NIA), June 2004.

Plan for the Future

No one ever plans to be sick or disabled. Yet it is just this kind of planning that can make all the difference in an emergency. Long before she fell, Louise had put all her important papers in one place and told her son where to find them. She gave him the name of her lawyer as well as a list of people he could contact at her bank, doctor's office, investment firm, and insurance company. She made sure he had copies of her Medicare and other health insurance cards. She added her son's name to her checking account, allowing him to write checks on her account. Finally, Louise made sure Medicare and her doctor had written permission to talk with her son about her health or any insurance claims.

On the other hand, because Ben always took care of family financial matters, he never talked about the details with Shirley. No one but Ben knew that his life insurance policy was in a box in the closet or that the car title and deed to the house were filed in his desk drawer. Ben never expected his wife would have to take over. His lack of planning has made a tough situation even tougher for Shirley.

Steps for Getting Your Affairs in Order

- Gather everything you can about your income, investments, insurance, and savings.

- Put your important papers and copies of legal documents in one place. You could set up a file, put everything in a desk or dresser drawer, or just list the information and location of papers in a notebook. If your papers are in a bank safe deposit box, keep copies in a file at home. Check each year to see if there's anything new to add.

- Tell a trusted family member or friend where you put all your important papers. You do not need to tell this friend or family member your personal business, but someone should know where you keep your papers in case of emergency. If you do not have a relative or friend you trust, ask a lawyer to help.

- Give consent in advance for your doctor or lawyer to talk with your caregiver as needed. There may be questions about your care, a bill, or a health insurance claim. Without your consent, your caregiver may not be able to get needed information. You can give permission in advance to Medicare, a credit card company, your bank, or your doctor. Sometimes you can give your approval over the telephone. Other times you may need to sign and return a form.

Legal Documents

There are many different types of legal documents that can help you plan how your affairs will be handled in the future.

Wills and trusts give you a way to say how you want the things you own given out after you die.

Advance directives describe your health care wishes in case you cannot speak for yourself. Advance directives such as a living will or durable power of attorney for health care can say how you want your health managed and may help avoid family conflict over your care. They also may make it easier for family members to make hard health care decisions on your behalf. For example, your aunt may not wish to have her life extended by being placed on a breathing machine (ventilator), or your brother may want to be an organ donor. Advance directives help people plan for these situations. Different States have different forms for advance directives.

Power of attorney lets you give someone the authority to act on your behalf. There are different types:

- *Standard power of attorney* lets you name another person to handle your personal or financial matters. This is useful only if you can still make your own decisions.

- *Durable power of attorney* lets you name another person to make decisions for you if you become unable to make your own decisions.

- *Durable power of attorney for health care* lets you name another person to make medical decisions for you if you are unable to make them yourself.

A living will says how you want your health care handled if you are in a life-threatening situation and cannot make medical decisions for yourself. It gives you the right to refuse certain types of care. It also gives those caring for you the legal right to follow your wishes. State laws vary, so check with your Area Office on Aging, a lawyer, or a financial planner about the rules and requirements in your State.

361

Important Papers

Important papers may be different for every family. The following lists can help you decide what is important for you. Remember, this is just a starting point. You may have other information to add. For example, if you have a pet, be sure to include the name and address of your vet or someone who could care for him or her.

Personal Records

- full legal name
- Social Security number
- legal residence
- date and place of birth
- names and addresses of spouse and children (or location of death certificates)
- location of living will or other advance directive
- location of birth certificate and certificates of marriage, divorce, citizenship, and adoption
- employers and dates of employment
- medications you take regularly
- education and military records
- your religion, name of church or synagogue, and names of clergy
- memberships in groups and awards received
- names and addresses of close friends, relatives, doctors, clergy, and lawyers or financial advisor

Financial Records

- sources of income and assets (pension funds, IRAs, 401Ks, interest, etc.)
- information about insurance policies, bank accounts, deeds, investments, and other valuables, such as jewelry or art
- Social Security and Medicare information
- investment income (stocks, bonds, property) and stock brokers' names and addresses

- insurance information (life, health, long-term care, home, and car) with policy numbers and agents' names
- name of your bank and bank account numbers (checking, savings, and credit union)
- location of safe deposit boxes
- copy of most recent income tax return
- copy of your will
- liabilities—what you owe, to whom, and when payments are due
- mortgages and debts—how and when paid
- location of deed of trust and car title
- credit card and charge account names and numbers
- property tax information
- location of all personal items, such as jewelry and family treasures

When Your Caregiver Lives Far Away

The person you choose to help you may live far away. In that case, a little more information can make it easier for him or her to help. For example, make sure she or he has the names, phone numbers, and e-mail addresses of people near you who could be helpful in an emergency, such as:

- family members, friends, and neighbors who live nearby
- your apartment manager
- your doctor and other health care providers
- your clergy
- your lawyer, accountant, or other advisors

Update this information every year.

Resources

You may want to talk with a lawyer about setting up a power of attorney, durable power of attorney, joint account, trust, or advance directive. Be sure to ask about the cost before you make an appointment. You should be able to find a directory of local lawyers at your library. An informed family member may be able to help you manage some of these issues.

Additional Information

American Association of Retired People (AARP)
601 E. Street, N.W.
Washington, DC 20049
Toll-Free: 888-687-2277
Website: http://www.aarp.org

National Association of Area Agencies on Aging
1730 Rhode Island Ave., N.W., Suite 1200
Washington, DC 20036
Phone: 202-872-0888
Fax: 202-872-0057
Website: http://www.n4a.org

National Association of State Units on Aging
1201 15th Street, N.W., Suite 350
Washington, DC 20005
Phone: 202-898-2578
Fax: 202-898-2583
Website: http://www.nasua.org
E-mail: info@nasua.org

National Institute on Aging (NIA)
NIA Information Center
P.O. Box 8057
Gaithersburg, MD 20898-8057
Toll-Free: 800-222-2225
Toll-Free TTY: 800-222-4225
Website: http://www.nia.nih.gov

Centers for Medicare and Medicaid Services
Toll-Free: 800-MEDICARE (800-633-4227)
Toll-Free TTY: 877-486-2048
Websites: http://www.medicare.gov or http://www.cms.hhs.gov

Chapter 46

Patients' Rights

Respecting Your Choices

Except under extraordinary circumstances, you have the legal right to make decisions about your body and your medical care. Ideally, these decisions should be made by capable, informed patients after discussion with their physicians and other health care providers. This underlying principle of informed consent is a legal and ethical practice that underlies medical care and research in the United States. It is based on our society's respect for independence and self-determination.

Informed Consent

Informed consent is a legal doctrine stating that you have the power to choose among medically reasonable plans for your care. Informed consent requires effective communication between you and your doctor. To be able to make informed choices, you need to discuss many things (as often as needed), including the following:

- your diagnosis
- the overall outlook (prognosis)

This chapter includes: Excerpts from "Ethical and Legal Issues," used with permission from the American Geriatrics Society Foundation for Health in Aging, http://www.healthinaging.org. © 2005. And, "What Does the HIPAA Privacy Rule Do?" and "Why was the HIPAA Privacy Rule consent requirement removed, and will it affect my privacy protections?" from U.S. Department of Health and Human Services (HHS), October 20, 2005.

- the nature of the recommended test or treatments
- the various alternatives
- the risks and benefits of each alternative
- likely outcomes of each alternative

Informed consent does not mean that you can or should dictate your care. If a person requests tests or treatments that the medical profession considers useless or harmful, physicians have no obligation to comply. Your health care providers have a duty to use their skills for your benefit and not to harm you. If you and your health care provider disagree about the type of care that you should receive, you should discuss the situation further so that your concerns are made clear and you can reach a decision that is mutually acceptable.

Decision Making Capability

The process of informed consent makes sense only for people who have the ability to make informed decisions. Adults are presumed to have this capacity when they reach the age of majority (usually 18 years of age). This does not change unless the individual is determined to be incompetent or incapacitated by a court of law. The terms incompetent or incapacitated are legal terms and apply specifically to legal cases in court.

In practical terms, physicians are sometimes asked to evaluate a person's capacity to make decisions. If a physician believes that a person lacks the ability to make informed decisions about medical care, that person is deemed incapable. This is significant because it means that decisions will then be made by someone other than the patient.

The term diminished capacity generally refers to specific types of decisions, rather than to overall inability to make any decision. For example, you may be capable of making decisions about medical care, but not about finances, or vice versa. This selective definition of capacity (often referred to as a sliding scale) affords people more protection and self-determination. Of course, people who are unconscious or severely mentally impaired may lack capacity to make any decisions.

Judging the Capacity to Make Decisions

Medical decisions:

- ability to understand relevant information

- ability to understand the consequences of the decision
- ability to communicate a decision

Decisions of self-care:

- ability to care for oneself or
- ability to accept the needed help to keep oneself safe

Finances:

- ability to manage bill payment
- ability to appropriately calculate and monitor funds

Last will and testament:

- ability to remember estate plans
- ability to express logic behind choices

Your capacity to make decisions about medical care requires that you realize that there are choices regarding the nature of the recommended care, the alternatives, the risks, benefits, and the likely consequences. This ability to understand the situation may change over time. For example, a person with delirium may be mentally clear in the morning but confused in the evening. Imagine having a high fever that clouds your thinking and makes you feel disoriented. When you are capable of making informed decisions, your choices should be respected. If there are times when you are not capable of making informed decisions, these decisions should be postponed if possible until you have regained your decision making capacity.

People may be given a formal test to gauge their mental status when their capacity is questionable. However, even if someone performs poorly on a mental status test or has impaired memory, they may still have the capacity to make informed decisions. In these situations, extra care may be needed to make sure the person understands the risks, benefits, and consequences of the alternative plans of care.

It is important not to confuse decision making capacity with so-called rational decisions. Decisions are often based on cultural, ethnic, or religious values and beliefs that vary from person to person. What is rational to one person might not seem rational to another. For example, a Jehovah's Witness may view a blood transfusion as unacceptable, even if the alternative is death. Requiring rationality would disqualify people who make highly personal or unconventional decisions. As one court declared in a case that involved the refusal of treatment, beliefs that are unwise, foolish, or ridiculous do not render a person incompetent.

Having Someone Make Decisions for You

If you lose the capacity to make decisions, someone will have to make decisions on your behalf. In this case, the person you designate as a stand-in (surrogate decision maker) should try to comply with any wishes you expressed while you were still capable of making decisions. Your expressed wishes are legally and ethically more important than what others want for you, even if they feel that they are acting in your best interests. Two common types of advance directives (advance care plans) that express your wishes are living wills and durable power of attorney for health care. (States have varying terms to designate durable power of attorney for health care, including health care proxy, health care declaration, etc.) It is also important to remember that advance directives have some limitations.

Acting in Your Best Interests

If you have not given advance directives or appointed a surrogate decision maker, health care providers may have to base decisions on what is in your best interest by weighing the benefits and possible problems of treatment. This is a complicated and often controversial process that requires dealing with such personal factors as pain and suffering, safety, and loss of independence, privacy, and dignity. Well-meaning third parties may disagree on how much weight to give to each of these factors, which are often summarized by the phrase quality of life. In addition, quality-of-life judgments based on assessments of third parties may be unfair or discriminatory, particularly if social worth or economic productivity is considered. For example, life situations that would be intolerable to young, healthy people may be acceptable to older, debilitated people, and vice versa.

Preventing Harm

Health care providers have a duty to use their expertise for the benefit of the people in their care. However, you retain the right to refuse treatments that your health care provider considers to be in your best interest. Again, good communication with your health care providers can improve your mutual understanding of risks, benefits, and underlying beliefs.

Placement Issues

Preventing harm to an individual is often raised in decisions to place someone in a nursing home. An older adult may wish to remain at home, but family member or caregivers may override this decision if they believe that living independently is not safe. However, the crucial ethical question is whether the older adult is capable of making an informed decision about where to live. If so, his or her decision should be respected, even if others believe that it is unwise or foolish, and even if it puts that person at greater risk. Caregivers can try to arrange for in-home supportive services that may greatly improve the situation and decrease risk.

Abuse of Older Adults

Family members or other caregivers can sometimes become abusive for a variety of reasons. These may include feeling overwhelmed and burnt out by caregiving responsibilities, lacking appropriate caregiving skills, or having no break from caregiving. The duty to protect older people often justifies intervening in these situations. Older adults may not be able to protect themselves or know how to get help. They may also fear retaliation or be ashamed to admit the abuse. Any concerned person who suspects abuse has an ethical duty to try to determine if the victim has the capacity to make decisions, is informed, and is not being coerced. Some states require physicians and caregivers to report suspected abuse to a protective service agency.

Guardianship

Some older people cannot manage their finances or provide themselves with food and shelter. Sometimes, relatives or friends make informal arrangements to help these individuals. In other cases, a capable person has executed a durable power of attorney that appointed another person to handle his or her affairs. In still other cases, it is necessary to ask the courts to appoint a guardian, as when property must be managed or sold to pay for long-term care.

In guardianship hearings, relatives or other petitioners (social service agencies or health care providers) must demonstrate that the person is no longer able to safely manage his or her affairs and needs. If the person is found incompetent or incapacitated, the court appoints a guardian.

All states allow the courts to establish limited guardianships (sometimes called conservatorships) and unlimited guardianships. A limited guardianship gives the guardian the power to take charge of a specific area that the older person is no longer able to manage (for example, finances). An unlimited guardianship strips the older person of all legal authority and gives the guardian the power to make all the decisions about the older person's life in matters that affect property, residence, medical care, and personal relationships. Most states prefer limited guardianships, because an unlimited guardianship requires that the court find that the person is legally incompetent or incapacitated in all areas of decision making.

Decisions for People in Nursing Homes

Nursing-home residents may need additional safeguards when decisions about life-sustaining treatments are made. These people may not have close relatives to act on their behalf, and their relationships with health care providers may be superficial. There are also fewer caregivers involved in decisions at nursing homes compared with hospitals. In addition, substandard care is sometimes a problem in nursing homes.

The decision to transfer a nursing-home resident to a hospital when their condition worsens is a common dilemma. This is because the goal of treatment for many residents is to relieve discomfort rather than to prolong life. If individuals or their surrogates turn down the transfer to a hospital, their wishes should be respected. It should be a routine part of nursing-home care to discuss these decisions well in advance.

Federal legislation now requires inquiry into advance directives for all patients in institutions (nursing homes) that receive federal funds. This leads to a more systematic approach to discussions about treatment status. Since this law was passed, nursing homes have transferred fewer patients to acute care hospitals, while maintaining patient and family satisfaction with care.

Life-Sustaining Treatments

Advances in medical technology have often created medical dilemmas. For example, health care providers may be able to successfully treat a sudden complication in a seriously ill person, but restoring function and improving the underlying disease may be impossible. In such a situation, treatment that only prolongs life may be appropriately withheld. In fact, the doctor may refuse treatment under a variety of situations:

- there is no specific medical rationale for the treatment
- the treatment has proved ineffective for the person
- the person is unconscious and will likely die in a matter of hours or days even if the treatment is given
- the expected survival is virtually none

The doctor's discretion in these matters may vary widely across the United States.

An informed person who is capable of making medical decisions may refuse life-sustaining treatment, such as cardiopulmonary resuscitation (CPR), intensive care, transfusions, antibiotics, and artificial feedings. An informed refusal should be respected, even if the person's life may be shortened as a result and even if the person is not terminally ill or in a coma. When people are not capable of making decisions, two questions need to be considered:

1. What standard should be used?

2. Who should make the decisions?

Do-Not-Resuscitate Orders

Cardiopulmonary resuscitation (CPR) may be an effective treatment for unexpected sudden death, but it is not effective for people whose death is expected. Older adults generally do poorly after CPR because of serious illnesses and decreased functional status. In fact, less than 10% of people over 70 survive to be discharged from the hospital after CPR.

When CPR is medically pointless and thus ethically not appropriate, a patient should not be offered the choice between CPR and no CPR. Instead, the physician should generally write a do-not-resuscitate order and explain why CPR is not indicated. In some settings, however, the law may require that physicians offer the option of CPR even when it would be pointless. When CPR might be of benefit, the physician must make sure that all concerned are aware that the likelihood of survival is low even if CPR is administered.

Many people with chronic illnesses do not want CPR, and their informed refusal should be respected. The attending physician should indicate the reasons for the order and plans for further care in the medical record. Note that a do-not-resuscitate order means that only CPR will not be performed—other treatments may still be given. Discussions with your health care providers about do-not-resuscitate orders are excellent opportunities to review your total plan of care, including supportive care and appropriate treatments that would be continued after the do-not-resuscitate order takes effect.

Withdrawing Treatment

Strange emotional feelings are a natural part of decisions to stop, withdraw, or withhold care. We are torn between the impending sense of loss of our loved ones and our desire that their suffering be relieved and their dignity maintained. Regardless, there is little point in continuing a treatment that is not effective.

Often, people make a distinction between stopping treatment and not starting it in the first place. For example, some people are willing to withhold mechanical support of breathing (for example, use of a ventilator), but are reluctant to discontinue it once it has been started. However, logically, ethically, and legally there is no difference between not starting treatment and stopping it. If you feel that there is an important emotional difference for you between stopping a treatment and not starting one, you should explicitly discuss this with your physician.

Health Insurance Portability and Accountability Act (HIPAA) Privacy Rule

What does the HIPAA Privacy Rule do?

The HIPAA Privacy Rule for the first time creates national standards to protect individuals' medical records and other personal health information.

- It gives patients more control over their health information.

- It sets boundaries on the use and release of health records.

- It establishes appropriate safeguards that health care providers and others must achieve to protect the privacy of health information.

- It holds violators accountable, with civil and criminal penalties that can be imposed if they violate patients' privacy rights.

- It strikes a balance when public responsibility supports disclosure of some forms of data—for example, to protect public health.

For Patients

HIPAA means being able to make informed choices when seeking care and reimbursement for care based on how personal health information may be used.

- It enables patients to find out how their information may be used, and about certain disclosures of their information that have been made.

- It generally limits release of information to the minimum reasonably needed for the purpose of the disclosure.

- It generally gives patients the right to examine and obtain a copy of their own health records and request corrections.

- It empowers individuals to control certain uses and disclosures of their health information.

Why was the consent requirement eliminated from the HIPAA Privacy Rule, and how will it affect individuals' privacy protections?

The consent requirement created the unintended effect of preventing health care providers from providing timely, quality health care to individuals in a variety of circumstances. The most troubling and pervasive problem was that health care providers would not have been able to use or disclose protected health information for treatment, payment, or health care operations purposes prior to the initial face-to-face encounter with the patient, which is routinely done to provide timely access to quality health care. The following are some examples of how the consent requirement would have posed barriers to health care:

- Pharmacists would not have been able to fill a prescription, search for potential drug interactions, determine eligibility, or verify coverage before the individual arrived at the pharmacy to pick up the prescription if the individual had not already provided consent under the Privacy Rule.

- Hospitals would not have been able to use information from a referring physician to schedule and prepare for procedures before the individual presented at the hospital for such procedure, or the patient would have had to make a special trip to the hospital to sign the consent form.

- Providers who do not provide treatment in person (such as a provider prescribing over the telephone) may have been unable to provide care because they would have had difficulty obtaining prior written consent to use protected health information at the first service delivery.

- Emergency medical providers were concerned that even if a situation was urgent they would have had to try to obtain consent to comply with the Privacy Rule, even if that would be inconsistent with the appropriate practice of emergency medicine.

- Emergency medical providers were also concerned that the requirement that they attempt to obtain consent as soon as reasonably practicable after an emergency would have required significant efforts and administrative burden which might have been viewed as harassing by patients, because these providers typically do not have ongoing relationships with individuals.

To eliminate such barriers to health care, mandatory consent was replaced with the voluntary consent provision that permits health care providers to obtain consent for treatment, payment, and healthcare operations at their option, and enables them to obtain consent in a manner that does not disrupt needed treatment. Although consent is no longer mandatory, the Rule still affords individuals the opportunity to engage in important discussions regarding the use and disclosure of their health information through the strengthened notice requirement, while allowing activities that are essential to quality health care to occur unimpeded. These modifications will ensure that the Rule protects patient privacy as intended without harming consumers' access to care or the quality of that care. Further, the individual's right to request restrictions on the use or disclosure of his or her protected health information is retained in the Rule as modified.

Chapter 47

Advance Directives, Health Care Power of Attorney, and Living Wills

Advance Preparation

Experience shows that a catastrophic medical event, such as an accident or a stroke, can leave a person incapacitated and unable to make decisions or to communicate with others. That leaves treatment decisions concerning what is in your best interest up to family members, significant others, health care providers, or the judicial system. In order to avoid this difficult situation, all adults—not just the adults with chronic diseases or other medical conditions—should plan for their future health care treatment preferences and complete an advance directive document that specifies personal preferences regarding acceptable and unacceptable medical treatments.

There is a fairly easy way to stay in control—to have your say—about these events that are often fraught with emotions. An advance directive document can provide specific guidance regarding a person's treatment preferences in a situation such as an irreversible coma following a debilitating stroke.

Typically, a person may not know what medical treatments he or she may prefer or reject. The advantage of preparing an advance directive is that the process serves as a guide for those who may need to make informed decisions regarding major treatments such as tube

"Having Your Say: Advance Directives, A Consumer's Guide," is reprinted with permission from the American Health Care Association, © 2004. For additional information, visit http://www.longtermcareliving.com.

feeding or ventilator care. You decide in different scenarios how you wish to be treated and if you wish to be treated. Since an advance directive prescribes your care plan if you are incapacitated, it may be wise to involve family, significant others, a religious advisor, your physician, other medical professionals or an attorney (however, an attorney may not be required to complete this document).

Each State government may regulate the preparation of an advance directive differently. This makes it important to work within a State's framework to ensure that health care providers, including nursing facilities and assisted living residences, honor your choices regarding, for example, situations involving permanent coma, persistent vegetative state, brain death, and comfort care.

Two Types of Advance Directives

There are two legal forms of an advance directive: a living will and a medical power of attorney (which may also be called a durable power of attorney for health care or health care proxy).

An advance directive allows you to state your choices for health care or to name someone to make those choices for you if you become unable to make decisions about your medical treatment or to communicate your preferences. It is best to complete an advance directive as part of a strategy for financial planning, retirement, or long-term health care. Preparation avoids having to deal with this matter in the event of unexpected serious illness or debilitation.

Living Will

A living will generally states the kind of medical care you prefer (or do not want) if you become unable to make your own decision or cannot communicate. It is called a living will because it takes effect while you are still living.

Most States have their own living will forms, each somewhat different. It may also be possible to complete and sign a preprinted living will form available in your own community, draw up your own form, or simply write a statement of your preferences for treatment. Generally a living will needs to be signed in the presence of two witnesses, and in some States it must also be notarized. You may also wish to speak to an attorney, your physician, health care or long-term health care provider to be certain the living will is properly prepared to ensure that your wishes are understood and followed. An advance directive should be completed prior to there being any question about competency of the individual, such as when Alzheimer disease or other dementias are present.

Medical Power of Attorney

A medical power of attorney is a signed, dated, and witnessed document—some States require notarization too—naming another person, such as a husband, wife, daughter, son, or significant other as your agent or proxy to make medical decisions for you if you are no longer capable of making them or unable to communicate your preferences. You can include instructions about any treatment you wish to avoid.

In selecting your health care agent, it is important to communicate with this person in advance and that they agree to the designation; they could be the ones making treatment decisions for you if future medical situations require it. The agent needs to have reached majority age for your jurisdiction, and not be a health care provider that is treating you. Be sure to verify any other exclusion in your jurisdiction.

Note that a medical power of attorney and the more commonly known power of attorney—often referred to as non-durable power of attorney—are not the same. Power of attorney allows a person to act on matters you specify, such as financial matters. Generally speaking, the person holding the power of attorney cannot also be designated as the medical power of attorney. Again, this information needs to be confirmed for your State.

Living Will Vs. Medical Power of Attorney

It might be best to have a living will and appoint a health care agent or proxy. However, in some States, laws may make it better to have one or the other. It may also be possible to combine both documents into a single document that describes treatment choices in a variety of situations—you might want to seek medical advice about these situations and choices—and names your health care agent.

Designating a health care agent as part of a medical power of attorney provides more flexibility for future decisions unanticipated in a living will. A health care agent, along with a written living will, can provide guidance in the absence of the health care agent or support decisions made by the health care agent based on knowledge of your wishes.

Modifying an Advance Directive

You may modify, update, or even cancel an advance directive at any time in accordance with State law. Any change or cancellation should be written, signed, and dated in accordance with State law, and copies should be given to your doctor or to others to whom you may have given copies of the original documents. Be sure to notify your health care agent of any changes. Some States allow an advance directive to be changed by oral statement, but if possible, it is always preferable to put your changes in writing.

If you change or cancel an advance directive while you are in any health care setting, the provider of those services should be advised of your decision with new documents to replace any outdated ones.

Even without a change in writing, your wishes stated verbally to your doctor may carry more weight than a living will or medical power of attorney, as long as you are competent to make decisions and can communicate your wishes. Again, be sure to clearly express your wishes and be sure that they are understood. It is always better if there are witnesses to your statements.

Retrieving the Advance Directive

Make sure that someone, such as a close family member or legal advisor, knows that you have an advance directive and knows where it is located. In the case of a health care proxy be sure that person has a current copy. If you spend a great deal of time in more than one State, you should consider having an advance directive in each State. Be sure to keep a copy in each location that you reside. You should also consider the following:

- If you have an advance directive—that is, a living will or medical power of attorney—give a copy to your health care agent or health care proxy among others.

- Give your physician and the long-term health care facility (a nursing facility or assisted living residence), or other health care provider, a copy of your advance directive and advise them to make it part of your permanent medical record.

- Keep a second copy of your advance directive in a safe place where it can be found easily if it is needed. However, do not keep in a safe deposit box, as that is not easily accessible to others.

- Keep a small card on your person that states that you have an advance directive, where it is located, and who your agent or proxy is if you have one.

Under federal law, when you are admitted to most health care settings you will be asked if you have an advance directive. If so, the facility will want a copy as part of your medical record.

Finally, as you've read in this chapter, an advance directive may prevent anguish and turmoil within families and provide clear guidance to health care and long-term care providers. An advance directive should be considered an essential component of future planning just as much as financial planning, life or disability insurance, or drawing up a will.

Additional Information on Advance Directives

For more information, contact personnel at a nursing facility, assisted living center, or residential care facility. Hospitals and other health care providers should also have information appropriate to your State.

Chapter 48

Financial Assistance at the End of Life

Income Support Programs

Federal and State governments and the private insurance industry offer a broad range of programs designed to ensure that disabled individuals have access to financial resources and health care and treatment programs. These programs provide support to people particularly those who find themselves without the ability to afford basic necessities, such as food, shelter, and clothing, let alone meet the high costs associated with the care and treatment of a debilitating illness.

Federal Social Security Programs

The Federal Social Security Administration (SSA) provides two types of income support programs for disabled individuals: Social Security Disability Insurance (SSDI) and Supplemental Security Income (SSI). Both programs provide financial support on a monthly basis to disabled individuals.

In order to be eligible for either SSI or SSDI a range of rules apply. For both programs an individual must be permanently and totally disabled. The SSA defines disability as a severe medical condition

Excerpts from *A Clinical Guide to Supportive and Palliative Care for HIV / AIDS 2003 Edition*, U.S. Department of Health and Human Services, 2003. Also, "Paying for Long-Term Care," March 31, 2005, Centers for Medicare and Medicaid Services.

(physical or mental) that prevents or is expected to prevent an individual from engaging in any substantial gainful activity for 12 or more consecutive months, or will result in death.

Social Security Disability Insurance (SSDI or SSD)

SSDI, often shortened to SSD, is a governmental disability insurance program. In addition to the eligibility requirement that an individual must be permanently and totally disabled as defined by the SSA, successful applicants must have a lawful immigration status and have a sufficient work history. Since SSDI is a federal insurance program and not a need-based program an individual's income or assets generally do not effect eligibility or monthly benefit payments.

The SSDI program pays a monthly benefit to disabled individuals who have made sufficient Social Security contributions through payroll deductions or self-employment tax premiums (under the Federal Insurance Contribution Act, or FICA). What qualifies as sufficient contributions depends upon an individual's age at the time she or he became disabled.

- Those 31 years of age or older must have paid sufficient taxes for at least 20 of the last 40 3-month periods or quarters.

- Those between the ages of 24 and 30 must have paid sufficient taxes for at least half of the quarters between their 24th birthday and the time of disability.

- Those under 24 must have paid sufficient taxes for at least six quarters during the 3 years before becoming disabled.

An individual's monthly SSDI benefit can range from a couple of hundred dollars a month to over $1500 per month. Monthly SSDI benefit levels vary greatly depending upon Social Security contributions, age at the onset of disability, and date of disability. A monthly benefit is also available for the dependent spouse or children of an SSDI recipient.

Supplemental Security Income (SSI)

SSI is a need-based program that provides monthly benefits to individuals who are disabled, blind, or over 65 years old, and who have limited income and assets. As with SSDI, once determined to be eligible for SSI, an individual is entitled to monthly payments until death or until the individual is no longer disabled.

Only the disabled person may receive SSI. There are no benefits available for spouses or dependent children of a disabled person, unless they are also disabled. The disability of one or more parents may, however, entitle the remaining family members to some other form of government assistance. It is very important that individuals apply for SSI as soon as possible since there are no retroactive SSI benefits.

In many States, recipients of SSI are automatically eligible for Medicaid. In other States, an SSI recipient must independently apply for Medicaid. In those States, Medicaid applications are generally successful as most States use the same criteria for determining Medicaid eligibility as the SSA uses for SSI eligibility.

Temporary Assistance to Needy Families (TANF)

TANF is an income assistance program funded and regulated by both the Federal and State governments. The program provides cash and automatic medical assistance to poor families so they can provide basic necessities for their children. Because TANF is administered by State welfare departments, eligibility, calculation of benefits, work requirements, and exemptions vary from State to State.

Generally, TANF provides assistance to eligible families consisting of a single parent and one or more minor children. Most States also provide assistance to families with two parents (where one parent is disabled or unemployed, or income is below a given level), families where a child lives with a relative who is not a parent, and pregnant women. Nearly all States will allow some children, exclusive of any parent or guardian, to qualify for assistance.

Families are eligible for cash assistance if their income is below the established standard. Most States also take assets, excluding the family home, into consideration. In some States, receipt of SSI benefits may affect eligibility. The maximum benefit amount varies according to family size, and is calculated according to State-determined guidelines.

One of TANF's key provisions is the time limit. Eligible families are permanently barred from the program after receiving assistance for 5 years. However, many States make exceptions for child-only cases, and families where a parent or guardian is disabled. The TANF standard of disability varies from State to State, although in many States it is an easier standard to meet than the SSI disability standard in that it only requires incapacity reducing or eliminating a parent's ability to work for at least 30 days.

TANF was created in 1996, to replace Aid to Families with Dependent Children (AFDC), under the Personal Responsibility and Work Opportunities Act of 1996 (often referred to as welfare reform). Families eligible for TANF may also be eligible for food stamps; women, infants and children (WIC); school breakfast and lunch; fuel assistance, and other programs available to low-income persons.

Other State-Run Income Support Programs

Many States provide need-based income support programs to individuals who for a variety of reasons are ineligible for SSI or TANF. These programs are wholly funded by States and therefore eligibility rules and program benefits vary from State to State. Several States operate programs that provide income support to individuals who do not meet the SSI or TANF disability requirements. In some States, citizenship or immigration status requirements are more flexible. In general, information on the programs that exist in your State is available through the State welfare office and/or community-based organizations.

Private Disability Insurance

Private disability insurance is designed to replace income lost as a result of a health condition that prevents an individual from working. The insurance coverage is generally either short-term (up to 2 years) or long-term (up to age 65 or for life). For those who have a private disability insurance policy, upon disability, the policy will generally pay a monthly income benefit equal to a percentage of an individual's pre-disability earnings or to a maximum dollar amount.

Life Insurance: Accelerated Benefits and Viatical Settlements

While life insurance polices are generally designed to provide income support to the survivors of a deceased life insurance policy holder, they can also provide much-needed income support to a person. Many life insurance policies include an accelerated benefits provision that allows a terminally ill person to obtain a portion of the life insurance proceeds that would normally be reserved for the surviving beneficiaries. The remaining proceeds go to the surviving beneficiaries upon the terminally ill person's death. In general, in accelerated benefits provisions, the definition of terminally ill is defined strictly as a life expectancy of one year or less.

In addition, private viatical settlement companies are often willing to purchase the life insurance of a person and pay a percentage of the value of the policy. The standard of what constitutes terminal illness is more flexible in viatication, but it is important to note that if a person's life expectancy is greater than two years the proceeds received will be taxable for Federal tax purposes. With viatication, the policyholder sells the policy to the viatical settlement company and upon the policyholder's death all of the life insurance proceeds are distributed to the company. An individual considering either an accelerated benefit or viatication should consult with an attorney or benefits expert. The viatical settlement industry, in particular, is largely unregulated and the transaction requires oversight to ensure that a person receives satisfactory terms of sale.

Health Care Support

Medicare

Medicare is government health insurance covering people over 65, the blind, and the disabled. Since it is a Federally administered program, Medicare rules are consistent throughout the country.

Medicare coverage consists of two parts: Part A (which is free) covers limited hospital care, skilled nursing care, and hospice care; and Part B (which is optional and requires a monthly premium) covers doctor's services, outpatient hospital services, and other medical services. If an individual elects Part B coverage, a monthly premium is deducted from the SSDI payment, although some States have a program that covers the cost for specified circumstances.

Some individuals who are covered by Medicare buy private insurance, called Medigap policies, to cover medical costs not covered by Medicare. Medigap policies vary greatly, but many cover the costs of Medicare deductibles and/or health services and pharmaceuticals not covered by Medicare. Several States have a program that will pay for the purchasing of a Medigap policy for a person living with HIV.

Medicare Hospice Benefit

The Medicare program also offers a hospice benefit for those who have a terminal illness with a life expectancy of 6 months or less. The hospice benefit provides a range of valuable services, all of which concentrate on improving an individual's quality of life as much as possible during the end stages of a terminal illness. The Medicare hospice benefit covers four categories of care: 1) routine home care, 2) continuous home-based nursing care, 3) respite care, and 4) general inpatient palliative care related to terminal illness. The hospice benefit includes services provided by a broad range of caregivers, including physicians, nurses, therapists, home health aides, clergy, social workers, and counselors. It also covers the purchase or rental of any durable medical equipment necessary to care for the individual in the home. In addition, the program covers the costs of services not typically covered by Medicare such as outpatient drugs, respite care, custodial care, and continuous nursing care in the home during medical emergencies. The Medicare hospice benefit generally covers all these programs and services in full.

Medicaid

Medicaid is government health insurance funded jointly by the Federal and State governments and administered by State government. Under State administration, States have many options regarding who is covered by the program and what services are provided. Medicaid rules vary greatly from State to State.

All States must provide the following Federally mandated Medicaid services: inpatient hospital services, outpatient hospital services, laboratory and x-ray services, skilled nursing facility services, physician's services, early and periodic screening, diagnosis and testing services, and family planning services and supplies.

Federally optional Medicaid services include the following: prescribed drugs; hospice services; home health care services; nursing home services and intermediate care facility services; durable medical goods; private day nursing services; clinical services; podiatry; dental services; physical, occupational and speech therapy; optometrists; and hearing aids.

Since the rules regarding access to Medicaid and the range of services provided vary greatly from State to State it is important to contact the State Medicaid office to determine the parameters of the program in your State and to obtain assistance with the application process.

Private Health Insurance

Many individuals have private health insurance policies that provide a range of health care benefits. In most cases, individuals have obtained private group health insurance through their jobs or are covered because a family member has group insurance coverage from work. In some instances, individuals have purchased their own individual policies. In either case, the types of polices offered can differ widely in terms of cost and coverage. Private insurance companies offer a broad range of plans so the particular terms will depend upon the plan selected.

Many health insurance policies include benefits limits, including specific limits on coverage or a maximum benefit for the policy as a whole. Others include co-payments, deductibles or other out-of-pocket expenses that an individual is responsible for paying. Some allow individuals to choose any doctor, whereas others restrict access to health care professionals under contract with the plan.

Understanding the specific health insurance terms under any individual policy is difficult. Often questions can be answered by customer service staff provided by the insurance company or through the human resources department of an employer who provides group health insurance. An in-depth analysis of the terms of a policy often requires obtaining a copy of the policy for review by an attorney or benefits expert.

Finally, many States operate programs that pay the private health insurance premiums for people living with HIV. It is, therefore, always important to see if such a buy-in program exists before an individual decides to terminate her private health insurance. The specific eligibility rules vary from State to State, but some cover individuals receiving and/or eligible for SSI, SSDI, private disability insurance, Medicaid, and Medicare. For many people living with HIV buy-in programs represent an opportunity to maintain their preferred choice of health care access and support.

The Consolidated Budget Reconciliation Act of 1985 (COBRA)

COBRA is a Federal law that requires employers who sponsor a group health plan to allow their employees and/or their dependents to remain covered under the group plan after they leave employment or are no longer qualified for coverage under the plan's rules. In general, continued coverage is available to employees who were covered under the plan and reduce their work hours, leave their employment, or are terminated for reasons other than gross misconduct. This continuation of coverage is also available to the spouse and/or dependent children of the employee if they were covered under the plan. This coverage is very important because access to group health insurance is generally cost-effective and provides a broader range of benefits than those typically found in individual policies.

Table 48.1. Comparison of Available Financing Options

Financing Option	Only Available for Long-Term Care Costs	Remaining Funds Available to Heirs	Rate of Asset Accumulation	Eligibility Requirement	Risk of Insufficient Funds
Family Support and Caregiving	No	No	None	No	Moderate: Family members may be unable or unwilling to provide care.
Personal Savings	No	Yes	Variable	No	High: Long-Term Care costs can exceed your personal savings.
Long-Term Care Insurance	Yes	No	Fixed	Yes	Moderate to Low: Long-Term Care costs could exceed original coverage amount.
Limited Long-Term Care Insurance	Yes	No	Fixed	Yes	Moderate to Low: Long-Term Care costs could exceed original coverage amount.
Life Settlement	Yes	No	Fixed	Yes	Moderate to Low: Amount received from benefit may not pay all long-term care costs.
Viatical Settlement	Yes	No	Fixed	Yes	Moderate to Low: Amount received from benefit may not pay all long-term care costs.
Accelerated Death Benefit	Yes	No	Fixed	Yes	Moderate to Low: Amount received from benefit may not pay all long-term care costs.

Reverse Mortgages	No	Yes	Variable	Yes	Moderate: Amount received from benefit may not pay all long-term care costs and home maintenance costs still exist.
Continuing Care Retirement Community	Yes	Yes	Variable	Yes	Low: Additional care provided as needed in CCRC assisted living or nursing facility.
Veterans Benefits	No	No	None	Yes	Moderate to High: Amount received from benefit may not pay all long-term care costs.
Medicare	No	No	None	Yes	Moderate to High: Amount received from Medicare may not pay all long-term care costs.
Medicaid	No	No	None	Yes	High: Amount received from Medicaid may not pay all long-term care costs and recovery of Medicaid may be made against estate.
PACE	Yes	No	None	Yes	Moderate to High: Amount received from benefit may not pay all long-term care costs.

For many disabled individuals leaving employment, COBRA offers the most cost-effective and comprehensive health insurance available. This is true despite the fact that individuals are generally required to pay the premiums or costs of this private group health insurance.

In the context of HIV, whether paid for through a government program or by an individual, COBRA offers much-needed insurance coverage to those ineligible for the need-based Medicaid program. For those eligible for Medicare through SSDI, COBRA can provide coverage during the 29-month Medicare waiting period.

In general, under Federal law, COBRA applies to employers who offer a group health care plan and employ 20 or more employees. Churches, small employers who employ less than 20 people, and the Federal government are generally exempt. COBRA does not apply to life insurance or disability insurance plans. Several States, however, have COBRA laws that cover employees with less than 20 employees, so it is important to check if your State has such a law.

COBRA coverage must be elected by the later of 60 days after leaving employment or within 60 days of receiving notice of COBRA rights by the employer. Employers are legally required to provide written notice of COBRA rights within 45 days after a person loses coverage.

The length of COBRA coverage depends upon several factors. In general, COBRA coverage lasts for 18 months. For those determined to be disabled by the Social Security Administration for SSI or SSDI purposes, at any time within the initial 18-month period, COBRA is extended to 29 months. In general, COBRA coverage is 36 months in the event of the death of a covered employee, for the loss of dependent child status under the plan, for divorce or legal separation of the covered employee, or when the covered employee becomes eligible for Medicare.

State-Run Health Care and Treatment Programs

Many States support health care programs for individuals living with HIV who have no other means of accessing treatment. Through a combination of Federal and State funding, including the Ryan White Comprehensive AIDS Resources Emergency (CARE) Act, many States operate programs that provide early intervention health care and access to medications. These programs are administered by States and, therefore, the services provided vary greatly. Information on the programs in your State is available through the State health department and/or community-based AIDS organizations.

Paying for Long-Term Care

The cost of long-term care can vary quite a bit depending on what kind of care you need, where you get the care, and where you live.

Additional Information

Social Security Administration
Office of Public Inquiries
Windsor Park Building
6401 Security Blvd.
Baltimore, MD 21235
Toll-Free: 800-772-1213
Toll-Free TTY: 800-325-0778
Website: http://www.ssa.gov

Chapter 49

Taxes and Social Security Issues after Death

Taxes Due after Death

Taxes due after a death can be complicated. Consult an attorney or certified public accountant (CPA) familiar with both federal estate tax laws and state inheritance taxes.

Estates in which all of the assets are bequeathed to a surviving spouse are generally not subject to estate tax upon the death of the first spouse. In addition, each individual can give assets away in specified amounts tax-free, subject to certain limits to any individual during his lifetime or at death. The Economic Growth and Tax Relief Reconciliation Act of 2001 raises the unified tax credit and gift tax exemption amount to $3.5 million in 2009.

After you have identified all assets belonging to the estate and determined its value, consult an attorney or CPA to determine if federal estate tax is due. Federal estate tax returns are generally due nine months after an individual's death. You can request an extension before that date if you need more time. You generally will not be charged a penalty for the extra time, but you will be subject to interest.

Many states impose inheritance taxes, often on estates valued well below the federal exemption limit. States may also impose inheritance taxes, with the rates depending on who inherits. States usually

This chapter includes: "Taxes Due after Death," © 2006 The USAA Educational Foundation. Reprinted with permission. All rights reserved. Also, "What to Do when a Beneficiary Dies," and "Burial Funds," from the Social Security Administration, August 16, 2005.

tax spouses, children, and parents at the lowest rate; siblings, other relatives, and non-family heirs pay a higher rate. An attorney or CPA will be able to guide you if state inheritance taxes are due.

Federal income tax returns and state income tax returns for the deceased are generally due on April 15 of the year following the death. If the estate generates income over a certain amount during that time, the estate itself may have to file an income tax return. You, as executor, are responsible for filing these returns. If the deceased had a tax attorney or CPA, that individual could be helpful in filing tax returns.

Property taxes (such as taxes on a home or other real estate) must be paid when they are typically due. Tax laws are complex and change frequently, so it is imperative that you speak with an attorney or CPA.

When a Social Security Beneficiary Dies

A family member or other person responsible for the beneficiary's affairs should do the following:

- Promptly notify the Social Security Administration (SSA) of the beneficiary's death by calling toll-free at 800-772-1213. (TTY 800-325-0778.)

- If monthly benefits were being paid via direct deposit, notify the bank or other financial institution of the beneficiary's death. Request that any funds received for the month of death and later be returned to Social Security as soon as possible.

- If benefits were being paid by check, do not cash any checks received for the month in which the beneficiary died or thereafter. Return the checks to Social Security as soon as possible.

One-Time Lump Sum Death Benefit

A one-time payment of $255 is payable to the surviving spouse if he or she was living with the beneficiary at the time of death, or if living apart, was eligible for Social Security benefits on the beneficiary's earnings record for the month of death. If there is no surviving spouse, the payment is made to a child who was eligible for benefits on the beneficiary's earnings record in the month of death.

Benefits for Survivors

Monthly survivor's benefits can be paid to certain family members, including the beneficiary's widow or widower, dependent children, and dependent parents. *Survivors Benefits* (Publication No. 05-10084) and *Social Security: Understanding the Benefits* (Publication No. 05-10024) are booklets available through the Social Security Administration which contain more information about filing for benefits.

Supplemental Security Income Burial Funds

What is a burial fund?

A burial fund is money set aside to pay for burial expenses. For example, this money can be in a bank account, other financial instrument, or a prepaid burial arrangement. Some states allow an individual to prepay their burial by contracting with a funeral home and paying in advance for their funeral. You should discuss this with your local Social Security office.

Does a burial fund count as a resource for supplemental security income (SSI)?

Generally, you and your spouse can set aside up to $1,500 each to pay for burial expenses. In most cases, this money will not count as a resource for SSI. If you (and your spouse) own life insurance polices or have other burial arrangements in addition to your $1,500 burial funds, some of the money in the burial fund may count toward the resource limit of $2,000 for an individual or $3,000 for a couple.

Does interest earned on your (and your spouse's) burial fund count as a resource or income for SSI?

No. Interest earned on your (or your spouse's) burial fund that you leave in the fund does not count as a resource or income for SSI and does not affect your SSI benefit.

Table 49.1. Unified Tax Credit and Gift Tax Exemptions

Year of Death	Exemption Amount
2006–2008	$2,000,000
2009	$3,500,000
2010	Not applicable/taxes repealed

Unless Congress provides otherwise, the Economic Growth and Tax Relief Reconciliation Act of 2001 will expire December 31, 2010.

How can you set up a burial fund?

Any account you set up must clearly show that the money is set aside to pay burial expenses. You can do this by:

- titling the account as a burial fund
- signing a statement saying—
  - how much has been set aside for burial expenses
  - for whose burial the money is set aside
  - how the money has been set aside
  - the date you first considered the money set aside for burial expenses

What happens when you spend money from a burial fund?

If you spend any money from a burial fund on items unrelated to burial expenses, there may be a penalty.

Additional Information

Social Security Administration
Office of Public Inquiries
Windsor Park Building
6401 Security Blvd.
Baltimore, MD 21235
Toll-Free: 800-772-1213
Toll-Free TTY: 800-325-0778
Website: http://www.ssa.gov

Chapter 50

Duties of an Executor

An executor, also called a personal representative, is the individual named in a will charged with executing or carrying out the will's instructions. Many people name their spouse, adult child, or other close family member as executor. Also, the will may name an institution, such as a bank, trust company, or an attorney, as executor or co-executor. Generally, an individual executor can settle a simple estate with minimal legal advice; the larger or more complicated the estate, the more likely the executor will need professional advice from an attorney, certified public accountant (CPA), or other professional advisers.

An executor is generally entitled to a fee for managing the estate, usually set by state law ranging from 1–5 percent of the value of the estate. If the executor is also a beneficiary, he usually waives this fee. The probate court usually requires that (unless the will provides otherwise) an executor be bonded to protect all interested parties against fraud, embezzlement, or negligence by the executor. When the executor is a spouse, adult child, or other close relative, the will often states that the executor may serve without bond, although the court may still require one.

If you are named executor of the estate, your responsibilities will usually include accumulating the assets of the estate, paying any debts or obligations owed by the decedent, distributing the remaining assets to heirs, and completing necessary tax returns.

Consult an attorney and/or CPA about your exact duties as executor. While it will typically be helpful to consult the deceased's own attorney and CPA, you are under no obligation to use their services on an ongoing basis. In most circumstances, insist on an hourly fee for legal and accounting services, not one based on a percentage of the estate's value.

Typical Duties of an Executor

File the Will and Initiate Probate

As executor, you will file the will with the appropriate state probate court.

Petition the Court for Letters of Testamentary

These letters provide proof that you are the legally-appointed executor. You will need several certified copies of the letters to submit for certain financial transactions for the estate.

Request at Least Ten Certified Copies of the Death Certificate

Companies and financial institutions will generally require them. In many places, you can order them from the county clerk's office in the county of the decedent's death. In other locations, you can procure them from the Health Department. The funeral director can advise you or may order the certificates for you.

Assemble and Inventory the Estate's Assets

- Include checking and savings accounts, real estate deeds, vehicle or boat titles, brokerage accounts, stock and bond certificates, and other property.

- If you are unfamiliar with the decedent's financial affairs (as is common when an adult child or friend serves as executor), it may be a challenge to identify all property.

- You will be responsible for determining the value of each asset at the time of death, which may require you to hire an appraiser.

- Locate important documents such as checking, savings, and brokerage accounts statements; employee benefits statements; previous tax returns; and marriage, divorce, and birth certificates of the decedent including joint accounts with any survivors, if applicable.

- Review the decedent's checkbook, previous tax returns, bank statements, and canceled checks looking for clues to the following:
  - insurance premiums
  - land contracts and mortgages
  - vehicle or other loans
  - payment of state and federal income taxes and property taxes
  - license fees for vehicle registration
  - safe deposit box rental fees
  - deposits of paychecks, retirement benefits, Social Security, veteran's benefits, or other income

Retitle Property as Necessary

- If real estate, vehicles, or boats are part of the estate, you will need to transfer these titles either to the beneficiary named to receive the property or to yourself as executor.
- If you hold the property in the estate for eventual distribution, the estate will have to pay taxes as they come due.
- If the decedent did not make specific bequests of tangible property, you may decide to sell the property and add proceeds to other cash in the estate.
- In some states, real estate passes directly to beneficiaries.
- Seek the advice of an attorney before selling or retitling property.
- If the decedent owned a business with other owners, you may need to check with others involved in the business about the existence of buy/sell agreements specifying the disposition of the business when an owner dies. These agreements may provide for the other owners to buy the decedent's share, or the decedent's share may go to the heirs or beneficiaries. Regardless of the situation, consult an attorney for assistance.

Manage and Protect the Estate's Property

- You must ensure that property is protected from theft or damage, manage investments, collect rent or other income produced by the estate, and keep insurance policies current.

List Liabilities Owed by the Estate

- As executor, you are responsible for paying any debts owed by the decedent at the time of death. The decedent's checkbook is a good place to begin.

- You will also want to review the mail, looking for bills as well as payment to the decedent. You must then notify all creditors of the death according to state law and invite them to submit claims against the estate. In particular, look for:

  - utility payments or bills

  - hospital, doctor and other medical expenses (you will also file any medical claims with the decedent's medical insurance carriers)

  - charitable contributions

  - payments on credit card accounts or loans

- Beware of con artists who submit counterfeit bills or claims to the estate hoping you will be unfamiliar with the decedent's affairs.

- Review all bills carefully and report any false claims to local law enforcement authorities.

Open and Inventory the Contents of All Safe Deposit Boxes

- Many banks seal safe deposit boxes immediately on the death of the owner.

- You may have to petition the court or the state for permission to open the box.

- Generally, a bank representative or state official will have to be present when you inventory the box.

- Determine whether under applicable state law any property in the box that was jointly owned by the decedent and another individual goes directly to that individual; other property normally becomes part of the estate and is subject to probate.

Arrange to Close Bank or Brokerage Accounts the Decedent Owned Solely

- Transfer those assets to new accounts you open for the estate.

- Generally, you will need to open a checking account for the estate to facilitate paying the estate's debts and other obligations.

Locate Insurance Policies and File Claims for Benefits

- Life insurance benefits are usually payable directly to named beneficiaries without becoming part of the estate considered in probate.

- Other sources of insurance or death benefits include group life insurance from employers, labor unions, fraternal or professional organizations, or other groups of which the decedent was a member; insurance on mortgage loans, credit card balances, vehicle loans, or other loans; accident insurance; and retirement plans either with an employer (for example, 401(k) or 403(b) plan), or in Keogh or Individual Retirement Accounts (IRAs).

- In many cases, unpaid wages or sick leave are paid directly to the surviving spouse or other designated beneficiaries and do not become part of the estate.

- The decedent's attorney or CPA may have copies of insurance policies. Otherwise, you will have to locate them.

- Look for policies, receipts, and canceled checks, then contact insurance brokers, employers, and union representatives. They will require:
  - policy numbers
  - full name of the decedent

Review Taxes Owed by the Decedent and the Estate

- As executor, you are responsible for filing federal, state, and local income tax returns for the decedent for the year in which he died.

- You may also need to file an income tax return for the estate, as well as federal estate tax returns and possibly state inheritance tax returns.

- Stay organized.

Keep Beneficiaries Informed of Your Progress

Final settlement will be easier if you keep detailed records of all your actions on behalf of the estate.

Contact the Nearest Social Security Office

- Eligible widows, widowers, minor children, and in some cases, dependent parents age 62 or older are eligible for survivor benefits.

- A special one-time payment of $255 can be made to the deceased's spouse or minor children if the deceased had enough work credits.

- Sometimes divorced spouses are also entitled to benefits; however, laws change frequently, so check with the Social Security office in your area.

- You may also call Social Security's toll-free number, 800-772-1213, for information. They will require:
  - certified copy of death certificate*
  - Social Security number of the decedent
  - the decedent's most recent W-2 forms or the most recent self-employment tax return
  - the decedent's employer
  - Social Security numbers of spouse and minor children
  - birth certificates of spouse and minor children*
  - marriage certificate*
  - divorce papers if a divorced spouse is applying for benefits*

Close the Estate and Distribute Remaining Assets to Beneficiaries

- Executors are responsible for ensuring claims against the estate are paid before distributing assets to beneficiaries.

- Usually, the state sets a time limit during which creditors must submit claims.

- Federal and generally state laws also require that all estate tax returns are usually due no later than nine months after a death.

- Many simple estates are settled within 1–2 months; more complicated ones may continue for months or even years, especially if anyone contests the provisions of the will.

*Must be either an original or a certified copy by the agency that issued the document.

Chapter 51

Understanding the Family and Medical Leave Act (FMLA)

The U.S. Department of Labor's Employment Standards Administration, Wage and Hour Division, administers and enforces the Family and Medical Leave Act (FMLA) for all private, state, and local government employees and some federal employees. Most federal and certain congressional employees are also covered by the law and are subject to the jurisdiction of the U.S. Office of Personnel Management or the Congress.

FMLA became effective on August 5, 1993, for most employers. FMLA entitles eligible employees to take up to 12 weeks of unpaid, job-protected leave in a 12-month period for specified family and medical reasons. The employer may elect to use the calendar year, a fixed 12-month leave, fiscal year, or a 12-month period prior to or after the commencement of leave as the 12-month period.

The law contains provisions on employer coverage; employee eligibility for the law's benefits; entitlement to leave, maintenance of health benefits during leave, and job restoration after leave; notice and certification of the need for FMLA leave; and, protection for employees who request or take FMLA leave. The law also requires employers to keep certain records.

This chapter includes excerpts from: "The Family and Medical Leave Act 1993," U.S. Department of Labor, 1995; and, "Family and Medical Leave Act Advisor: Frequently Asked Questions and Answers," U.S. Department of Labor, (http://www.dol.gov/elaws/esa/fmla/faq.asp) accessed March 1, 2006.

Employer Coverage

FMLA applies to all:

- public agencies, including state, local and federal employers, local education agencies (schools), and

- private-sector employers who employed 50 or more employees in 20 or more workweeks in the current or preceding calendar year, and who are engaged in commerce or in any industry or activity affecting commerce—including joint employers and successors of covered employers.

Employee Eligibility

To be eligible for FMLA benefits, an employee must:

1. work for a covered employer;

2. have worked for the employer for a total of 12 months*;

3. have worked at least 1,250 hours over the previous 12 months*; and

4. work at a location in the United States or in any territory or possession of the United States where at least 50 employees are employed by the employer within 75 miles.

*There are special rules for returning reservists under the Uniformed Services Employment and Reemployment Rights Act.

Leave Entitlement

A covered employer must grant an eligible employee up to a total of 12 workweeks of unpaid leave during any 12-month period for one or more of the following reasons:

- for the birth and care of the newborn child of the employee

- for placement with the employee of a son or daughter for adoption or foster care

- to care for an immediate family member (spouse, child, or parent) with a serious health condition

- to take medical leave when the employee is unable to work because of a serious health condition

Spouses employed by the same employer are jointly entitled to a combined total of 12 workweeks of family leave for the birth and care of the newborn child, for placement of a child for adoption or foster care, and to care for a parent who has a serious health condition.

Leave for birth and care, or placement for adoption or foster care must conclude within 12 months of the birth or placement.

Under some circumstances, employees may take FMLA leave intermittently—which means taking leave in blocks of time, or by reducing their normal weekly or daily work schedule.

- If FMLA leave is for birth and care or placement for adoption or foster care, use of intermittent leave is subject to the employer's approval.

- FMLA leave may be taken intermittently whenever medically necessary to care for a seriously ill family member, or because the employee is seriously ill and unable to work.

Also, subject to certain conditions, employees or employers may choose to use accrued paid leave (such as sick or vacation leave) to cover some or all of the FMLA leave.

The employer is responsible for designating if an employee's use of paid leave counts as FMLA leave, based on information from the employee.

Maintenance of Health Benefits

A covered employer is required to maintain group health insurance coverage for an employee on FMLA leave whenever such insurance was provided before the leave was taken and on the same terms as if the employee had continued to work. If applicable, arrangements will need to be made for employees to pay their share of health insurance premiums while on leave. In some instances, the employer may recover premiums it paid to maintain health coverage for an employee who fails to return to work from FMLA leave.

Job Restoration

Upon return from FMLA leave, an employee must be restored to the employee's original job, or to an equivalent job with equivalent pay, benefits, and other terms and conditions of employment.

In addition, an employee's use of FMLA leave cannot result in the loss of any employment benefit that the employee earned or was entitled to before using FMLA leave, nor be counted against the employee under a no fault attendance policy.

Under specified and limited circumstances where restoration to employment will cause substantial and grievous economic injury to its operations, an employer may refuse to reinstate certain highly-paid key employees after using FMLA leave during which health coverage was maintained. In order to do so, the employer must:

- notify the employee of his/her status as a key employee in response to the employee's notice of intent to take FMLA leave;**

- notify the employee as soon as the employer decides it will deny job restoration, and explain the reasons for this decision;

- offer the employee a reasonable opportunity to return to work from FMLA leave after giving this notice; and

- make a final determination as to whether reinstatement will be denied at the end of the leave period if the employee then requests restoration.

**A key employee is a salaried eligible employee who is among the highest paid ten percent of employees within 75 miles of the work site.

Notice and Certification

Employees seeking to use FMLA leave are required to provide 30-day advance notice of the need to take FMLA leave when the need is foreseeable and such notice is practicable.

Employers may also require employees to provide:

- medical certification supporting the need for leave due to a serious health condition affecting the employee or an immediate family member;

- second or third medical opinions (at the employer's expense) and periodic recertification; and

- periodic reports during FMLA leave regarding the employee's status and intent to return to work.

When intermittent leave is needed to care for an immediate family member or the employee's own illness, and is for planned medical treatment, the employee must try to schedule treatment so as not to unduly disrupt the employer's operation.

Covered employers must post a notice approved by the Secretary of Labor explaining rights and responsibilities under FMLA. An employer that willfully violates this posting requirement may be subject to a fine of up to $100 for each separate offense.

Also, covered employers must inform employees of their rights and responsibilities under FMLA, including giving specific written information on what is required of the employee and what might happen in certain circumstances, such as if the employee fails to return to work after FMLA leave.

Unlawful Acts

It is unlawful for any employer to interfere with, restrain, or deny the exercise of any right provided by FMLA. It is also unlawful for an employer to discharge or discriminate against any individual for opposing any practice, or because of involvement in any proceeding, related to FMLA.

Enforcement

The Wage and Hour Division investigates complaints. If violations cannot be satisfactorily resolved, the U.S. Department of Labor may bring action in court to compel compliance. Individuals may also bring a private civil action against an employer for violations.

Frequently Asked Questions and Answers about FLMA

Does the law guarantee paid time off?

No. The FMLA only requires unpaid leave. However, the law permits an employee to elect, or the employer to require the employee, to use accrued paid leave such as vacation or sick leave for some or all of the FMLA leave period. When paid leave is substituted for unpaid FMLA leave, it may be counted against the 12-week FMLA leave entitlement if the employee is properly notified of the designation when the leave begins.

Does workers' compensation leave count against an employee's FMLA leave entitlement?

It can. FMLA leave and workers' compensation leave can run together, provided the reason for the absence is due to a qualifying serious illness or injury, and the employer properly notifies the employee in writing that the leave will be counted as FMLA leave.

If an employer fails to tell employees that the leave is FMLA leave, can the employer count the time they have already been off against the 12 weeks of FMLA leave?

In most situations, the employer cannot count leave as FMLA leave retroactively. The employee must be notified in writing that an absence is being designated as FMLA leave. If the employer was not aware of the reason for the leave, leave may be designated as FMLA leave retroactively only while the leave is in progress or within two business days of the employee's return to work.

Who is considered an immediate family member for purposes of taking FMLA leave?

An employee's spouse, children (son or daughter), and parents (not parents-in-law) are immediate family members for purposes of FMLA. The terms son or daughter do not include individuals age 18 or over unless they are incapable of self-care because of mental or physical disability that limits one or more of the major life activities as those terms are defined in regulations issued by the Equal Employment Opportunity Commission (EEOC) under the Americans with Disabilities Act (ADA).

Which employees are eligible to take FMLA leave?

Employees are eligible to take FMLA leave if they have worked for their employer for at least 12 months, and have worked for at least 1,250 hours over the previous 12 months, and work at a location where at least 50 employees are employed by the employer within 75 miles.

Do the 12 months of service with the employer have to be continuous or consecutive?

No. The 12 months do not have to be continuous or consecutive; all time worked for the employer is counted.

Do the 1,250 hours include paid leave time or other absences from work?

No. The 1,250 hours include only those hours actually worked for the employer. Paid leave and unpaid leave, including FMLA leave, are not included.

How do I determine if I have worked 1,250 hours in a 12-month period?

Your individual record of hours worked would be used to determine whether 1,250 hours had been worked in the 12 months prior to the commencement of FMLA leave. As a rule of thumb, the following may be helpful for estimating whether this test for eligibility has been met;

- 24 hours worked in each of the 52 weeks of the year; or

- over 104 hours worked in each of the 12 months of the year; or

- 40 hours worked per week for more than 31 weeks (over seven months) of the year.

Do I have to give my employer my medical records for leave due to a serious health condition?

No. You do not have to provide medical records. The employer may, however, request that for any leave taken due to a serious health condition, you provide a medical certification confirming that a serious health condition exists.

Can my employer require that I return to work before I exhaust my leave?

Subject to certain limitations, your employer may deny the continuation of FMLA leave due to a serious health condition if you fail to fulfill any obligations to provide supporting medical certification. The employer may not, however, require you to return to work early by offering you a light duty assignment.

Are there any restrictions on how I spend my time while on leave?

Employers with established policies regarding outside employment while on paid or unpaid leave may uniformly apply those policies to employees on FMLA leave. Otherwise, the employer may not restrict your activities. The protections of FMLA will not, however, cover situations where the reason for leave no longer exists, where the employee has not provided required notices or certifications, or where the employee has misrepresented the reason for leave.

Can my employer make inquiries about my leave during my absence?

Yes, but only to you. Your employer may ask you questions to confirm whether the leave needed or being taken qualifies for FMLA purposes, and may require periodic reports on your status and intent to return to work after leave. Also, if the employer wishes to obtain another opinion, you may be required to obtain additional medical certification at the employer's expense, or rectification during a period of FMLA leave. The employer may have a health care provider representing the employer contact your health care provider, with your permission, to clarify information in the medical certification or to confirm that it was provided by the health care provider. The inquiry may not seek additional information regarding your health condition or that of a family member.

Can my employer refuse to grant me FMLA leave?

If you are an eligible employee who has met FMLA's notice and certification requirements (and you have not exhausted your FMLA leave entitlement for the year), you may not be denied FMLA leave.

Will I lose my job if I take FMLA leave?

Generally, no. It is unlawful for any employer to interfere with or restrain or deny the exercise of any right provided under this law. Employers cannot use the taking of FMLA leave as a negative factor in employment actions, such as hiring, promotions, or disciplinary actions; nor can FMLA leave be counted under no fault attendance policies. Under limited circumstances, an employer may deny reinstatement to work—but not the use of FMLA leave—to certain highly-paid, salaried (key) employees.

Are there other circumstances in which my employer can deny me FMLA leave or reinstatement to my job?

In addition to denying reinstatement in certain circumstances to key employees, employers are not required to continue FMLA benefits or reinstate employees who would have been laid off or otherwise had their employment terminated had they continued to work during the FMLA leave period as, for example, due to a general layoff.

Employees who give unequivocal notice that they do not intend to return to work lose their entitlement to FMLA leave.

Employees who are unable to return to work and have exhausted their 12 weeks of FMLA leave in the designated 12 month period no longer have FMLA protections of leave or job restoration.

Under certain circumstances, employers who advise employees experiencing a serious health condition that they will require a medical certificate of fitness for duty to return to work may deny reinstatement to an employee who fails to provide the certification, or may delay reinstatement until the certification is submitted.

Can my employer fire me for complaining about a violation of FMLA?

No. Nor can the employer take any other adverse employment action on this basis. It is unlawful for any employer to discharge or otherwise discriminate against an employee for opposing a practice made unlawful under FMLA.

Does an employer have to pay bonuses to employees who have been on FMLA leave?

The FMLA requires that employees be restored to the same or an equivalent position. If an employee was eligible for a bonus before taking FMLA leave, the employee would be eligible for the bonus upon returning to work. The FMLA leave may not be counted against the employee. For example, if an employer offers a perfect attendance bonus, and the employee has not missed any time prior to taking FMLA leave, the employee would still be eligible for the bonus upon returning from FMLA leave.

On the other hand, FMLA does not require that employees on FMLA leave be allowed to accrue benefits or seniority. For example, an employee on FMLA leave might not have sufficient sales to qualify for a bonus. The employer is not required to make any special accommodation for this employee because of FMLA. The employer must, of course, treat an employee who has used FMLA leave at least as well as other employees on paid and unpaid leave (as appropriate) are treated.

Under what circumstances is leave designated as FMLA leave and counted against the employee's total entitlement?

In all circumstances, it is the employer's responsibility to designate leave taken for an FMLA reason as FMLA leave. The designation must be based upon information furnished by the employee. Leave may not be designated as FMLA leave after the leave has been completed and the employee has returned to work, except if;

- the employer is awaiting receipt of the medical certification to confirm the existence of a serious health condition;

- the employer was unaware that leave was for an FMLA reason, and subsequently acquires information from the employee such as when the employee requests additional or extensions of leave; or,

- the employer was unaware that the leave was for an FMLA reason, and the employee notifies the employer within two days after return to work that the leave was FMLA leave.

Additional Information

U.S. Department of Labor

Frances Perkins Building
200 Constitution Ave., N.W.
Washington, DC 20210
Toll-Free: 866-4-USWAGE (487-9243)
Toll-Free TTY: 877-889-5627
Website: http://www.dol.gov

The final rule implementing FMLA is contained in the January 6, 1995, Federal Register. For more information, please contact the nearest office of the Wage and Hour Division, listed in most telephone directories under U.S. Government, Department of Labor.

Part Eight

Final Arrangements

Chapter 52

Funerals: A Consumer Guide

When a loved one dies, grieving family members and friends often are confronted with dozens of decisions about the funeral—all of which must be made quickly and often under great emotional duress. What kind of funeral should it be? What funeral provider should you use? Should you bury or cremate the body, or donate it to science? What are you legally required to buy? What other arrangements should you plan? And, as callous as it may sound, how much is it all going to cost?

Each year, Americans grapple with these and many other questions as they spend billions of dollars arranging more than two million funerals for family members and friends. The increasing trend toward pre-need planning—when people make funeral arrangements in advance—suggests that many consumers want to compare prices and services so that ultimately, the funeral reflects a wise and well-informed purchasing decision, as well as a meaningful one.

A Consumer Product

Funerals rank among the most expensive purchases many consumers will ever make. A traditional funeral, including a casket and vault, costs about $6,000, although extras like flowers, obituary notices, acknowledgment cards, or limousines can add thousands of dollars to the bottom line. Many funerals run well over $10,000.

Federal Trade Commission, June 2000. The information offered is still pertinent despite the date of this document.

Yet even if you're the kind of person who might haggle with a dozen dealers to get the best price on a new car, you're likely to feel uncomfortable comparing prices or negotiating over the details and cost of a funeral, either pre-need or at the time of need. Compounding this discomfort is the fact that some people overspend on a funeral or burial because they think of it as a reflection of their feelings for the deceased.

Pre-Need and Planning

To help relieve their families of some of these decisions, an increasing number of people are planning their own funerals, designating their funeral preferences, and sometimes even paying for them in advance. They see funeral planning as an extension of will and estate planning.

Thinking ahead can help you make informed and thoughtful decisions about funeral arrangements. It allows you to choose the specific items you want and need and compare the prices offered by several funeral providers. It also spares your survivors the stress of making these decisions under the pressure of time and strong emotions.

You can make arrangements directly with a funeral establishment or through a funeral planning or memorial society—a nonprofit organization that provides information about funerals and disposition but doesn't offer funeral services. If you choose to contact such a group, recognize that while some funeral homes may include the word "society" in their names, they are not nonprofit organizations.

One other important consideration when pre-planning a funeral is where the remains will be buried, entombed, or scattered. In the short time between the death and burial of a loved one, many family members find themselves rushing to buy a cemetery plot or grave—often without careful thought or a personal visit to the site. That's why it is in the family's best interest to buy cemetery plots before you need them.

You may wish to make decisions about your arrangements in advance, but not pay for them in advance. Keep in mind that over time, prices may go up and businesses may close or change ownership. However, in some areas with increased competition, prices may go down over time. It is a good idea to review and revise your decisions every few years, and to make sure your family is aware of your wishes. It's a good idea to review and revise your decision every few years.

Put your preferences in writing, give copies to family members and your attorney, and keep a copy in a handy place. Do not designate your preferences in your will, because a will often is not found or read until after the funeral. Avoid putting the only copy of your preferences in a safe deposit box because your family may have to make arrangements on a weekend or holiday, before the box can be opened.

Prepaying

Millions of Americans have entered into contracts to prearrange their funerals and prepay some or all of the expenses involved. Laws of individual states govern the prepayment of funeral goods and services; various states have laws to help ensure that these advance payments are available to pay for the funeral products and services when they are needed. But protections vary widely from state to state, and some state laws offer little or no effective protection. Some state laws require the funeral home or cemetery to place a percentage of the prepayment in a state-regulated trust or to purchase a life insurance policy with the death benefits assigned to the funeral home or cemetery.

If you're thinking about prepaying for funeral goods and services, it is important to consider these issues before putting down any money:

- What are you are paying for? Are you buying only merchandise, like a casket and vault, or are you purchasing funeral services as well?

- What happens to the money you have prepaid? States have different requirements for handling funds paid for prearranged funeral services.

- What happens to the interest income on money that is prepaid and put into a trust account?

- Are you protected if the firm you dealt with goes out of business?

- Can you cancel the contract and get a full refund if you change your mind?

- What happens if you move to a different area or die while away from home? Some prepaid funeral plans can be transferred, but often at an added cost.

Be sure to tell your family about the plans you have made; let them know where the documents are filed. If your family is not aware that you have made plans, your wishes may not be carried out. And if family members do not know that you have prepaid the funeral costs, they could end up paying for the same arrangements. You may wish to consult an attorney on the best way to ensure that your wishes are followed.

The Funeral Rule

Most funeral providers are professionals who strive to serve their clients' needs and best interests, but some are not. They may take advantage of their clients through inflated prices, overcharges, double charges, or unnecessary services. Fortunately, there is a federal law that makes it easier for you to choose only those goods and services you want or need and to pay only for those you select, whether you are making arrangements pre-need or at the time of need.

The Funeral Rule, enforced by the Federal Trade Commission, requires funeral directors to give you itemized prices in person and, if you ask, over the phone. The Rule also requires funeral directors to give you other information about their goods and services. For example, if you ask about funeral arrangements in person, the funeral home must give you a written price list to keep that shows the goods and services the home offers. If you want to buy a casket or outer burial container, the funeral provider must show you descriptions of the available selections and the prices before actually showing you the caskets.

Many funeral providers offer various packages of commonly selected goods and services that make up a funeral. But when you arrange for a funeral, you have the right to buy individual goods and services. That is, you do not have to accept a package that may include items you do not want.

According to the Funeral Rule:

- You have the right to choose the funeral goods and services you want (with some exceptions).

- The funeral provider must state this right in writing on the general price list.

- If state or local law requires you to buy any particular item, the funeral provider must disclose it on the price list, with a reference to the specific law.

- The funeral provider may not refuse, or charge a fee, to handle a casket you bought elsewhere.

- A funeral provider that offers cremations must make alternative containers available.

Choosing a Funeral Provider

Many people do not realize that they are not legally required to use a funeral home to plan and conduct a funeral. However, because they have little experience with the many details and legal requirements involved and may be emotionally distraught when it is time to make the plans, many people find the services of a professional funeral home to be a comfort.

Consumers often select a funeral home or cemetery because it is close to home, has served the family in the past, or has been recommended by someone they trust. But people who limit their search to just one funeral home may risk paying more than necessary for the funeral or narrowing their choice of goods and services.

Comparison shopping need not be difficult, especially if it is done before the need for a funeral arises. Sometimes it's more convenient and less stressful to price shop funeral homes by telephone. The Funeral Rule requires funeral directors to provide price information over the phone to any caller who asks for it. In addition, many funeral homes are happy to mail you their price lists, although that is not required by law.

When comparing prices, be sure to consider the total cost of all the items together, in addition to the costs of single items. Every funeral home should have price lists that include all the items essential for the different types of arrangements it offers.

In addition, there is a growing trend toward consolidation in the funeral home industry, and many neighborhood funeral homes are thought to be locally owned when in fact, they're owned by a national corporation. If this issue is important to you, you may want to ask if the funeral home is locally owned.

Funeral Costs

Basic Services Fee for the Funeral Director and Staff

The Funeral Rule allows funeral providers to charge a basic services fee that customers cannot decline to pay. The basic services fee includes services that are common to all funerals, regardless of the specific arrangement. These include funeral planning, securing the necessary permits and copies of death certificates, preparing the notices, sheltering the remains, and coordinating the arrangements with the cemetery, crematory or other third parties. The fee does not include charges for optional services or merchandise.

Charges for Other Services and Merchandise

These are costs for optional goods and services such as transporting the remains; embalming and other preparation; use of the funeral home for the viewing, ceremony or memorial service; use of equipment and staff for a graveside service; use of a hearse or limousine; a casket, outer burial container or alternate container; and cremation or interment.

Cash Advances

These are fees charged by the funeral home for goods and services it buys from outside vendors on your behalf, including flowers, obituary notices, pallbearers, officiating clergy, organists, and soloists. Some funeral providers charge you their cost for the items they buy on your behalf. Others add a service fee to their cost. The Funeral Rule requires those who charge an extra fee to disclose that fact in writing, although it does not require them to specify the amount of their markup. The Rule also requires funeral providers to tell you if there are refunds, discounts or rebates from the supplier on any cash advance item.

Calculating the Actual Cost

The funeral provider must give you an itemized statement of the total cost of the funeral goods and services you have selected when you are making the arrangements. If the funeral provider does not know the cost of the cash advance items at the time, he or she is required to give you a written good faith estimate. This statement also must disclose any legal, cemetery, or crematory requirements that you purchase any specific funeral goods or services. The Funeral Rule does not require any specific format for this information. Funeral providers may include it in any document they give you at the end of your discussion about funeral arrangements.

Services and Products

Embalming

Many funeral homes require embalming if you are planning a viewing or visitation. But embalming generally is not necessary or legally required if the body is buried or cremated shortly after death. Eliminating this service can save you hundreds of dollars. Under the Funeral Rule, a funeral provider:

- may not provide embalming services without permission;

- may not falsely state that embalming is required by law;

- must disclose in writing that embalming is not required by law, except in certain special cases;

- may not charge a fee for unauthorized embalming unless embalming is required by state law;

- must disclose in writing that you usually have the right to choose a disposition, such as direct cremation or immediate burial, that does not require embalming if you do not want this service;

- must disclose in writing that some funeral arrangements, such as a funeral with viewing, may make embalming a practical necessity and if so, a required purchase.

Caskets

For a Traditional, Full-Service Funeral

A casket often is the single most expensive item you will buy if you plan a traditional, full-service funeral. Caskets vary widely in style and price and are sold primarily for their visual appeal. Typically, they are constructed of metal, wood, fiberboard, fiberglass, or plastic. Although an average casket costs slightly more than $2,000, some mahogany, bronze, or copper caskets sell for as much as $10,000.

When you visit a funeral home or showroom to shop for a casket, the Funeral Rule requires the funeral director to show you a list of caskets the company sells, with descriptions and prices, before showing you the caskets. Industry studies show that the average casket shopper buys one of the first three models shown, generally the middle-priced of the three. So it is in the seller's best interest to start out by showing you higher-end models. If you have not seen some of the lower-priced models on the price list, ask to see them—but do not be surprised if they are not prominently displayed, or not on display at all.

Traditionally, caskets have been sold only by funeral homes. But with increasing frequency, showrooms and websites operated by third-party dealers are selling caskets. You can buy a casket from one of these dealers and have it shipped directly to the funeral home. The Funeral Rule requires funeral homes to agree to use a casket you bought elsewhere, and does not allow them to charge you a fee for using it.

No matter where or when you are buying a casket, it is important to remember that its purpose is to provide a dignified way to move the body before burial or cremation. No casket, regardless of its qualities or cost, will preserve a body forever. Metal caskets frequently are described as protective or sealer caskets. These terms mean that the casket has a rubber gasket or some other feature that is designed to delay the penetration of water into the casket and prevent rust. The Funeral Rule forbids claims that these features help preserve the remains indefinitely because they do not. They just add to the cost of the casket.

Most metal caskets are made from rolled steel of varying gauges—the lower the gauge, the thicker the steel. Some metal caskets come with a warranty for longevity. Wooden caskets generally do not have gaskets or a warranty for longevity. They can be hardwood like mahogany, walnut, cherry, oak, or softwood like pine. Pine caskets are a less expensive option, but funeral homes rarely display them. Manufacturers of both wooden and metal caskets usually warranty workmanship and materials.

Cremation Casket Needs

Many families that opt to have their loved ones cremated rent a casket from the funeral home for the visitation and funeral, eliminating the cost of buying a casket. If you opt for visitation and cremation, ask about the rental option. For those who choose a direct cremation without a viewing or other ceremony where the body is present, the funeral provider must offer an inexpensive unfinished wood box or alternative container, a non-metal enclosure—pressboard, cardboard or canvas—that is cremated with the body.

Under the Funeral Rule, funeral directors who offer direct cremations:

- may not tell you that state or local law requires a casket for direct cremations, because none do;

- must disclose in writing your right to buy an unfinished wood box or an alternative container for a direct cremation; and

- must make an unfinished wood box or other alternative container available for direct cremations.

Burial Vaults or Grave Liners

Burial vaults or grave liners, also known as burial containers, are commonly used in traditional, full-service funerals. The vault or liner is placed in the ground before burial, and the casket is lowered into it at burial. The purpose is to prevent the ground from caving in as the casket deteriorates over time. A grave liner is made of reinforced concrete and will satisfy any cemetery requirement. Grave liners cover only the top and sides of the casket. A burial vault is more substantial and expensive than a grave liner. It surrounds the casket in concrete or another material and may be sold with a warranty of protective strength.

State laws do not require a vault or liner, and funeral providers may not tell you otherwise. However, keep in mind that many cemeteries require some type of outer burial container to prevent the grave from sinking in the future. Neither grave liners nor burial vaults are designed to prevent the eventual decomposition of human remains. It is illegal for funeral providers to claim that a vault will keep water, dirt, or other debris from penetrating into the casket if that is not true. Before showing you any outer burial containers, a funeral provider is required to give you a list of prices and descriptions. It may be less expensive to buy an outer burial container from a third-party dealer than from a funeral home or cemetery. Compare prices from several sources before you select a model.

Preservative Processes and Products

As far back as the ancient Egyptians, people have used oils, herbs, and special body preparations to help preserve the bodies of their dead. Yet, no process or products have been devised to preserve a body in the grave indefinitely. The Funeral Rule prohibits funeral providers from telling you that it can be done.

Cemetery Sites

When you are purchasing a cemetery plot, consider the location of the cemetery and whether it meets the requirements of your family's religion. Other considerations include what, if any, restrictions the cemetery places on burial vaults purchased elsewhere, the type of monuments or memorials it allows, and whether flowers or other remembrances may be placed on graves.

Cost is another consideration. Cemetery plots can be expensive, especially in metropolitan areas. Most, but not all, cemeteries require you to purchase a grave liner, which will cost several hundred dollars. Note that there are charges—usually hundreds of dollars—to open a grave for interment and additional charges to fill it in. Perpetual care on a cemetery plot sometimes is included in the purchase price, but it is important to clarify that point before you buy the site or service. If it is not included, look for a separate endowment care fee for maintenance and groundskeeping.

If you plan to bury your loved one's cremated remains in a mausoleum or columbarum, you can expect to purchase a crypt and pay opening and closing fees, as well as charges for endowment care and other services. The FTC's Funeral Rule does not cover cemeteries and mausoleums unless they sell both funeral goods and funeral services, so be cautious in making your purchase to ensure that you receive all pertinent price and other information, and that you're being dealt with fairly.

Veterans Cemeteries

All veterans are entitled to a free burial in a national cemetery and a grave marker. This eligibility also extends to some civilians who have provided military-related service and some Public Health Service personnel. Spouses and dependent children also are entitled to a lot and marker when buried in a national cemetery. There are no charges for opening or closing the grave, for a vault or liner, or for setting the marker in a national cemetery. The family generally is responsible for other expenses, including transportation to the cemetery. For more information, visit the Department of Veterans Affairs' website at http:// www.cem.va.gov. To reach the regional Veterans office in your area, call 800-827-1000.

In addition, many states have established state veterans cemeteries. Eligibility requirements and other details vary. Contact your state for more information.

Beware of commercial cemeteries that advertise so-called veterans' specials. These cemeteries sometimes offer a free plot for the veteran, but charge exorbitant rates for an adjoining plot for the spouse, as well as high fees for opening and closing each grave. Evaluate the bottom-line cost to be sure the special is as special as you may be led to believe.

For More Information

Most states have a licensing board that regulates the funeral industry. You may contact the board in your state for information or help. If you want additional information about making funeral arrangements and the options available, you may want to contact interested business, professional, and consumer groups. Some of the biggest are:

Funeral Consumers Alliance
33 Patchen Road
South Burlington, VT 05403
Toll-Free: 800-765-0107
Website: http://www.funerals.org

FCA, a nonprofit, educational organization that supports increased funeral consumer protection, is affiliated with the Funeral and Memorial Society of America (FAMSA). Funeral Consumer's Alliance can offer advice to resolve complaints.

International Cemetery and Funeral Association
107 Carpenter Dr., Suite 100
Sterling, VA 20164
Toll-Free: 800-645-7700
Phone: 703-391-8400
Fax: 703-391-8416
Website: http://www.icfa.org

ICFA is a nonprofit association of cemeteries, funeral homes, crematories, and monument retailers that offers informal mediation of consumer complaints through its Cemetery Consumer Service Council.

National Funeral Directors Association
Funeral Service Consumer Assistance Program
13625 Bishop's Drive
Brookfield, WI 53005-6607
Toll-Free: 800-228-6332
Phone: 262-789-1880
Fax: 262-789-6977
Website: http://www.nfda.org
E-mail: nfda@nfda.org

FSCAP is a nonprofit consumer service of the National Funeral Directors Association designed to help people understand funeral service and related topics and to help them resolve funeral service concerns. FSCAP service representatives and an intervener assist consumers in identifying needs, addressing complaints, and resolving problems. Free brochures on funeral related topics are available.

Federal Trade Commission
Consumer Response Center
600 Pennsylvania Ave., N.W.
Washington, DC 20580

Toll-Free: 877-FTC-HELP (382-4357)
Toll-Free TDD: 866-653-4261
Website: http://www.ftc.gov

Although the Commission cannot resolve individual problems for consumers, it can act against a company if it sees a pattern of possible law violations.

Chapter 53

Planning Funeral or Memorial Services

Planning your funeral will ease the emotional burden on your sur-vivors and ensure that your wishes are completed. The three basic types of funerals are traditional full-service, direct burial, and direct cremation.

Traditional Funeral Service

Traditional full-service funerals include the following:

- a viewing or visitation

- a formal funeral service

- the use of a hearse to transport the body to the funeral site and cemetery

- a burial, entombment or the cremation of the remains

If you choose a traditional full-service funeral, consider the follow-ing:

- Do you prefer an open or closed casket?

- Are there special types of clothing and jewelry that you prefer to be buried in?

- Would you like a service? If so, would you like it to be indoors, graveside, or both?

- If you would like an indoor service, would you prefer it to be at the funeral home or your place of worship?

- Who would you prefer to conduct the services?

- Are there specific individuals you would like to serve as pallbearers?

- Would you like someone to speak at the service?

- Do you want music? If so, which selections?

- Do you want live or recorded music?

Direct Burial

- The body is buried shortly after death and usually in a simple container.

- There is no viewing or visitation; the body is not embalmed.

- If desired, a memorial service may be held at the graveside.

Direct Cremation

- The body is cremated shortly after death; the body is not embalmed.

- The cremains are placed in an urn or other type of container.

- There is no viewing or visitation; a memorial service may be held with or without the cremains.

- The cremains may be kept by a family member, scattered in a favorite location or buried in a grave or mausoleum. Check with state or local laws if you choose to have your cremains scattered.

Editor's Note: Memorial services held in lieu of a traditional funeral service may be at a time and place convenient for the family, and may include all aspects of a traditional funeral service or be unique to the deceased person and family preferences. Such services have been held in parks, churches, graveyards, or family homes usually within a few weeks of the death, but occasionally as long as several months or a year after the death.

Additional Information

Consumer Resource Guide
International Cemetery and Funeral Association
107 Carpenter Dr., Suite 100
Sterling, VA 20164
Toll-Free: 800-645-7700
Phone: 703-391-8400
Fax: 703-391-8416
Website: http://www.icfa.org/consumer.html

National Funeral Directors Association
Funeral Service Consumer Assistance Program
13625 Bishop's Drive
Brookfield, WI 53005-6607
Toll-Free: 800-228-6332
Phone: 262-789-1880
Fax: 262-789-6977
Website: http://www.nfda.org
E-mail: nfda@nfda.org

Chapter 54

Common Funeral Myths

Myth: Embalming is required by law

Embalming is never required for the first 24 hours. In many states, it is not required at all under any circumstances. Refrigeration is almost always an alternative to embalming if there will be a delay before final disposition.

Myth: Embalming protects the public health

There is no public health purpose served by embalming. In fact, the embalming process may create a health hazard by exposing embalmers to disease and toxic chemicals. In many cases, disease can still be found in an embalmed body. A dead body is less of a threat to public health than a live one that is still coughing and breathing.

Myth: An embalmed body will last like the beautiful picture forever

Mortuary-type embalming is meant to hold the body only for a week or so. Ultimately, the body will decompose even if it has been embalmed. Temperature and climate are more influential factors affecting the rate of decomposition.

Myth: *Viewing is necessary for closure after a death*

When the death has been anticipated, family members have already started their good-byes. There is relatively little need to see the body to accept the reality of death. In fact, according to a 1990 Wirthlin study commissioned by the funeral industry, 32% of those interviewed found the viewing experience an unpleasant one for various reasons.

Myth: *Protective caskets help to preserve the body*

While caskets with gaskets may keep out air, water, and other outside elements for a while, the body will decompose regardless. In fact, a gasket or sealed casket interferes with the natural dehydration that would otherwise occur. Fluids are released from the body as it begins to decompose, and the casket is likely to rust out from the inside.

Myth: *Protective or sealed vaults help to preserve the body*

Nothing the traditional funeral industry sells will preserve the body forever. If there is a flood, however, such vaults have popped out of the ground and floated away. (Mass graves after the plague in England were ultimately found to be without health problems, according to the 1995 British health journal *Communicable Disease Report*. Burial in containers, however, often kept the disease encapsulated.)

Myth: *Coffin vaults are required by law*

No state has a law requiring burial vaults. Most cemeteries, however, do have such regulations because the vault keeps the grave from sinking in after decomposition of the body and casket, reducing maintenance for the cemetery workers. Grave liners are usually less expensive than vaults. New York state forbids cemeteries from requiring vaults or liners, in deference to religious traditions that require burial directly in the earth. Those who have started green burial grounds do not permit vaults or metal caskets.

Myth: *Vaults are required for the interment of cremated remains*

Alas, with the increasing cremation rate, many cemeteries are making this claim, no doubt to generate more income. There is no similar safety reason as claimed for using a casket vault. Any cemetery trying to force such a purchase should be reported to the Federal Trade Commission for unfair marketing practices: 877-FTC-HELP (382-4357).

Myth: What is left after the cremation process are ashes

When people think of ashes they envision what you would find in the fireplace or what is left over after a campfire. However, what remains after the cremation process are bone fragments, like broken seashells. These are pulverized to a small dimension, not unlike aquarium gravel.

Myth: Cremated remains must be placed in an urn and interred in a cemetery lot or niche

There is no reason you cannot keep the cremated remains in the cardboard or plastic box that comes from the crematory. In all states, it is legal to scatter or bury cremated remains on private property (with the landowner's permission). Cremation is considered final disposition because there is no longer any health hazard. There are no cremains police checking on what you do with cremated remains.

Myth: It is a good idea to prepay for a funeral to lock in prices

Funeral directors selling pre-need funerals expect the interest on your money to pay for any increase in prices. They would not let you prepay unless there was some benefit for the funeral home, such as capturing more market share or being allowed to pocket some of your money now. Prepaid funeral money is not well-protected against embezzlement in most states. Furthermore, if you were to move, die while traveling, or simply change your mind—from body burial to cremation, perhaps—you may not get all your money back or transferred to a new funeral home. The interest on your money, in a pay-on-death account at your own bank, should keep up with inflation and will let you stay in control. Please note: There are more low-cost, low-overhead funeral operations opening up, so prices may go down in the future in areas with open price competition.

Myth: With a pre-need contract, I took care of everything

There are over 20 items found on many final funeral bills that cannot be included in a pre-need contract because these items are purchased from third parties and cannot be calculated prior to death. Extra charges after an autopsy, clergy honoraria, obituary notices, flowers, the crematory fee or grave opening are typical examples. All such items will be paid for by the decedent's estate or family in addition to what has already been paid for in the pre-need contract.

Myth: Insurance is a good way to pay for a funeral

Interest accrued by an insurance policy may be outpaced by funeral inflation and is generally less than what is earned by money in a trust. When a funeral is paid for with funeral insurance, either the funeral director will absorb the loss (and many reluctantly do)—or figure out a way for your survivors to pay a little more: "The casket your mother picked out is no longer available. You'll have to pick out a new one, and the price has gone up."

If what you have is life insurance, not funeral insurance, it may be considered an asset when applying for Medicaid. In that case, you will have to cash it in, getting pennies on the dollar. The same may be true if you are making time payments on your funeral insurance, and, in hard times, you decide to stop making payments. In fact, the company may be able to keep everything you paid, as liquidated damages.

Chapter 55

Cremation Explained

What is cremation?

It is the process of reducing the body to ashes and bone fragments through the use of intense heat. The process usually takes two to four hours. Depending on the size of the body, the cremated remains weigh about three to nine pounds.

Is there a trend toward cremation?

Yes. The percentage of cremations in the United States is rapidly rising each year because of the considerable expense of traditional funerals, the diminishing space available for cemeteries, and increasing environmental concerns. In a number of areas in the nation, particularly on the West Coast and in Florida, cremation is the preferred method of disposition.

Over 90% of Funeral Consumer Alliance (FCA) members throughout the U.S. choose cremation because they seek a simple, dignified, and affordable option. In England and Japan, where cemetery space is at a premium, the cremation rate is also close to 90%.

Is a casket required for cremation?

No, a casket is never required for cremation. However, most crematories do require that the body be enclosed in some form of rigid container. Under the Federal Trade Commission Rule of 1984, all mortuaries must make available to the customer an unfinished wooden box or similar inexpensive cremation container. Customers may make or furnish their own suitable container.

How much does cremation cost?

If an undertaker is used to transport the body, obtain permits, and file the death certificate, the fee for services may run well over $1,000. If a visitation or a funeral service is held before cremation, the charges will be higher.

Many FCA affiliates offer members cremation services provided by licensed funeral homes at costs considerably less than the national average. Families who care for their own dead can use crematories directly at charges from $100 to $300.

Since 1984, all undertakers are required to explain the firm's charges in detail before a funeral purchase. You also may ask for these prices over the phone.

Do I have to hire an undertaker?

Possibly not. Most states permit religious groups or private citizens to obtain the necessary death certificate and permits for transit and disposition.

Is a funeral service necessary?

Although visitation and a funeral service with a body present may be held before cremation, many have found it more helpful to have a memorial service without the body present. It is less costly and family and friends will appreciate an opportunity to pay tribute to the memory of a special person.

Can a casket be rented?

In many parts of the country, mortuaries will rent an attractive casket to a family that wants to have the body present for visitation or for a funeral service preceding cremation. After the service, the body is transferred to an inexpensive cremation container. Significant savings may be realized by using a rental casket.

What can be done with cremated remains?

Several choices exist: they can be placed in a niche in a columbarium, buried, scattered, or kept by the family. Cremated remains are sterile and pose no health hazard. In fact, new options are being offered each year, such as artificial reefs in the ocean into which cremated remains have been mixed.

A columbarium is an assembly of niches designed to hold containers of cremated remains. It is most often located in a mausoleum with a cemetery. Some churches provide niches within the church or as a part of a garden wall.

Earth burial can be in a cemetery, either in a regular grave or in a special urn garden. Many cemeteries will permit two or three containers in one adult-size plot. However, the family, if so inclined, can bury the cremains anywhere it wishes, with the property owner's permission.

Scattering cremains over some area that had significance to the deceased has an appeal for many and is legal in most jurisdictions. Although there are commercial firms which will handle the cremated remains for a fee, most families prefer to do this themselves. Remains should be processed by the crematory to reduce all fragments to fine particles.

Must an urn be purchased?

No. Crematories return the cremated remains in a metal, plastic, or cardboard container that is perfectly adequate for burial, shipping, or placing in a columbarium. The family may prefer an aesthetic or other appropriate receptacle. Urns usually cost in excess of $150, but alternative containers are equally suitable.

Are cremation societies the same as memorial societies?

No. The most important difference is that memorial societies are not-for-profit consumer groups which are democratically controlled, whereas direct cremation societies operate for profit. They masquerade as nonprofit by using society in their name and by charging a membership fee. If there is no memorial society (or Funeral Consumers Alliance) in your area, you may find some of the direct cremation firms considerably less expensive than their competition.

How do religious groups view cremation?

Most religions permit cremation. Since Vatican II Council in 1964, the Code of Canon Law allows Roman Catholics a choice between burial and cremation. The Greek and Jewish Orthodox faiths oppose cremation, as do some others.

Chapter 56

Medical Certification of Death

A significant number of the deaths occurring in the United States must be investigated and certified by a medical-legal officer. Although state laws vary in specific requirements, deaths that typically require investigation are those due to unusual or suspicious circumstances, violence (accident, suicide, or homicide), those due to natural disease processes when the death occurred suddenly and without warning, when the decedent was not being treated by a physician, or the death was unattended.

In those cases where death is not the result of accident, suicide, or homicide, some states include in their laws a specific time period regarding how recently treatment must have been provided by a physician for that physician to be authorized to complete the medical certification of cause of death. These time limits vary from state to state. In some states where no time limit is specified, it is left to interpretation or local custom to determine whether the cause of death should be completed by a physician or by the medical examiner or coroner. The medical-legal officer should investigate the case and ensure that the medical certification of cause of death is properly completed. State laws, regulations, and customs vary significantly regarding which cases must be investigated by a medical-legal officer. If there is any doubt as to jurisdiction, the medical-legal officer should assume jurisdiction.

Excerpts from "Medical Examiners' and Coroners' Handbook on Death Registration and Fetal Death Reporting," Centers for Disease Control and Prevention (CDC), 2003.

Importance of Death Registration and Fetal Death Reporting

The death certificate is a permanent record of the fact of death and may be needed to get a burial permit. The information in the record is considered as *prima facie* evidence of the fact of death that can be introduced in court as evidence. State law specifies the required time for completing and filing the death certificate.

The death certificate provides important personal information about the decedent and about the circumstances and cause of death. This information has many uses related to the settlement of the estate and provides family members' closure, peace of mind, and documentation of the cause of death.

The death certificate is the source for state and national mortality statistics. Because statistical data derived from death certificates can be no more accurate than the information provided on the certificate, it is very important that all persons concerned with the registration of deaths strive not only for complete registration, but also for accuracy and promptness in reporting these events. Furthermore, the potential usefulness of detailed specific information is greater than more general information.

Confidentiality of Vital Records

State laws and supporting regulations define which persons have authorized access to vital records. Some states have few restrictions on access to death certificates. However, there are restrictions on access to death certificates in the majority of states. Legal safeguards to the confidentiality of vital records have been strengthened over time in some states.

The fetal death report is designed primarily to collect information for statistical and research purposes. In many states these records are not maintained in the official files of the state health department. Most states never issue certified copies of these records; the other states issue certified copies very rarely.

Responsibility of the Medical Examiner or Coroner in Death Registration

The principal responsibility of the medical examiner or coroner in death registration is to complete the medical part of the death certificate.

Before delivering the death certificate to the funeral director, he or she may add some personal items for proper identification such as name, residence, race, and sex. Under certain circumstances and in some jurisdictions, he or she may provide all the information, medical and personal, required on the certificate.

The funeral director, or other person in charge of interment, will otherwise complete those parts of the death certificate that call for personal information about the decedent. He or she is also responsible for filing the certificate with the registrar where the death occurred. Each state prescribes the time within which the death certificate must be filed with the registrar.

In general, the duties of the medical examiner or coroner are to:

- complete relevant portions of the death certificate

- deliver the signed or electronically authenticated death certificate to the funeral director promptly so that the funeral director can file it with the state or local registrar within the state's prescribed time period

- assist the state or local registrar by answering inquiries promptly

- deliver a supplemental report of cause of death to the state vital statistics office when the autopsy report or further investigation reveals the cause of death to be different from what was originally reported

When the cause of death cannot be determined within the statutory time limit, a death certificate should be filed with the notation that the report of cause of death is deferred pending further investigation. A permit to authorize disposal or removal of the body may then be obtained. If there are other reasons for a delay in completing the medical portion of the certificate, the registrar should be given written notice of the reason for the delay.

When the circumstances of death (accident, suicide, or homicide) cannot be determined within the statutory time limit, the cause-of-death section should be completed and the manner of death should be shown as pending investigation. As soon as the cause of death and circumstances or manner of death are determined, the medical examiner or coroner should file a supplemental report with the registrar or correct or amend the death certificate according to state and local regulations regarding this procedure.

Medical Certification of Death

The medical examiner or coroner's primary responsibility in death registration is to complete the medical part of the death certificate. The medical certification includes:

- date and time pronounced dead
- date and time of death
- if the case was referred to the medical examiner or coroner
- cause of death, manner of death, tobacco use, and pregnancy status
- injury items for cases involving injuries
- certifier section with signatures

The proper completion of this section of the certificate is of utmost importance to the efficient working of a medical-legal investigative system.

Cause of Death

The cause-of-death section is designed to elicit the opinion of the medical certifier. Causes of death on the death certificate represent a medical opinion that might vary among individual medical-legal officers. A properly completed cause-of-death section provides an etiological explanation of the order, type, and association of events resulting in death. The initial condition that starts the etiological sequence is specific if it does not leave any doubt as to why it developed. For instance, sepsis is not specific because a number of different conditions may have resulted in sepsis, whereas human immunodeficiency virus (HIV) infection is specific.

In certifying the cause of death, any disease, abnormality, injury, or poisoning, if believed to have adversely affected the decedent, should be reported. If the use of alcohol and/or other substance, a smoking history, or a recent pregnancy, injury, or surgery was believed to have contributed to death, then this condition should be reported. The conditions present at the time of death may be completely unrelated, arising independently of each other; or they may be causally related to each other, that is, one condition may lead to another which in turn leads to a third condition, and so forth. Death may also result from the combined effect of two or more conditions.

The mechanism of death, such as cardiac or respiratory arrest, should not be reported as it is a statement not specifically related to the disease process, and it merely attests to the fact of death. The mechanism of death therefore provides no additional information on the cause of death. The cause-of-death section consists of two parts. The first part is for reporting the sequence of events leading to death, proceeding backwards from the final disease or condition resulting in death. The second part includes other significant conditions that contributed to the death, but did not lead to the underlying cause.

In addition, there are questions relating to autopsy, manner of death (for example, accident), and injury. The cause of death should include information provided by the pathologist if an autopsy or other type of postmortem examination is done. For deaths that have microscopic examinations pending at the time the certificate is filed, the additional information should be reported as soon as it is available.

The completion of the cause-of-death section for a medical-legal case requires careful consideration due to special problems that may be involved. The medical-legal case may depend upon toxicological examination for its ultimate cause-of-death certification (a situation not encountered as frequently in ordinary medical practice). Occasionally the medical examiner or coroner must deal with death certifications in which the cause of death is not clear, even after autopsy and toxicological examination. Despite these special problems that the medical examiner or coroner may encounter in dealing with causes of death, it is important that the medical certification be as accurate and complete as circumstances allow.

For statistical and research purposes, it is important that the causes of death and, in particular, the underlying cause of death be reported as specifically and as precisely as possible. Careful reporting results in statistics for both underlying and multiple causes of death (for example, all conditions mentioned on a death certificate) reflecting the best medical opinion. Statistically, mortality research focuses on the underlying cause of death because public health interventions seek to break the sequence of causally related medical conditions as early as possible. However, all cause information reported on death certificates is important and is analyzed.

Changes to Cause of Death

Should additional medical information or autopsy findings become available that would change the cause or causes of death originally reported, the original death certificate should be amended by the

443

medical-legal officer by immediately reporting the revised cause of death to the state vital records office or local registrar.

Chapter 57

If Death Occurs while Traveling

Death Away from Home

Death in the U.S.

Even if you believe your traveling companion is already dead, it is a good idea to call 911 or the operator. An unexpected death will likely mean the involvement of a medical examiner or coroner to investigate the cause of death. Consequently, this may delay for several days any arrangements for body disposition, time you may appreciate.

Once death has been pronounced, you will need to notify close relatives, even if the hour is late when you call. Studies show that most will feel left out if they are not told right away, so do not feel you have to wait until morning unless there are special circumstances. Those calls—including calls to clergy—may provide needed support for you, too. Be sure to give a phone number where you can be reached later.

Unless there is a reason to have services with the body present in the area where death occurred (a summer cottage, perhaps, where there are established friends), you will usually save money by working through the hometown funeral director if the body is to be shipped back home. If cremation is the chosen method of disposition—without

This chapter includes: "Death Away from Home," reprinted with permission from http://www.funerals.org. © 2005 Funeral Consumers Alliance. All rights reserved. Also, "Consular Report of Death of a U.S. Citizen Abroad," U.S. Department of State, current as of February 25, 2006; and "Return of Remains of Deceased Americans," U.S. Department of State, 2003.

445

any services prior to cremation—check with local funeral directors or the local hospital for referrals.

Medical Emergencies Outside the U.S.

If you are a Medicare beneficiary and are traveling outside the United States and its territories (including Puerto Rico, U.S. Virgin Islands, Guam, American Samoa, Northern Mariana Islands), and need medical services, you should be aware of the following: Generally, Medicare does not pay for hospital or medical services outside the United States. For specific information regarding exceptions, call your Medicare office before planning your trip.

You may want to buy special short-term insurance for foreign travel. If you have other health insurance in addition to Medicare, check to see if health care in a foreign country is covered. Medicare will pay for care in qualified Canadian or Mexican hospitals if you are in the U.S. when an emergency occurs (or traveling between Alaska and another state) and a Canadian or Mexican hospital is closer to or substantially more accessible than the nearest U.S. hospital.

Death Outside the U.S.

When a U.S. citizen dies abroad, making arrangements for disposition can become very involved and expensive. The Department of State makes several suggestions:

1. Call the nearest U.S. Embassy or Consulate before calling the family. A cablegram is sent from the overseas post directly to the next-of-kin with official notification of the death and an outline of options available, along with costs.

2. Be certain that the name of a person to be contacted in the event of an emergency is included in your passport.

3. Your preference for body disposition should also be attached to your passport.

4. If needed, money should be wired to the Department of State which will then wire it on to the Embassy. Working through the banks takes too long. The Department of State can be reached at 888-407-4747, or 202-647-4000 (ask for the overseas citizen duty officer). There are no U.S. Government funds appropriated for the repatriation of a deceased U.S. citizen.

Options for Foreign Body Disposition

Local Burial. Although usually the least expensive option in some places, a few countries do not allow the burial of foreigners. The Consular Officer will be able to tell you.

Cremation. This option is available in most countries, although it may be prohibited in predominantly Catholic or Moslem countries. (It is now being done more often in Italy because of the limited cemetery space.) Some countries have only one crematory, causing greater cost and delay in returning the cremated remains.

Body donation. There is an urgent need of body donors in many countries. The Consular Officer should be able to assist with arrangements.

Return of an embalmed body to the U.S. Preparation and shipment are according to local laws, regulations, and customs. Embalming is not widely practiced in most foreign countries. There are other methods of preparation for shipment, but they will preclude viewing. (The body may be wrapped in a chemically-saturated shroud.) Charges for these services are high and vary widely from one location to another. After receipt of the necessary funds, there may be a 3–10 day interval until actual shipment. You will need to notify your funeral director in the U.S. who can assist with arrangements.

Bereavement Airfares

Bereavement airfares are available for both domestic and international travel; however, are not always the least expensive seats. Check for the lowest available fares before asking if there are bereavement seats available. Only certain classes of seats are marked for the bereavement discount.

Return of Remains of Deceased Americans

One of the tasks of the Department of State and of U.S. embassies and consulates abroad is to provide assistance to families of U.S. citizens who die abroad. The U.S. consular officer in the foreign country will assist the family in making arrangements with local authorities for preparation and disposition of the remains, following the family's instructions in accordance with local law. The authority and responsibilities of a U.S. consular officer concerning return of remains of a deceased U.S. citizen abroad are based on U.S. laws (22 U.S.C. 4196; 22 CFR 72.1), treaties, and international practice. Options available to a family depend upon local law and practice in the foreign country. Certain documents are required by U.S. and foreign law before remains can be sent from one country to another. These requirements may vary depending on the circumstances of the death.

Consular Mortuary Certificate

A U.S. consular mortuary certificate is required to ensure orderly shipment of remains and to facilitate U.S. Customs clearance. The certificate is in English and confirms essential information concerning the cause of death. The U.S. consular officer will prepare the certificate and ensure that the foreign death certificate (if available), affidavit of the foreign funeral director, and transit permit, together with the consular mortuary certificate accompany the remains to the United States.

Affidavit of Foreign Funeral Director and Transit Permit

The U.S. consular officer will ensure that the required affidavit is executed by the local (foreign) funeral director. This affidavit attests to the fact that the casket contains only the remains of the deceased and the necessary clothing and packing materials. The affidavit may also state that the remains have been embalmed or otherwise prepared. In addition, the U.S. consular officer ensures that a transit permit accompanies the remains. The transit permit is issued by local health authorities at the port of embarkation.

U.S. Entry Requirements for Quarantine and Customs

In general, if remains have been embalmed, the documentation which accompanies the consular mortuary certificate will satisfy U.S. public health requirements. If the foreign death certificate is not available at the time the remains are returned, the consular mortuary certificate will include reference to the fact that the deceased did not die from a quarantinable disease and that the remains have been embalmed. The affidavit of the funeral director which is attached to the consular mortuary certificate complies with the U.S. Customs requirement that the casket and the packing container for the casket contain only the remains. If the remains are not accompanied by a passenger, a bill of lading must be issued by the airline carrier company to cover the transport. The customs house permit for entry to the United States is obtained by the airline carrier at the point of departure.

Shipment of Remains Which Are Not Embalmed

If the remains are not embalmed, the U.S. consular officer should alert U.S. Customs and the U.S. Public Health Service at point of entry in advance, faxing copies of the consular mortuary certificate, local death certificate (if available), affidavit of foreign funeral director, and a formal statement from competent foreign authorities stating that the individual did not die from a communicable disease. This statement generally is required even if the exact cause of death is unknown in order for unembalmed remains to enter the United States.

Consular Report of Death of a U.S. Citizen Abroad

Foreign Death Certificate

Foreign death certificates are issued by the local registrar of deaths or similar local authority. The certificates are written in the language of the foreign country and prepared in accordance with the laws of the foreign country. Although authenticated copies of the foreign death certificate can be obtained, since the documents are written in the language of the foreign country they are sometimes unacceptable in the United States for insurance and estate purposes. In the United States, a "Report of Death of an American Citizen Abroad" issued by the U.S. consular officer is generally used in lieu of a foreign death certificate as proof of death.

Report of Death of a U.S. Citizen Abroad

The consular "Report of Death of an American Citizen Abroad" is a report that provides the essential facts concerning the death of a U.S. citizen, disposition of remains, and custody of the personal effects of a deceased citizen. This form is generally used in legal proceedings in the United States in lieu of the foreign death certificate. The Report of Death is based on the foreign death certificate, and cannot be completed until the foreign death certificate has been issued. This can sometimes take from four to six weeks or longer after the date of the death, depending on how long it takes local authorities to complete the local form. U.S. Embassies and Consulates work with local authorities to see that this time is as short as possible.

Legal Authority

U.S. insurance companies and other agencies sometimes inquire regarding the authority for issuance of Reports of Death. See 22 U.S. Code 4196; 22 Code of Federal Regulations 72.1.

Copies of the Report of Death

The U.S. consular officer will send the family up to 20 certified copies of the Report of Death at the time the initial report is issued. These are provided at no fee. Additional copies can be obtained subsequently by contacting the

Passport Vital Records Office
1111 19th Street, N.W., Suite 510
Washington, D.C. 20036
Phone: 202-955-0307
Website: http://travel.state.gov

Submit a notarized, written request including all pertinent facts along with a photocopy of the requester's driver license or picture identification, and their return address and telephone number. Effective June 1, 2002, there is a $30 fee for a certified copy of Reports of Death, and a $20 fee for each additional copy provided at the same time. Call to be certain of current fees as requests cannot be honored without the correct fee included.

Chapter 58

Loss, Grief, and Bereavement

People cope with the loss of a loved one in many ways. For some, the experience may lead to personal growth, even though it is a difficult and trying time. There is no right way of coping with death. The way a person grieves depends on the personality of that person and the relationship with the person who has died. How a person copes with grief is affected by their experience with illness, the way the disease progressed, the person's cultural and religious background, coping skills, mental history, support systems, and the person's social and financial status.

The terms grief, bereavement, and mourning are often used in place of each other, but they have different meanings.

Grief is the normal process of reacting to the loss. Grief reactions may be felt in response to physical losses (death) or in response to symbolic or social losses (divorce or loss of a job). Each type of loss means the person has had something taken away. As a family goes through a cancer illness, many losses are experienced, and each triggers its own grief reaction. Grief may be experienced as a mental, physical, social, or emotional reaction. Mental reactions can include anger, guilt, anxiety, sadness, and despair. Physical reactions can

Excerpted from "Loss, Grief, and Bereavement (PDQ®): Supportive Care–Patient," PDQ® Cancer Information Summary, National Cancer Institute; Bethesda, MD. Updated September 2005, available at: http://cancer.gov. Accessed March 1, 2006.

include sleeping problems, changes in appetite, physical problems, or illness. Social reactions can include feelings about taking care of others in the family, seeing family or friends, or returning to work. As with bereavement, grief processes depend on the relationship with the person who died, the situation surrounding the death, and the person's attachment to the person who died. Grief may be described as the presence of physical problems, constant thoughts of the person who died, guilt, hostility, or a change in the way one normally acts.

Bereavement is the period after a loss during which grief is experienced and mourning occurs. The time spent in a period of bereavement depends on how attached the person was to the person who died, and how much time was spent anticipating the loss.

Mourning is the process by which people adapt to a loss. Mourning is also influenced by cultural customs, rituals, and society's rules for coping with loss.

Grief work includes the processes that a mourner needs to complete before resuming daily life. These processes include separating from the person who died, readjusting to a world without him or her, and forming new relationships. To separate from the person who died, a person must find another way to redirect the emotional energy that was given to the loved one. This does not mean the person was not loved or should be forgotten, but that the mourner needs to turn to others for emotional satisfaction. The mourner's roles, identity, and skills may need to change to readjust to living in a world without the person who died. The mourner must give other people or activities the emotional energy that was once given to the person who died in order to redirect emotional energy.

People who are grieving often feel extremely tired because the process of grieving usually requires physical and emotional energy. The grief they are feeling is not just for the person who died, but also for the unfulfilled wishes and plans for the relationship with the person. Death often reminds people of past losses or separations. Mourning may be described as having the following three phases:

- the urge to bring back the person who died

- disorganization and sadness

- reorganization

The Pathway to Death

People who are dying may move towards death over longer or shorter periods of time and in different ways. Different causes of death result in different paths toward death.

The pathway to death may be long and slow, sometimes lasting years, or it may be a rapid fall towards death (for example, after a car accident) when the chronic phase of the illness, if it exists at all, is short. The peaks and valleys pathway describes the patient who repeatedly gets better and then worse again (for example, a patient with AIDS or leukemia). Another pathway to death may be described as a long, slow period of failing health and then a period of stable health (for example, patients whose health gets worse and then stabilizes at a new, more limiting level). Patients on this pathway must readjust to losses in functioning ability.

Deaths from cancer often occur over a long period of time, and may involve long-term pain and suffering, and/or loss of control over one's body or mind. Deaths caused by cancer are likely to drain patients and families physically and emotionally because they occur over a long period of time.

Anticipatory Grief

Anticipatory grief is the normal mourning that occurs when a patient or family is expecting a death. Anticipatory grief has many of the same symptoms as those experienced after a death has occurred. It includes all of the thinking, feeling, cultural, and social reactions to an expected death that are felt by the patient and family.

Anticipatory grief includes depression, extreme concern for the dying person, preparing for the death, and adjusting to changes caused by the death. Anticipatory grief gives the family more time to slowly get used to the reality of the loss. People are able to complete unfinished business with the dying person. Anticipatory grief may not always occur. Anticipatory grief does not mean that before the death, a person feels the same kind of grief as the grief felt after a death. There is not a set amount of grief that a person will feel. The grief experienced before a death does not make the grief after the death last a shorter amount of time.

Grief that follows an unplanned death is different from anticipatory grief. Unplanned loss may overwhelm the coping abilities of a person, making normal functioning impossible. Mourners may not be able to realize the total impact of their loss. Even though the person recognizes that the loss occurred, he or she may not be able to accept the loss mentally and emotionally. Following an unexpected death, the mourner may feel that the world no longer has order and does not make sense.

Some people believe that anticipatory grief is rare. To accept a loved one's death while he or she is still alive may leave the mourner feeling that the dying patient has been abandoned. Expecting the loss often makes the attachment to the dying person stronger. Although anticipatory grief may help the family, the dying person may experience too much grief causing the patient to become withdrawn.

Phases of Grief

The process of bereavement may be described as having four phases.

1. **Shock and numbness:** Family members find it difficult to believe the death; they feel stunned and numb.

2. **Yearning and searching:** Survivors experience separation anxiety and cannot accept the reality of the loss. They try to find and bring back the lost person and feel ongoing frustration and disappointment when this is not possible.

3. **Disorganization and despair:** Family members feel depressed and find it difficult to plan for the future. They are easily distracted and have difficulty concentrating and focusing.

4. **Reorganization.**

Treatment

Most of the support that people receive after a loss comes from friends and family. Doctors and nurses may also be a source of support. For people who experience difficulty in coping with their loss, grief counseling or grief therapy may be necessary.

Grief counseling helps mourners with normal grief reactions work through the tasks of grieving. Grief counseling can be provided by professionally trained individuals or in self-help groups where bereaved people help other bereaved people. All of these services may be available in individual or group settings.

The goals of grief counseling include helping the bereaved to:

• accept the loss by helping him or her to talk about the loss

- identify and express feelings related to the loss (for example, anger, guilt, anxiety, helplessness, and sadness)

- live without the person who died and to make decisions alone

- separate emotionally from the person who died and to begin new relationships

- find support and time to focus on grieving at important times such as birthdays and anniversaries

- describe normal grieving and the differences in grieving among individuals

- find continuous support

- understand his or her methods of coping

- identify coping problems and making recommendations for professional grief therapy

Grief therapy is used with people who have more serious grief reactions. The goal of grief therapy is to identify and solve problems the mourner may have in separating from the person who died. When separation difficulties occur, they may appear as physical or behavior problems, delayed or extreme mourning, conflicted or extended grief, or unexpected mourning (although this is seldom present with cancer deaths).

Grief therapy may be available as individual or group therapy. A contract is set up with the individual that establishes the time limit of the therapy, the fees, the goals, and the focus of the therapy. In grief therapy, the mourner talks about the deceased and tries to recognize whether he or she is experiencing an expected amount of emotion about the death. Grief therapy may allow the mourner to see that anger, guilt, or other negative or uncomfortable feelings can exist at the same time as more positive feelings about the person who died.

Human beings tend to make strong bonds of affection or attachment with others. When these bonds are broken, as in death, a strong emotional reaction occurs. After a loss occurs, a person must accomplish certain tasks to complete the process of grief. These basic tasks of mourning include accepting that the loss happened, living with and feeling the physical and emotional pain of grief, adjusting to life without the loved one, and emotionally separating from the loved one and going on with life without him or her. It is important that these tasks are completed before mourning can end.

Six Goals of Grief Therapy

1. Develop the ability to experience, express, and adjust to painful grief-related changes.

2. Find effective ways to cope with painful changes.

3. Establish a continuing relationship with the person who died.

4. Stay healthy and keep functioning.

5. Re-establish relationships and understand that others may have difficulty empathizing with the grief they experience.

6. Develop a healthy image of oneself and the world.

Complications in grief may come about due to uncompleted grief from earlier losses. The grief for these earlier losses must be managed in order to handle the current grief. Grief therapy includes dealing with the blockages to the mourning process, identifying unfinished business with the deceased, and identifying other losses that result from the death. The bereaved is helped to see that the loss is final and to picture life after the grief period.

Complicated Grief

Complicated grief reactions require more complex therapies than uncomplicated grief reactions. Adjustment disorders (especially depressed and anxious mood or disturbed emotions and behavior), major depression, substance abuse, and even post-traumatic stress disorder are some of the common problems of complicated bereavement. Complicated grief is identified by the extended length of time of the symptoms, the interference caused by the symptoms, or by the intensity of the symptoms (for example, intense suicidal thoughts or acts).

Complicated or unresolved grief may appear as a complete absence of grief and mourning, an ongoing inability to experience normal grief reactions, delayed grief, conflicted grief, or chronic grief. Factors that contribute to the chance that one may experience complicated grief include the suddenness of the death, the gender of the person in mourning, and the relationship to the deceased (for example, an intense, extremely close, or very contradictory relationship). Grief reactions that turn into major depression should be treated with both drug and psychological therapy. One who avoids any reminders of the person who died, who constantly thinks or dreams about the person who died, and who gets scared and panics easily at any reminders of the person who died may be suffering from post-traumatic stress disorder. Substance abuse may occur in an attempt to avoid painful feelings about the loss or in an attempt to handle symptoms (such as sleeplessness).

Culture and Response to Grief and Mourning

Grief felt for the loss of a loved one, the loss of a treasured possession, or a loss associated with an important life change, occurs across all ages and cultures. However, the role that cultural heritage plays in an individual's experience of grief and mourning is not well understood. Attitudes, beliefs, and practices regarding death must be described according to myths and mysteries surrounding death within different cultures.

Individual, personal experiences of grief are similar in different cultures. This is true even though different cultures have different mourning ceremonies, traditions, and behaviors to express grief. Helping families cope with the death of a loved one includes showing respect for the family's cultural heritage and encouraging them to decide how to honor the death. Important questions that should be asked of people who are dealing with the loss of a loved one include:

- What are the cultural rituals for coping with dying, the deceased person's body, the final arrangements for the body, and honoring the death?
- What are the family's beliefs about what happens after death?
- What does the family feel is a normal expression of grief and the acceptance of the loss?
- What does the family consider to be the roles of each family member in handling the death?
- Are certain types of death less acceptable (for example, suicide), or are certain types of death especially hard to handle for that culture (for example, the death of a child)?

Death, grief, and mourning spare no one and are normal life events. All cultures have developed ways to cope with death. Interfering with these practices may interfere with the necessary grieving processes.

Chapter 59

How to Help Grieving People

What You Can Say, What You Can Do

Relatives, friends and neighbors are supportive at the time of a death, during the wake and funeral. Food, flowers, and physical presence are among the many thoughtful expressions. After the funeral, however, many grieving people wonder what happened to their friends.

They need their support and caring even more when the reality begins to hit and the long process of grief begins. Their help is essential since immediate family members have their hands full of grief and may find it difficult to give support to one another, or may not live nearby. Your help and understanding can make a significant difference in the healing of another's grief.

Unresolved grief can lead to physical or mental illness, suicide, or premature death. A grieving person needs friends willing to cry with them, sit with them, care, listen, have creative ideas for coping, be honest, help them feel loved and needed, and believe they will make it through their grief. Ways of helping grieving people are as limitless as your imagination.

- Read about the various phases of grief so you can understand and help the bereaved to understand.

459

- All that is necessary is a hand squeeze, a kiss, a hug, your presence. If you want to say something, "I'm sorry" or "I care" is sufficient.

- It is not necessary to ask questions about how the death happened. Let the bereaved tell you as much as they want when they are ready. A helpful question might be, "Would you like to talk about the death? I'll listen." Do not say, "I know just how you feel."

- The bereaved may ask "Why?" It is often a cry of pain rather than a question. It is not necessary to answer, but if you do, you may reply, "I don't know why. Maybe we'll never know (this side of heaven)."

- Don't use platitudes like "Life is for living," or "It's God's will." Explanations rarely console. It is better to say nothing.

- Recognize the bereaved may be angry. They may be angry at God, the person who died, the clergy, doctors, rescue teams, or other family members. Encourage them to acknowledge their anger and to find ways of handling it.

- It is good to cry. Crying is a release. People should not say, "Don't cry."

- Be available to listen frequently. Most bereaved want to talk about the person who has died. Encourage them to talk about the deceased. Do not change the conversation or avoid mentioning the person's name. Talking about the pain slowly lessens its sting. Your concern and effort can make a big difference in helping someone recover from grief.

- Be patient. Do not say, "You'll get over it in time." Mourning may take a long time. They will never stop missing the person who has died, but time will soften the hurt. The bereaved need you to stand by them for as long as possible. Encourage them to be patient with themselves as there is no timetable for grieving.

- Offer to help with practical matters such as errands, fixing food, caring for children. Inquire about specific items you could pick up at the store. It is not helpful to say, "Call me if there is anything I can do."

- Accept whatever feelings are expressed. Do not tell people how they should feel or not feel. This attitude puts pressure on the bereaved to push down their feelings. Encourage them to express their feelings—cry, hit a pillow, scream.

- Be aware the average person's self-esteem, on a scale of 100, is in the 70s. A bereaved person's self-esteem may be in the teens or lower.

- When someone feels guilty and is filled with "if only" statements, it merely adds to their negative view of themselves to say, "Don't feel guilty." They would handle it better if they could. Listen with true concern.

- Depression is often part of grief. It is a scary feeling. To be able to talk things over with an understanding friend or loved one is one factor that may help a person not to become severely depressed.

- Give special attention to the children in the family. Do not tell them not to cry or not to upset the adults. Do not shield the children from the grieving of others. It is important to have them express their own feelings, as the adults in the family have their hands full with their own grief.

- Suggest the bereaved person keep a daily journal.

- The bereaved may appear to be getting worse. This is often due to the reality of death hitting them.

- Physical reactions to the death (lack of appetite, sleeplessness, headaches, inability to concentrate) affect a person's coping ability, energy, and recovery.

- Be aware of the use of drugs and alcohol. Often they only delay the grief response. Medication should only be taken under the supervision of a physician.

- Sometimes the pain of bereavement is so intense that thoughts of suicide occur. Do not be shocked, instead try to be a truly confiding friend.

- Do not say, "It has been four months (six months, a year). You must be over it by now." Life will never be the same.

- Encourage counseling if grief is getting out of hand.

- Suggest grieving people take part in support groups such as Hope for Widowed, Hope for Bereaved Parents, and Hope for Survivors, or Those whom Suicide Leaves Behind. Sharing similar experiences helps. Offer to attend a support group meeting with them. The meetings are not morbid. They offer understanding, friendship, and suggestions for coping and hope.

- Suggest major decisions be postponed (moving, or giving everything away) if possible. Later they may regret hasty decisions. It is best to keep decision-making to a minimum.

- Suggest exercise to help work off bottled-up tension and anger, to relax, and to aid sleep. Offer to join them in activities such as tennis, aerobic exercise classes, swimming, or walking.

- Encourage the bereaved to balance life (rest, reading, work, prayer, and recreation).

- Encourage good nutrition. If they have trouble sleeping, suggest avoiding cola, coffee, tea, or aspirin-based remedies containing caffeine.

- Help the bereaved to not have unrealistic expectations as to how they should feel and when they will be better. It is helpful, when appropriate, to say, "I don't know how you do as well as you do."

- Do not avoid the bereaved. It adds to their loss. As the widowed often say, "I not only lost my spouse, but my friends as well."

- Be aware that weekends, holidays, and evenings may be more difficult.

- Consider sending a note at the time of their loved one's birthday, anniversary of death, special days.

- Practice continuing acts of thoughtfulness—a note, visit, plant, helpful book on grief, plate of cookies, phone call, invitation for lunch, dinner, coffee. Take the initiative in calling the bereaved.

Chapter 60

Working through Grief

Helping Yourself through Grief

Grief is experienced whenever you lose something important to you. Grief is so powerful that people sometimes look for ways to go around it rather than experience it. This approach will not work. The best thing you can do for yourself is to work through grief and express your feelings. The following are specific ways to help you work through grief.

Basic Health Concerns

Grief is exhausting and it is important to continue your daily health routines.

1. Try to eat regular, nourishing meals. If it is too difficult to eat three regular meals, try four or five small ones. Have nourishing food available to nibble on rather than chips and candy.

2. Rest is important. Try to develop regular bedtime routines. If you are having a hard time getting to sleep, try a glass of

warm milk or some soft, easy-listening music to soothe your thoughts.

3. Continue your exercise program and develop a manageable routine.

4. Meditation, perhaps in the form of prayer or yoga, can help you get the rest you need.

5. Make sure your family doctor knows what has happened so he or she can help monitor you health.

Outside Support

Grief does not have to be as isolating as it seems.

1. Look for a support group, lecture, or seminar that pertains to your situation.

2. Continue attending church services and stay in contact with this "family," if that has been a source of support to you.

3. Let your friends and other family members know what your emotional or physical needs are. The more they know what to do to help you, the more available they will be.

Feelings

1. Read books or articles of the process of grief so you can identify what you are feeling and have some ideas on how to help yourself.

2. Allow your feelings to be expressed appropriately.

3. Crying is good. You feel lighter after you have had a good cry. Consider sharing your tears with other loved ones. We laugh together; why not cry together as well?

4. Find friends or family members to share your feelings with.

5. Be careful not to use alcohol, drugs, or tranquilizers. These will only mask the pain and could lead to problems.

6. Keeping a journal is a good way to identify feelings and also to see progress.

7. Holidays and anniversaries need special planning. They are impossible to ignore. Look for a workshop on dealing with the holidays and make plans with your family and friends.

Be Kind to Yourself

1. If you desire some alone time, take it as often as you need to.

2. Give yourself rewards along the way as something to look forward to.

3. Look for small ways to pamper yourself, such as bubble baths, new cologne, soft pajamas, or a new hair cut.

4. A short trip can be a good break from grief, but be aware that upon your return, the pain of grief will be waiting for you. However, you will have had a rest and the knowledge that you can enjoy some things in life again.

5. Look for some new interests, perhaps a new hobby or resuming an old one.

6. Carry a special letter, poem, or quote with you to read when the going gets tough.

7. Try to enjoy the good days and don't feel guilty for doing so.

8. Reach out to help someone else.

9. Learn to have patience with yourself. Remember, grief takes time.

10. Know that you will get better and there will be a time when you can look forward to getting up in the morning and be glad you are alive.

Help for Your Marriage and Relationships

1. Good communication is necessary. People cannot read your mind. They may not know that this particular day is difficult or they may not know how to help you.

2. Talk about what is helpful to you and what is not helpful to you.

3. Be sensitive to the needs of your partner. Grief is different for each person.

4. By reviewing past losses together, you can understand how your partner may react to the recent one.

5. Avoid competition in who is hurting most. Each person will have difficult issues to cope with. Grief is hard for everybody.

6. Consult each other regarding birthdays, holidays, and anniversaries. It is a mistake to hope the holiday will slip by unnoticed. Make plans and discuss them.

7. Try not to expect too much from your partner. People do not operate at 100 percent during the grieving period. The dishes may not get done or the yard may not be mown as regularly as before. Many chores can wait. Hire someone to help you catch-up.

8. Read and educate yourself about the grief process. Go to the library and get an armload of books. Read ones in which you feel the author is speaking to you and return the others. Grief books do not need to be read cover to cover. Look for a book with a detailed table of contents that will enable you to select certain parts as you need them.

9. Consider the gender differences. Men and women grieve differently. Usually women are more comfortable expressing their emotions. Men often get busy, burying themselves at work or taking on projects at home.

10. Avoid pressuring your partner about decisions that can wait. Of course, some decisions cannot be postponed, and those will have to be dealt with. However, many can be put off for a day or a week or even longer.

11. Take a short trip to re-group. If a child has died, it is very important to re-acquaint yourself with the new family structure. Getting away from the telephone and memories for a few days can help you do this.

12. Seek professional guidance, especially if you feel your loss is interfering with your marriage or relationships.

© 2000 American Hospice Foundation. All Rights Reserved. Despite the date of this document, the guidelines described are deemed pertinent.

You Know You Are Getting Better When...

The progress through grief is so slow and so often of a "one-step forward and two-steps backwards" motion, that it is difficult to see signs of improvement. The following are clues that will help you to see that you are beginning to work through your grief:

- You are in touch with the finality of the death. You now know in your heart that your loved one is truly gone and will never return to this earth.

- You can review both pleasant and unpleasant memories. In early grief, memories are painful because they remind you of how much you have lost. Now it feels good to remember, and you look for people to share memories with.

- You can enjoy time alone and feel comfortable. You no longer need to have someone with you all the time or look for activities to keep you distracted.

- You can drive somewhere by yourself without crying the whole time. Driving seems to be a place where many people cry, which can be dangerous for you and other drivers.

- You are less sensitive to some of the comments people make. You realize that painful comments made by family or friends are made in ignorance.

- You look forward to holidays. Once dreaded occasions can now be anticipated with excitement, perhaps through returning to old traditions or creating new ones.

- You can reach out to help someone else in a similar situation. It is healing to be able to use your experience to help others.

- The music you shared with the one you lost is no longer painful to hear. Now, you may even find it comforting.

- You can sit through a church service without crying.

- Some time passes in which you have not thought of your loved one. When this first happens, you may panic, thinking, "I am forgetting." This is not true. You will never forget. You are giving yourself permission to go on with your life and your loved one would want you to do this.

- You can enjoy a good joke and have a good laugh without feeling guilty.

- Your eating, sleeping, and exercise patterns return to what they were beforehand.

- You no longer feel tired all the time.

- You have developed a routine or a new schedule in your daily life that does not include your loved one.

- You can concentrate on a book or favorite television program. You can even retain information you have just read or viewed.

- You no longer have to make daily or weekly trips to the cemetery. You now feel comfortable going once a month or only on holidays or other special occasions.

- You can find something to be thankful for. You always knew there were good things going on in your life, but they didn't matter much before.

- You can establish new and healthy relationships. New friends are now part of your life, and you enjoy participating in activities with them.

- You feel confident again. You are in touch with your new identity and have a stronger sense of what you are going to do with the rest of your life.

- You can organize and plan your future.

- You can accept things as they are and not keep trying to return things to what they were.

- You have patience with yourself through grief attacks. You know they are becoming further apart and less frightening and painful.

- You look forward to getting up in the morning.

- You stop to smell the flowers along the way and enjoy experiences in life that are meant to be enjoyed.

- The vacated roles that your loved one filled in your life are now being filled by yourself or others. When a loved one dies he or she leaves many holes in your life. Now those holes are being filled with other people and activities, although some will remain empty. You are more at ease with these changes.

- You can take the energy and time spent thinking about your loss and put those energies elsewhere, perhaps by helping others in similar situations or making concrete plans with your own life.

- You acknowledge your new life and even discover personal growth from experiencing grief.

Additional Information

American Hospice Foundation
2120 L Street N.W., Suite 200
Washington, DC 20037
Phone: 202-223-0204
Fax: 202-223-0208
Website: http://www.americanhospice.org
E-mail: ahf@americanhospice.org

Part Nine

Mortality Statistics

Chapter 61

Global Mortality Trends

Chapter Contents

Section 61.1

Life Expectancy Improves—But Not for All

Excerpted from "The World Health Report: 2003: Shaping the Future."
© 2003 World Health Organization. Reprinted with permission.

Over the past fifty years, average life expectancy at birth has increased globally by almost 20 years, from 46.5 years in 1950–1955 to 65.2 years in 2002. This represents a global average increase in life expectancy of four months per year across this period. On average, the gain in life expectancy was nine years in developed countries (including Australia, European countries, Japan, New Zealand and North America), 17 years in the high-mortality developing countries (with high child and adult mortality levels), including most African countries and poorer countries in Asia, the Eastern Mediterranean Region, and Latin America; and 26 years in the low-mortality developing countries. The large life expectancy gap between the developed and developing countries in the 1950s has changed to a large gap between the high-mortality developing countries and others.

Life expectancy at birth in 2002 ranged from 78 years for women in developed countries to less than 46 years for men in sub-Saharan Africa, a 1.7-fold difference in total life expectancy. Exceptions to the life expectancy increases in most regions of the world in the last fifty years are Africa and countries of eastern Europe formerly in the Soviet Union. In the latter case, male and female life expectancies at birth declined, by 2.9 years and one year, respectively, over the period 1990 to 2000.

The increases in life expectancy that occurred in the first half of the 20th century in developed countries were the result of rapid declines in mortality, particularly infant and maternal mortality and that caused by infectious diseases in childhood and early adulthood. Access to better housing, sanitation and education, a trend to smaller families, growing incomes, and public health measures such as immunization against infectious diseases all contributed greatly to this epidemiological transition. In many developed countries, this shift started approximately 100 to 150 years ago. In a number of countries, such as Japan, the transition started later but proceeded much more quickly. In many developing countries, the transition started even later and has not yet been completed. In developed countries, improvements in life expectancy now come mainly from reductions in death rates among adults.

Global Mortality Patterns

Almost 57 million people died in 2002, 10.5 million (or nearly 20%) of whom were children of less than five years of age. Of these child deaths, 98% occurred in developing countries. Over 60% of deaths in developed countries occur beyond age 70, compared with about 30% in developing countries. A key point is the comparatively high number of deaths in developing countries at younger adult ages (15–59 years). Just over 30% of all deaths in developing countries occur at these ages, compared with 20% in richer regions. This vast premature adult mortality in developing countries is a major public health concern.

Developing countries themselves are a very heterogeneous group in terms of mortality. A contrast between low-mortality developing countries such as China (with more than one-sixth of the world's population) and high-mortality countries in Africa (with one-tenth of the global population) illustrates the extreme diversity in health conditions among developing countries. Less than 10% of deaths in China occur below five years of age compared with 40% in Africa. Conversely, 48% of deaths in China occur beyond age 70, compared with only 10% in Africa.

Although risk of death is the simplest comparable measure of health status for populations, there has been increasing interest in describing, measuring, and comparing health states of populations. Mortality statistics, in particular, substantially underestimate the burden from noncommunicable adult disease because they exclude non-fatal health outcomes such as depression and visual impairment. A useful method of formulating a composite summary of disease burden is to calculate disability-adjusted life years (DALYs), which combine years of life lost (YLLs) through premature death with years lived with disability (YLDs). One DALY can be thought of as one lost year of healthy life and the measured disease burden is the gap between a population's health status and that of a normative global reference population with high life expectancy lived in full health. In terms of DALYs, 36% of total lost years of healthy life for the world in 2002 were a result of disease and injury in children aged less than 15 years, and almost 50% as a result of disease and injury in adults aged 15–59 years.

473

Child survival continues to be a major focus of the international health agenda for developing countries. Nearly 90% of global deaths under age 15 occur before the age of five. In contrast, the international effort to understand the magnitude of challenges to adult health in developing countries is still in its early stages. Even at present, there remains a perception that adult health is of great concern only in wealthy countries, where premature mortality among children has been substantially reduced. However there is a high proportion of burden of disease and injury suffered by adults in developing countries, a growing burden that requires urgent action by the global public health community.

Section 61.2

Surviving the First Five Years of Life

Excerpted from "The World Health Report: 2003: Shaping the Future."
© 2003 World Health Organization. Reprinted with permission.

Although approximately 10.5 million children under five years of age still die every year in the world, progress has been made since 1970, when the figure was more than 17 million. These reductions did not take place uniformly across time and regions, but the success stories in developing countries demonstrate clearly that low mortality levels are attainable in those settings. The effects of such achievements are not to be underestimated. If the whole world were able to share the current child mortality experience of Iceland (the lowest in the world in 2002), over 10 million child deaths could be prevented each year.

Today nearly all child deaths occur in developing countries, almost half of them in Africa. While some African countries have made considerable strides in reducing child mortality, the majority of African children live in countries where the survival gains of the past have been wiped out, largely as a result of the human immunodeficiency virus/acquired immune deficiency syndrome (HIV/AIDS) epidemic.

Across the world, children are at higher risk of dying if they are poor. The most impressive declines in child mortality have occurred in developed countries, and in low-mortality developing countries whose economic situation has improved. In contrast, the declines observed in countries with higher mortality have occurred at a slower rate, stagnated, or even reversed. Owing to the overall gains in developing regions, the mortality gap between the developing and developed world has narrowed since 1970. However, because the better-off countries in developing regions are improving at a fast rate, and many of the poorer populations are losing ground, the disparity between the different developing regions is widening.

Child Mortality: Global Contrasts

Regional child mortality levels are indicated in Table 61.1. Of the 20 countries in the world with the highest child mortality (probability of death under five years of age), 19 are in Africa, the exception being Afghanistan.

Table 61.1. Child Mortality in the Six WHO Regions, 2002

Region	Deaths per 1,000 live births
Africa	168
Americas	25
South-East Asia	80
Europe	20
Eastern Mediterranean	92
Western Pacific	36
World	80

A baby born in Sierra Leone is three and a half times more likely to die before its fifth birthday than a child born in India, and more than a hundred times more likely to die than a child born in Iceland or Singapore. Fifteen countries, mainly European but including Japan and Singapore, had child mortality rates in 2002 of less than five per 1000 live births.

Child Mortality: Gender and Socioeconomic Differences

Throughout the world, child mortality is higher in males than in females, with only a few exceptions. In China, India, Nepal, and Pakistan, mortality in girls exceeds that of boys. This disparity is particularly noticeable in China, where girls have a 33% higher risk of dying than their male counterparts. These inequities are thought to arise from the preferential treatment of boys in family health care-seeking behavior and in nutrition.

There is considerable variability in child mortality across different income groups within countries. Data collected by 106 demographic and health surveys in more than 60 countries show that children from poor households have a significantly higher risk of dying before the age of five years than the children of richer households. The identification of poor and non-poor populations uses a global scale based on an estimate of permanent income constructed from information on ownership of assets, availability of services, and household characteristics. This approach has the advantage of allowing comparison of socioeconomic levels across countries. It implies that the individuals defined as poor in Bangladesh have the same economic status as the population defined as poor in Bolivia or Niger.

There are significant differences in child mortality risks by poverty status in all countries, although the size of the gap varies; the risk of dying in childhood is approximately 13 percentage points higher for the poor than for the non-poor in Niger but less than 3 percentage points higher in Bangladesh.

Child mortality rates among the poor are much higher in Africa than in any other region despite the same level of income used to define poverty. The probability of poor children in Africa dying is almost twice that of poor children in the Americas. Likewise, better-off children in Africa have double the probability of dying than their counterparts in the Americas. Moreover, better-off children in Africa have a higher mortality risk (16%) than poor children in the Americas, whose risk of death is 14%.

Child Survival: Improvements for Some

The last three decades have witnessed considerable gains in child survival worldwide. Global child mortality decreased from 147 per 1000 live births in 1970 to about 80 per 1000 live births in 2002. The reduction in child mortality has been particularly compelling in certain countries of the Eastern Mediterranean and South-East Asia Regions, and Latin America, while that of African countries was more modest. Gains in child survival have also occurred in rich industrialized nations, where levels of mortality were already low.

Although child mortality has fallen in most regions of the world, the gains were not consistent across time and regions. The greatest reductions in child mortality across the world occurred 20–30 years ago, though not in the African or the Western Pacific Regions, where the decline slowed down during the 1980s, nor in some eastern European countries, where mortality actually increased in the 1970s. Over the past decade, only countries of the South-East Asia Region and the higher mortality countries in Latin America have further accelerated their reduction in child mortality.

The most impressive gains in child survival over the past 30 years occurred in developing countries where child mortality was already relatively low, whereas countries with the highest rates had a less pronounced decline. Despite an overall decline in global child mortality over the past three decades, the gap between and within developing regions has widened.

Although the chances of child survival among less developed regions of the world are becoming increasingly disparate, the gaps in child mortality among affluent nations have been closing over the past 30 years, largely as a result of medical-technological advances, particularly in the area of neonatal survival.

In 16 countries (14 of which are in Africa) current levels of under-five mortality are higher than those observed in 1990. In nine countries (eight of which are in Africa) current levels exceed even those observed over two decades ago. HIV/AIDS has played a large part in these reversals.

Analyses from the demographic and health surveys show that while child mortality has increased in many of the African countries surveyed, the gap between poor and non-poor populations has remained constant over time in this setting. In contrast, there has been a widening of the mortality gap between poor and better-off groups in the Americas, where overall child mortality rates have fallen. This indicates that survival gains in many regions have benefited the better-off. The reduction in child mortality has been much slower in rural areas, where poor people are concentrated, than in urban areas. These analyses suggest that health interventions implemented in the past decade have not been effective in reaching poor people.

Losses in child survival in the countries described are at odds with impressive gains in some African countries. Despite the ravages of the HIV/AIDS epidemic in Africa, eight countries in the region have reduced child mortality by more than 50% since 1970. Among these are Gabon, Gambia, and Ghana.

Overall, at least 169 countries, 112 of them developing countries, have shown a decline in child mortality since 1970. Oman has had the most striking reduction, from 242 per 1000 live births in 1970 to its current rate of 15 per 1000 live births, which is lower than that of many countries in Europe. Overall, the lower mortality countries of the Eastern Mediterranean Region experienced an impressive decline in child mortality, which has been accompanied by a reduction in the gap between countries' child mortality levels since 1970.

Child mortality has also declined substantially in the Americas. The most striking proportional reductions in mortality have been seen in Chile, Costa Rica, and Cuba, where child mortality has decreased by over 80% since 1970. There have also been large absolute reductions in child mortality in Bolivia, Nicaragua, and Peru. In contrast, Haitian child mortality rates are still 133 per 1000: almost double the mortality rate of Bolivia, the next highest country in the Americas.

An interesting pattern of child mortality trends has been observed in several eastern European countries. Here, child mortality initially increased or remained constant during the 1970s, only to decline after 1980. This may to some extent be attributed to a more complete registration of child and infant deaths during that period. Interestingly, while adult mortality levels increased in the early 1990s, child mortality continued to decline. There is no other region where this particular pattern of mortality has occurred in such a systematic manner, and the reasons for the trend remain poorly understood.

Causes of Death in Children

Infectious and parasitic diseases remain the major killers of children in the developing world, partly as a result of the HIV/AIDS epidemic. Although notable success has been achieved in certain areas (for example, polio), communicable diseases still represent seven out of the top 10 causes of child deaths, and account for about 60% of all child deaths. Overall, the 10 leading causes represent 86% of all child deaths.

Many countries of the Eastern Mediterranean Region and in Latin America and Asia have partly shifted towards the cause-of-death pattern observed in developed countries. Here, conditions arising in the perinatal period, including birth asphyxia, birth trauma, and low birth weight, have replaced infectious diseases as the leading cause of death and are now responsible for one-fifth to one-third of deaths. Such a shift in the cause-of-death pattern has not occurred in sub-Saharan Africa, where perinatal conditions rank in fourth place. Here, undernutrition, malaria, lower respiratory tract infections, and diarrheal diseases continue to be among the leading causes of death in children, accounting for 45% of all deaths.

About 90% of all HIV/AIDS and malaria deaths in children in developing countries occur in sub-Saharan Africa, where 23% of the world's births and 42% of the world's child deaths are observed. The immense surge of HIV/AIDS mortality in children in recent years means that HIV/AIDS is now responsible for 332,000 child deaths in sub-Saharan Africa, nearly 8% of all child deaths in the region.

There are 14 countries in WHO's African Region in which child mortality has risen since reaching its lowest level in 1990. About 34% of the population under five years of age in sub-Saharan Africa is now exposed to this disturbing trend. Only two countries outside Africa observed similar setbacks in the same period—countries that experienced armed conflict or economic sanctions. Eight of the 14 countries are in southern Africa, which boasted some of the most notable gains in child survival during the 1970s and 1980s. Those promising gains have been wiped out in a mere decade.

The indirect effects of HIV/AIDS in adults contribute to the tragedy. Children who lose their mothers to HIV/AIDS are more likely to die than children with living mothers, irrespective of their own HIV status. The diversion of already stretched health resources away from child health programs into care of people living with AIDS further compounds the situation, in the presence of increasing malaria mortality, civil unrest, or social anarchy.

Table 61.2. Leading Causes of Death in Children in Developing Countries, 2002

Rank	Cause	Numbers (000)	% of all deaths
1	Perinatal conditions	2,375	23.1
2	Lower respiratory infections	1,856	18.1
3	Diarrheal diseases	1,566	15.2
4	Malaria	1,098	10.7
5	Measles	551	5.4
6	Congenital anomalies	386	3.8
7	HIV/AIDS	370	3.6
8	Pertussis	301	2.9
9	Tetanus	185	1.8
10	Protein-energy malnutrition	138	1.3
	Other causes	1,437	14.0
	Total	10,263	100

Some progress has been observed in the areas of diarrheal diseases and measles. While incidence is thought to have remained stable, mortality from diarrheal diseases has fallen from 2.5 million deaths in 1990 to about 1.6 million deaths in 2002, now accounting for 15% of all child deaths. There has also been a modest decline in deaths from measles, although more than half a million children under five years of age still succumb to the disease every year. Malaria causes around a million child deaths per year, of which 90% are children under five years of age. In this age group the disease accounts for nearly 11% of all deaths.

The overall number of child deaths in India has fallen from approximately 3.5 million in 1990 to approximately 2.3 million in 2002. This impressive decline is a result of a reduction in overall child mortality rates of about 30%, and a decline in total fertility rates of around 10%. The cause-of-death pattern has remained fairly stable, with the exception of perinatal conditions whose proportion has notably increased. There were some declines in the proportion of deaths from diarrheal diseases, measles, and tetanus, which may be the result of increased use of oral rehydration therapy and improved coverage of routine vaccination, as well as intensive immunization campaigns.

A similar picture is emerging in China, where the number of child deaths has decreased by 30% since 1990, owing to a reduction in child mortality of 18% and a 6% decline in total fertility. As in India, the most notable change in the cause-of-death pattern in China over the past decade is an increase in the proportion of perinatal deaths.

The challenge of reducing child mortality is widely recognized and effective interventions are available. The issue now is urgent implementation.

Section 61.3

Adult Mortality Rates and Patterns

Excerpted from "The World Health Report: 2003: Shaping the Future."
© 2003 World Health Organization. Reprinted with permission.

Adult Health at Risk: Slowing Gains and Widening Gaps

Adult mortality rates have been declining in recent decades in most regions of the world. Life expectancy at age 15 has increased by between two and three years for most regions over the last 20 years. The notable exceptions are the high-mortality countries in Africa, where life expectancy at age 15 decreased by nearly 7 years between 1980 and 2002, and the high-mortality countries, mainly those of the former Soviet Union, in eastern Europe, where life expectancy at age 15 decreased over the same period by 4.2 years for males and 1.6 years for females.

Of the 45 million deaths among adults aged 15 years and over in 2002, 32 million, or almost three-quarters, were caused by noncommunicable diseases which killed almost four times as many people as communicable diseases and maternal, perinatal, and nutritional conditions combined (8.2 million, or 18% of all causes). Injuries killed a further 4.5 million adults in 2002—one in 10 of the total adult deaths. More than 3 million of these injury deaths—almost 70% of them—concern males, whose higher risk is most pronounced for road traffic injuries (three times higher) and for violence and war (more than four times higher). The relative importance of these causes varies markedly across regions. Thus in Africa, only about one in three adult deaths is caused by noncommunicable diseases, compared with nearly nine out of ten in developed countries. It is of concern that three in four adult deaths in Latin America and in the developing countries of Asia and the Western Pacific Region are caused by noncommunicable disease, reflecting the relatively advanced stage of the epidemiological transition achieved in these populations and the emergence of the double burden of disease.

481

Global Patterns of Premature Mortality Risk

The probability of premature adult death varies widely between regions. For example, the probability of premature adult death in some parts of sub-Saharan Africa is much higher—nearly four times higher—than that observed in low-mortality countries of the Western Pacific Region. Even within developed regions there are wide variations. Men in some eastern European countries are three to four times more likely to die prematurely than men in other developed regions. Furthermore, male adult mortality in eastern Europe is much greater than in developing countries of the Americas, Asia, and the Eastern Mediterranean Region. In all regions, male mortality is higher than female, and the discrepancy between the two sexes in mortality risk is much larger than that seen among children. The variation in the proportion of women dying prematurely is much less dramatic.

Adult Mortality Trends: 15–59 Years of Age

There have been impressive gains in the health status of adults worldwide in the past five decades. The risk of death between ages 15 and 60 has declined substantially from a global average of 354 per 1000 in 1955, to 207 per 1000 in 2002. The recent slowdown in the rate of decline is a clear warning that continued reductions in adult mortality, particularly in developing countries, will not be easily achieved.

There is substantial variation in the pace and magnitude of declining trends in premature adult mortality across both sexes and global regions. The global slowdown of the pace is primarily a result of a shift in trends in adult mortality in a few regions. Among the signs of deteriorating adult health, the most disturbing is the fact that adult mortality in Africa has reversed, shifting in 1990 from a state of steady decline into a situation characterized by rapidly increasing mortality. The reversal in parts of sub-Saharan Africa has been so drastic that current adult mortality rates today exceed the levels of three decades ago. In Zimbabwe, upturns in reported adult deaths were significantly greater in 1991–1995 than in 1986–1990. Older childhood and older adult mortality have changed little. Without human immunodeficiency virus/acquired immune deficiency syndrome (HIV/AIDS), life expectancy at birth in the African Region would have been almost 6.1 years higher in 2002. The reduction in life expectancy varies significantly across the African Region. The greatest impact has been in Botswana,

Lesotho, Swaziland, and Zimbabwe where HIV/AIDS has reduced male and female life expectancies by more than 20 years.

The fragile state of adult health in the face of social, economic, and political instability is also apparent in regions outside Africa. Male mortality in some countries in eastern Europe has increased substantially and is approaching the level of adult mortality in some African countries. As a result, for the European Region as a whole, average adult mortality risk for men between 15 and 60 years is 230 per 1000, which is similar to the rate observed in the 1980s. This contrasts with the continuously declining trend for women in this region as a whole. Their risk has declined from 130 in 1970, to 98 in 2002. The probability of death from injury among adults aged 15–59 years in the high-mortality countries of eastern Europe is nearly six times higher than in neighboring western European countries.

Adult Mortality: Widening Gaps

Continuously declining adult mortality in low-mortality regions, combined with trend reversals in high-mortality areas, have resulted in widening gaps in adult mortality worldwide. The gap between the lowest and highest regional adult mortality risk between ages 15 and 60 has now increased to a level of 340 per 1000 in 2002. Regional aggregation of adult mortality also hides enormous and sobering disparities between countries. For example, within the Eastern Mediterranean Region, adult mortality risk between ages 15 and 60 among women in Djibouti was seven times higher than that of women in Kuwait in 2002. Overall, there is an almost 12-fold difference between the world's lowest and highest adult mortality at country level.

HIV/AIDS: The Leading Health Threat

Tables 61.3 and 61.4 show the leading causes of death and DALYs among adults worldwide for 2002. Despite global trends of declining communicable disease burden in adults, HIV/AIDS has become the leading cause of mortality and the single most important contributor to the burden of disease among adults aged 15–59 years.

Nearly 80% of the almost 3 million global deaths from HIV/AIDS in 2002 occurred in sub-Saharan Africa. As stated earlier, HIV/AIDS is the leading cause of death in this region. It causes more than 6000 deaths every day and accounts for one in two deaths of adults aged 15–59 years. It has reversed mortality trends among adults in this region and turned previous gains in life expectancy into a continuous decline in life expectancy since 1990.

Mortality and Disease among Older Adults

In developing countries, 42% of adult deaths occur after 60 years of age, compared with 78% in developed countries. Globally, 60-year-olds have a 55% chance of dying before their 80th birthday. Regional variations in risk of death at older ages are smaller, ranging from around

Table 61.3. Leading Causes of Mortality among Adults Aged 15–59

Rank	Cause	Deaths (000)
1	HIV/AIDS	2279
2	Ischemic heart disease	1332
3	Tuberculosis	1036
4	Road traffic injuries	814
5	Cerebrovascular disease	783
6	Self-inflicted injuries	672
7	Violence	473
8	Cirrhosis of the liver	382
9	Lower respiratory infections	352
10	Chronic obstructive pulmonary disease	343

Table 61.4. Leading Causes of Mortality among Adults Aged 60 and Older

Rank	Cause	Deaths (000)
1	Ischemic heart disease	5825
2	Cerebrovascular disease	4689
3	Chronic obstructive pulmonary disease	2399
4	Lower respiratory infections	1396
5	Trachea, bronchus, lung cancers	928
6	Diabetes mellitus	754
7	Hypertensive heart disease	735
8	Stomach cancer	605
9	Tuberculosis	495
10	Colon and rectum cancers	477

40% in the developed countries of western Europe to 60% in most developing regions and 70% in Africa. Historical data from countries such as Australia and Sweden show that life expectancy at age 60 changed slowly during the first six to seven decades of the 20th century but, since around 1970, has started to increase substantially. Life expectancy at age 60 has now reached 25 years in Japan. From 1990 onwards, eastern European countries such as Hungary and Poland have started to experience similar improvements in mortality for older people, but others, such as the Russian Federation, have not, and are experiencing worsening trends. The leading causes of mortality and burden of disease in older people have not changed greatly over the past decade.

With old-age dependency ratios increasing in virtually all countries of the world, the economic contributions and productive roles of older people will assume greater importance. Supporting people to remain healthy and ensure a good quality of life in their later years is one of the greatest challenges for the health sector in both developed and developing countries.

Cardiovascular diseases account for 13% of the disease burden among adults over 15 years of age. Ischemic heart disease and cerebrovascular disease (stroke) are the two leading causes of mortality and disease burden among older adults (over age 60). In developed countries, ischemic heart disease and cerebrovascular disease are together responsible for 36% of deaths, and death rates are higher for men than women. The increase in cardiovascular mortality in eastern European countries has been offset by continuing declines in many other developed countries. In contrast, the mortality and burden resulting from cardiovascular diseases are rapidly increasing in developing regions.

Of the 7.1 million cancer deaths estimated to have occurred in 2002, 17% were attributable to lung cancer alone and of these, three-quarters occurred among men. There were an estimated 1.2 million lung cancer deaths in 2000, an increase of nearly 30% in the 10 years from 1990, reflecting the emergence of the tobacco epidemic in low-income and middle-income countries. Stomach cancer, which until recently was the leading cause of cancer mortality worldwide, has been declining in all parts of the world where trends can be reliably assessed, and now causes 850 000 deaths each year, or about two-thirds as many as lung cancer. Liver and colon/rectum cancers are the third and fourth leading causes. More than half of all liver cancer deaths are estimated to occur in the Western Pacific Region. Among women, the leading cause of cancer deaths is breast cancer. During the past decade, breast cancer survival rates have been improving, though the chance of survival varies according to factors such as coverage and access to secondary prevention.

Conclusion

This chapter is a reminder that children are among the most vulnerable members of societies around the world. Despite considerable achievements, much still needs to be done, urgently, to avert child deaths from preventable causes. The success stories in many poor countries in all regions demonstrate clearly that much progress can be made with limited resources. Tragically, many other countries, particularly in Africa, have lost the ground gained in previous decades. The gaps in mortality between rich and poor populations are widening, leaving 7% of the world's children and 35% of Africa's children at higher risk of death today than they were 10 years ago.

In the last five decades, there have been impressive gains in adult health status worldwide. The average figures, however, mask disparities in population health. Of great concern are the reversals in adult mortality in the 1990s in sub-Saharan Africa caused by HIV/AIDS and in parts of eastern Europe attributable to a number of noncommunicable diseases (particularly cardiovascular and alcohol-related diseases) and injuries.

Demographic trends and health transitions, along with changes in the distribution of risk factors, have accelerated the epidemic of noncommunicable disease in many developing countries. Infectious diseases such as HIV/AIDS and tuberculosis have serious socioeconomic consequences in both the developed and the developing worlds. Thus, the majority of developing countries are facing a double burden from both communicable and noncommunicable diseases. In addition, contrary to common perceptions, disabilities tend to be more prevalent in developing regions, as the disease burden is often skewed towards highly vulnerable sub-populations. The global public health community is now faced with a more complex and diverse pattern of adult disease than previously expected. It has been estimated that 47% of premature deaths and 39% of the total disease burden result from 20 leading risk factors for childhood and adult diseases and injuries and that removal of these risks would increase global healthy life expectancy by 9.3 years, ranging from 4.4 years in industrialized countries of the Western Pacific Region to 16.1 years in parts of sub-Saharan Africa.

Historically unprecedented increases in life expectancy at older ages in developed countries have already exceeded earlier predictions of maximum population life expectancy. With such increases, the nonfatal burden of disease plays an increasingly important role, and it will be a major goal of health policy worldwide to ensure that longer life is accompanied by greater health and less disability.

Chapter 62

Mortality Trends in the United States

Health Status and Its Determinants

Life expectancy in the United States continues to show a long-term upward trend, although the most dramatic increases were in the early part of the 20th century. In 2003, American men could expect to live three years longer, and women more than one year longer, than they did in 1990. Infant mortality and mortality from heart disease, stroke, and cancer continued to decline in recent years. In 2002 the infant mortality rate in the United States increased for the first time since 1958; preliminary data indicate a small, but not statistically significant, decline in 2003.

Of particular concern in recent years has been the increase in overweight and obesity, which are risk factors for many chronic diseases and disabilities including heart disease, hypertension, and back pain. The rising number of children and adolescents who are overweight, and the high percentage of Americans who are not physically active raise additional concerns about Americans' future health.

Decreased cigarette smoking among adults is a prime example of a trend that has contributed to overall declines in mortality. However, the rapid drop in cigarette smoking in the two decades following the first Surgeon General's Report in 1964 has slowed in recent years. About 24 percent of men and 19 percent of women were current smokers in 2003. Prevalence of risky behaviors has also improved over time,

Excerpts from *Health, United States, 2005*, Centers for Disease Control and Prevention (CDC), DHHS Publication No. 2005–1232, November 2005.

including the percent of high school students in grades 9–12 who rode with a driver who had been drinking alcohol. This statistic decreased from 40 percent to 30 percent between 1991 and 2003, yet further reductions are certainly necessary.

Disparities in Risk Factors, Access, and Utilization

Efforts to improve Americans' health in the 21st century will be shaped by important changes in demographics. Ours is a Nation that is growing older and becoming more racially and ethnically diverse. In 2004 nearly one-third of adults and about two-fifths of children were identified as black, Hispanic, Asian, or American Indian, or Alaska Native. Fourteen percent of Americans in 2004 identified themselves as Hispanic, twelve percent as black, and four percent as Asian.

Health, United States, 2005, identifies major disparities in health and health care that exist by socioeconomic status, race, ethnicity, and insurance status. Persons living in poverty are considerably more likely to be in fair or poor health and to have disabling conditions, and less likely to have used many types of health care.

Large disparities in infant mortality rates remain among racial and ethnic groups. The gap in life expectancy between the black and white populations has narrowed, but persists. Disparities in risk factors, access to health care, and morbidity also remain. Hispanic and American Indian persons under 65 years are more likely to be uninsured than those in other racial and ethnic groups. Obesity, a major risk factor for many chronic diseases, varies by race and ethnicity. In 2003, the rate of recent mammogram screening for white and black women was similar, but rates for Asian and Hispanic women remained at a lower level.

Many aspects of the health of the Nation have improved, but the health of some racial and ethnic groups has improved less than others. The large differences in health status by race and Hispanic origin documented may be explained by factors including socioeconomic status, health practices, psychosocial stress and resources, environmental exposures, discrimination, and access to health care. Socioeconomic and cultural differences among racial and ethnic groups in the United States will likely continue to influence future patterns of disease, disability, and health care use.

Mortality Trends

In 2003, the preliminary infant mortality rate was 6.9 infant deaths per 1,000 live births, similar to the rate in 2002 (7.0 per 1,000). In

2002, the infant mortality rate increased for the first time in more than 40 years. The rise in infant mortality in 2002 was concentrated among neonatal deaths occurring in the first week of life, due largely to an increase in the number of infants born weighing less than 750 grams (1 pound 10.5 ounces).

Between 1950 and 2003 the age-adjusted death rate for the total population declined 43 percent to 831 deaths per 100,000 population (preliminary data). This reduction was driven largely by declines in mortality from heart disease, stroke, and unintentional injury.

Mortality from heart disease, the leading cause of death, declined almost four percent in 2003 (preliminary data), continuing a long-term downward trend. The 2003 age-adjusted death rate for heart disease was 60 percent lower than the rate in 1950.

Mortality from cancer, the second leading cause of death, decreased more than two percent in 2003 (preliminary data), continuing the decline that began in 1990. Overall cancer age-adjusted death rates rose from 1960 to 1990 and then reversed direction.

Mortality from stroke, the third leading cause of death, declined almost five percent in 2003 (preliminary data). Between 1950 and 2003, the age-adjusted death rate for stroke declined 70 percent.

In 2003, mortality from chronic lower respiratory diseases (CLRD), the fourth leading cause of death, decreased almost five percent from its peak in 1999 (preliminary data). Age-adjusted death rates for CLRD generally rose between 1980 and 1999, mainly as a result of steadily increasing death rates for females, most noticeably for females age 55 years and over.

Mortality from unintentional injuries, the fifth leading cause of death, decreased more than two percent in 2003 (preliminary data). Age-adjusted death rates for unintentional injuries generally declined from 1950 until 1992 and then increased slightly.

Disparities in Mortality

As overall death rates have declined, racial and ethnic disparities in mortality persist, but the gap in life expectancy between the black and white populations has narrowed. Disparities in mortality also persist among persons of different education levels.

Large disparities in infant mortality rates among racial and ethnic groups continue. In 2002, infant mortality rates were highest for infants of non-Hispanic black mothers (13.9 deaths per 1,000 live births), Hawaiian mothers (9.6 per 1,000), American Indian mothers (8.6 per 1,000), and Puerto Rican mothers (8.2 per 1,000), and lowest for infants of mothers of Chinese origin (3.0 per 1,000 live births) and Cuban mothers (3.7 per 1,000).

Infant mortality increases as mother's level of education decreases among infants of mothers 20 years of age and over. In 2002 the mortality rate for infants of mothers with less than 12 years of education was 58 percent higher than for infants of mothers with 13 or more years of education. This disparity was more marked among non-Hispanic white infants, for whom mortality among infants of mothers with less than a high school education was more than twice that for infants of mothers with more than a high school education.

Between 1990 and 2003, life expectancy at birth increased 3.0 years for males and 1.3 years for females (preliminary data). The gap in life expectancy between males and females narrowed from 7.0 years in 1990 to 5.3 years in 2003.

Between 1990 and 2003, mortality from lung cancer declined for men and increased for women. Although these trends reduced the sex differential for this cause of death, the age-adjusted death rate for lung cancer was still 74 percent higher for men than for women in 2003 (preliminary data).

Since 1990, mortality from chronic lower respiratory diseases remained relatively stable for men while it increased for women. These trends reduced the gap between the sexes for this cause of death. In 1990, the age-adjusted death rate for males was more than 100 percent higher than for females. In 2003 (preliminary data), the difference between the rates had been reduced to 38 percent.

Between 1990 and 2003, life expectancy at birth increased more for the black than for the white population, thereby narrowing the gap in life expectancy between these two racial groups. In 1990, life expectancy at birth for the white population was 7.0 years longer than for the black population. By 2003, the difference had narrowed to 5.2 years, based on preliminary data.

Overall mortality was 30 percent higher for black Americans than for white Americans in 2003 (preliminary data) compared with 37 percent higher in 1990. In 2003, age-adjusted death rates for the black population exceeded those for the white population by 43 percent for stroke, 31 percent for heart disease, 23 percent for cancer, and almost 750 percent for HIV disease.

The 5-year survival rate for black females diagnosed in 1992–2000 with breast cancer was 14 percentage points lower than the five-year survival rate for white females (74 percent compared with 88 percent).

In 2003, breast cancer mortality for black females was 37 percent higher than for white females (preliminary data), compared with less than 15 percent higher in 1990 (based on age-adjusted death rates).

Homicide rates among young black males 15–24 years of age and young Hispanic males were about 50 percent lower in 2002 than in 1992 and 1993 when homicide rates peaked for these groups. Despite these downward trends, homicide was still the leading cause of death for young black males and the second leading cause for young Hispanic males in 2002, and their homicide rates remained substantially higher than for young non-Hispanic white males.

HIV disease mortality peaked in 1995 and then fell sharply with the advent of new drug therapies. However, the decline in HIV disease mortality has slowed in recent years. Between 1999 and 2003 (preliminary data), age-adjusted death rates for HIV disease declined about four percent per year on average for males and were unchanged for females.

In 2002, the death rate for motor vehicle-related injury for young American Indian males 15–24 years of age was almost 40 percent higher and the suicide rate was almost 60 percent higher than the rates for those causes for young white males. Death rates for the American Indian population are known to be underestimated.

In 2002, death rates for stroke for Asian males 45–54 and 55–64 years of age were about 15 percent higher than for white males of those ages. Since 1990, stroke mortality for Asian males and females 45–74 years of age has generally exceeded that for white males and females of those ages. Death rates for the Asian population are known to be underestimated.

Death rates vary by educational attainment. In 2002, the age-adjusted death rate for persons 25–64 years of age with fewer than 12 years of education was 2.7 times the rate for persons with at least one year of college.

Occupational Health

In 2003, 5,043 occupational injury deaths occurred in the private sector or 4.7 fatal occupational injuries per 100,000 employed private sector workers. Natural resources and mining had the highest fatality rate (55.7 per 100,000). Natural resources industries include agriculture, forestry, fishing, and hunting. The next highest fatality rates were for the construction (14.3 per 100,000) and trade, transportation, and utilities industries (5.6 per 100,000).

A total of 2,715 pneumoconiosis deaths, for which pneumoconiosis was either the underlying or cause of death, occurred in 2002, compared with 4,151 deaths in 1980. Pneumoconiosis is primarily associated with workplace exposures to dusts, including asbestos and dust in coal mines.

Chapter 63

Leading Causes of Death in the United States

Chapter Contents

Section 63.1

Total Deaths for the 15 Leading Causes of Death

Excerpts from "Deaths: Final Data for 2003," National Center for Health Statistics, Centers for Disease Control and Prevention (CDC), January 19, 2006.

This information from the Centers for Disease Control and Prevention's (CDC) National Center for Health Statistics (NCHS) provides selected key findings for the 2003 final mortality data for the United States. The findings come from information reported on death certificates completed by funeral directors, attending physicians, medical examiners, and coroners.

Mortality Experience in 2003

- In 2003, a total of 2,448,288 deaths occurred in the United States.

- The age-adjusted death rate, which takes the aging of the population into account, was 832.7 deaths per 100,000 U.S. standard population.

- Life expectancy at birth was 77.5 years.

Infant Mortality Rate

In 2003, the infant mortality rate was 6.85 infant deaths per 1,000 live births. The 10 leading causes of infant death were:

- congenital malformations, deformations, and chromosomal abnormalities (congenital malformations);

- disorders relating to short gestation and low birthweight, not elsewhere classified (low birthweight);

- sudden infant death syndrome (SIDS);

- newborn affected by maternal complications of pregnancy (maternal complications);

Table 63.1. Percentage of total deaths, death rates,** age-adjusted death rates for 2003, percentage change in age-adjusted death rates from 2002 to 2003, and ratio of age-adjusted death rates by race and sex for the 15 leading causes of death for the total population in 2003: United States.

Rank[1]	Cause of death (Based on the Tenth Revision International Classification of Diseases, 1992)	Number	Percent of total deaths	Age-adjusted death rate 2003	Percent change 2002 to 2003
	All causes	2,448,288	100.0	832.7	-1.5
1	Diseases of heart (I00–I09, I11, I13, I20–I51)	685,089	28.0	232.3	-3.5
2	Malignant neoplasms (cancer) (C00–C97)	556,902	22.7	190.1	-1.8
3	Cerebrovascular diseases (stroke) (I60–I69)	157,689	6.4	53.5	-4.8
4	Chronic lower respiratory diseases (J40–J47)	126,382	5.2	43.3	-0.5
5	Accidents (unintentional injuries) (V01–X59, Y85–Y86)	109,277	4.5	37.3	1.1
6	Diabetes mellitus (E10–E14)	74,219	3.0	25.3	-0.4
7	Influenza and pneumonia (J10–J18)	65,163	2.7	22.0	-2.7
8	Alzheimer disease (G30)	63,457	2.6	21.4	5.9
9	Nephritis, nephrotic syndrome and nephrosis (kidney disease) (N00–N07, N17–N19, N25–N27)	42,453	1.7	14.4	1.4
10	Septicemia (A40–A41)	34,069	1.4	11.6	-0.9
11	Intentional self-harm (suicide) (*U03, X60–X84, Y87.0)	31,484	1.3	10.8	-0.9
12	Chronic liver disease and cirrhosis (K70, K73–K74)	27,503	1.1	9.3	-1.1
13	Essential (primary) hypertension and hypertensive renal disease (I10, I12)	21,940	0.9	7.4	5.7
14	Parkinson disease (G20–G21)	17,997	0.7	6.2	5.1
15	Assault (homicide) (U01–*U02, X85–Y09, Y87.1)	17,732	0.7	6.0	-1.6
	All other causes (Residual)	416,932	17.0		

*The asterisks preceding the cause-of-death codes indicate that they are not part of the *International Classification of Diseases, Tenth Revision (ICD-10)*].

**Death rates on an annual basis per 100,000 population: age-adjusted rates per 100,000 U.S. standard population.

[1] Rank based on number of deaths.

- newborn affected by complications of placenta, cord, and membranes (cord and placental complications);

- accidents (unintentional injuries);

- respiratory distress of newborn;

- bacterial sepsis of newborn;

- neonatal hemorrhage;

- diseases of the circulatory system (circulatory diseases).

Trends

- The age-adjusted death rate in 2003 was a record low and 1.5 percent less than the 2002 rate.

- Life expectancy was 77.5 years, a record high that surpassed the previous highest value recorded in 2002 by 0.2 years. Record high life expectancy was attained by the total population, as well as by each of the black and white populations. Both males and females in each of the two major race groups attained record high levels.

- For the most part, the 15 leading causes of death in 2003 remained the same as in 2002. Age-adjusted death rates decreased from 2002 to 2003 for four of the 15 leading causes of death and increased for five of the 15 leading causes of death. Decreasing trends for heart disease, cancer, and stroke, the three leading causes, continued. Increasing trends for Alzheimer disease continued.

- Differences in mortality between men and women continued to narrow. The age-adjusted death rate for men was 41 percent greater than that for women (down from 42 percent greater in 2002), and life expectancy for men was less than that for women by 5.3 years, the smallest difference since 1948.

- Differences in mortality between the black and white populations persisted even though there was a trend toward convergence. The age-adjusted death rate was 1.3 times greater, the infant mortality rate 2.4 times greater, and maternal mortality rate 3.5 times greater for the black population than that for the white population. Life expectancy for the white population exceeded that for the black population by 5.3 years.

- The number of maternal deaths increased by 138 deaths between 2002 and 2003 resulting in a maternal mortality rate of 12.1 deaths per 100,000 live births. The increase, in part, reflects that an increasing number of states use a separate item on pregnancy status on the death certificate to help identify these deaths.

- The infant mortality rate decreased significantly in 2003; infant mortality had increased for the first time in over four decades in 2002.

Technical Notes

Nature and Sources of Data

Data in this report are based on information from all death certificates filed in the fifty states and the District of Columbia and are processed by the CDC's NCHS. Data for 2003 are based on records of deaths that occurred during 2003 and were received as of February 28, 2005. The U.S. Standard Certificate of Death—which is used as a model by the states—was revised in 2003. Prior to 2003, the Standard Certificate of Death had not been revised since 1989. This report includes data for five areas (California, Idaho, Montana, New York City, and New York state), which implemented the 2003 revision of the U.S. Standard Certificate of Death in 2003 and for the remaining 46 states and the District of Columbia that collected and reported death data in 2003 based on the 1989 revision of the U.S. Standard Certificate of Death.

Since most of the items presented in this report appear largely comparable despite changes to item wording and format in the 2003 revision, data from both groups of states are combined unless otherwise stated.

Race and Hispanic origin

The 2003 revision of the U.S. Standard Certificate of Death allows the reporting of more than one race (multiple races). This change was implemented to reflect the increasing diversity of the population of the United States and to be consistent with the decennial census.

Maternal Mortality

Maternal mortality rates are computed on the basis of the number of live births. The maternal mortality rate indicates the likelihood of a pregnant woman dying of maternal causes. They are calculated by dividing the number of maternal deaths in a calendar year by the number of live births registered for the same period and are presented as rates per 100,000 live births. The number of live births used in the denominator is an approximation of the population of pregnant women who are at risk of a maternal death.

Maternal deaths are defined by the World Health Organization as "the death of a woman while pregnant or within 42 days of termination of pregnancy, irrespective of the duration and the site of the pregnancy, from any cause related to or aggravated by the pregnancy or its management, but not from accidental or incidental causes." Included in these deaths are ICD-10 codes A34, O00–O95, and O98–O99.

Population Bases for Computing Rates

Populations used for computing death rates and life tables shown in this report represent the population residing in the United States, enumerated as of April 1 for census years and estimated as of July 1 for all other years.

Death rates, shown in this report, for 1991–2003 are based on populations that are consistent with the 2000 census levels. These estimates were produced under a collaborative arrangement with the U.S. Census Bureau and are based on the 2000 census counts by age, race, and sex, modified to be consistent with race categories as of 1977 and historical categories for death data.

Section 63.2.

Leading Causes of Death for Men by Age and Race

"Leading Causes of Death, Males—United States, 2002,"
Centers for Disease Control and Prevention (CDC), March 31, 2005.

Heart disease and cancer are the top leading causes of death in males for all ages and races. The following tables show the top ten leading causes of death for all ages of men by race.

Table 63.2. Leading Causes of Death, Males, All Races, All Ages, U.S. 2002

Rank	Cause of death	Percent*
1	Heart disease	28.4
2	Cancer	24.1
3	Unintentional injuries	5.8
4	Stroke	5.2
5	Chronic lower respiratory diseases	5.1
6	Diabetes	2.9
7	Influenza and pneumonia	2.4
8	Suicide	2.1
9	Kidney disease	1.6
10	Chronic liver disease	1.5

*Percent of total deaths in the race category due to the disease indicated.

Table 63.3. Leading Causes of Death, White Males, All Ages, U.S. 2002

Rank	Cause of death	Percent*
1	Heart disease	29.0
2	Cancer	24.4
3	Unintentional injuries	5.7
4	Chronic lower respiratory diseases	5.4
5	Stroke	5.2
6	Diabetes	2.7
7	Influenza and pneumonia	2.5
8	Suicide	2.2
9	Alzheimer disease	1.5
10	Kidney disease	1.5

*Percent of total deaths in the race category due to the disease indicated.

Table 63.4. Leading Causes of Death, Black Males, All Ages, U.S. 2002

Rank	Cause of death	Percent*
1	Heart disease	25.3
2	Cancer	22.2
3	Unintentional injuries	5.9
4	Stroke	5.3
5	Homicide	4.7
6	HIV disease	3.6
7	Diabetes	3.5
8	Chronic lower respiratory diseases	3.0
9	Kidney disease	2.3
10	Influenza and pneumonia	1.9

*Percent of total deaths in the race category due to the disease indicated.

Table 63.5. Leading Causes of Death, American Indian or Alaska Native Males, All Ages, U.S. 2002

Rank	Cause of death	Percent*
1	Heart disease	20.9
2	Cancer	16.0
3	Unintentional injuries	14.9
4	Diabetes	5.0
5	Chronic liver disease	4.7
6	Suicide	3.8
7	Stroke	3.5
8	Chronic lower respiratory diseases	3.3
9	Homicide	2.7
10	Influenza and pneumonia	2.0

*Percent of total deaths in the race category due to the disease indicated.

Table 63.6. Leading Causes of Death, Asian or Pacific Islander Males, All Ages, U.S. 2002

Rank	Cause of death	Percent*
1	Heart disease	27.0
2	Cancer	25.4
3	Stroke	7.8
4	Unintentional injuries	5.7
5	Chronic lower respiratory diseases	3.6
6	Diabetes	3.2
7	Influenza and pneumonia	3.1
8	Suicide	2.3
9	Kidney disease	1.6
10	Homicide	1.4

*Percent of total deaths in the race category due to the disease indicated.

Table 63.7. Leading Causes of Death, Hispanic Males, All Ages, U.S. 2002

Rank	Cause of death	Percent*
1	Heart disease	22.5
2	Cancer	18.6
3	Unintentional injuries	11.7
4	Stroke	4.6
5	Diabetes	4.2
6	Homicide	4.0
7	Chronic liver disease	3.7
8	Suicide	2.5
9	Chronic lower respiratory diseases	2.5
10	HIV disease	2.2

*Percent of total deaths in the race category due to the disease indicated.

Section 63.3

Leading Causes of Death for Women by Age and Race

This section includes: "Leading Causes of Death," U.S. Department of Health and Human Services, Health Resources and Services Administration. *Women's Health USA 2005*. Rockville, Maryland: U. S. Department of Health and Human Services, 2005. Also, "Leading Causes of Death Females—U.S., 2002," Centers for Disease Control and Prevention (CDC), March 31, 2005.

In 2002, there were over 1.2 million deaths among females. Of these deaths, more than half were attributed to diseases of the heart and malignant neoplasms (cancer). Heart disease represented 356,014 deaths (28.6 percent), while 268,503 (21.6 percent) were from cancer. The next two leading causes of death were cerebrovascular diseases (stroke), which accounted for 8.0 percent of all female deaths. This was followed by chronic lower respiratory diseases which accounted for 5.2 percent.

Crude death rates varied for women by race and ethnic group. For non-Hispanic White, non-Hispanic Black, and Hispanic women, the leading cause of death was heart disease, with 292.3, 211.6, and 69.7 deaths per 100,000 females, respectively. In contrast, among American Indian/Alaska Native and Asian/Pacific Islander women, the leading cause of death was malignant neoplasms (cancer), accounting for 71.0 and 72.6 deaths per 100,000 females, respectively.

Table 63.8. Leading Causes of Death, Females, All Races, All Ages, U.S. 2002

Rank	Cause of death	Percent*
1	Heart disease	28.6
2	Cancer	21.6
3	Stroke	8.0
4	Chronic lower respiratory diseases	5.2
5	Diabetes	3.4
6	Alzheimer disease	3.1
7	Unintentional injuries	3.0
8	Influenza and pneumonia	3.0
9	Kidney disease	1.7
10	Septicemia	1.5

*Percent of total deaths due to the cause indicated.

Table 63.9. Leading Causes of Death, White Females, All Ages, U.S. 2002

Rank	Cause of death	Percent*
1	Heart disease	28.8
2	Cancer	21.6
3	Stroke	8.1
4	Chronic lower respiratory diseases	5.6
5	Alzheimer disease	3.6
6	Influenza and pneumonia	3.1
7	Unintentional injuries	3.0
8	Diabetes	2.8
9	Kidney disease	1.6
10	Septicemia	1.4

*Percent of total deaths due to the cause indicated.

Table 63.10. Leading Causes of Death, Black Females, All Ages, U.S. 2002

Rank	Cause of death	Percent*
1	Heart disease	28.3
2	Cancer	20.9
3	Stroke	7.7
4	Diabetes	5.2
5	Kidney disease	2.8
6	Unintentional injuries	2.7
7	Chronic lower respiratory diseases	2.4
8	Septicemia	2.4
9	Influenza and pneumonia	2.2
10	HIV disease	1.8

*Percent of total deaths due to the cause indicated.

Table 63.11. Leading Causes of Death, American Indiana or Alaska Native Females, All Ages, U.S. 2002

Rank	Cause of death	Percent*
1	Cancer	19.3
2	Heart disease	18.6
3	Unintentional injuries	8.6
4	Diabetes	7.2
5	Stroke	5.8
6	Chronic lower respiratory diseases	4.1
7	Chronic liver disease	4.0
8	Influenza and pneumonia	2.9
9	Kidney disease	2.2
10	Septicemia	1.8

*Percent of total deaths due to the cause indicated.

Table 63.12. Leading Causes of Death, Asian or Pacific Islander Females, All Ages, U.S. 2002

Rank	Cause of death	Percent*
1	Cancer	26.9
2	Heart disease	25.0
3	Stroke	10.8
4	Diabetes	4.0
5	Unintentional injuries	3.9
6	Influenza and pneumonia	3.0
7	Chronic lower respiratory diseases	2.2
8	Kidney disease	1.8
9	Alzheimer disease	1.3
10	Hypertension	1.2

*Percent of total deaths due to the cause indicated.

Table 63.13. Leading Causes of Death, Hispanic Females, All Ages, U.S. 2002

Rank	Cause of death	Percent*
1	Heart disease	25.4
2	Cancer	21.2
3	Stroke	6.7
4	Diabetes	6.1
5	Unintentional injuries	4.7
6	Chronic lower respiratory diseases	2.8
7	Influenza and pneumonia	2.8
8	Perinatal conditions	2.0
9	Alzheimer disease	2.0
10	Chronic liver disease	1.9

*Percent of total deaths due to the cause indicated.

Chapter 64

Life Expectancy at Birth

Life Expectancy Hits Record High

Life expectancy for Americans has reached an all-time high, according to the U.S. mortality statistics released in February 2005 by the Centers for Disease Control and Prevention (CDC). The report, "Deaths: Preliminary Data for 2003," prepared by CDC's National Center for Health Statistics (NCHS), shows life expectancy at 77.6 years in 2003, up from 77.3 in 2002.

The gap between male and female life expectancy closed from 5.4 years in 2002 to 5.3 years in 2003, continuing a trend toward narrowing since the peak gap of 7.8 years in 1979. Record-high life expectancies were found for white males (75.4 years) and black males (69.2 males), as well as for white females (80.5 years) and black females (76.1 years).

Other findings in the report include:

- The preliminary age-adjusted death rate in the U.S. reached an all-time low in 2003 of 831.2 deaths per 100,000.

- Age-adjusted death rates declined for eight of the 15 leading causes of death. Declines were seen for heart disease (down 3.6

This chapter includes: "Life Expectancy Hits Record High," Centers for Disease Control and Prevention (CDC), February 27, 2005; and excerpts from "United States Life Tables, 2002," *National Vital Statistics Reports,* Volume 53, Number 6, Centers for Disease Control and Prevention (CDC), November 10, 2004; and "Table 27," from *Health, United States, 2005*, Centers for Disease Control and Prevention (CDC), 2005.

percent) and cancer (down 2.2 percent), the two leading causes of death which account for more than half of all deaths in the United States each year. Declines were also documented for stroke (4.6 percent), suicide (3.7 percent), flu/pneumonia (3.1 percent), chronic liver disease and cirrhosis (2.1 percent), and accidents/ unintentional injuries (2.2. percent).

- After the first infant mortality rate increase in 44 years in 2002, the rate for 2003 did not change significantly (6.9 deaths per 1,000 live births in 2003 compared to a rate of 7.0 per 1,000 in 2002.)

- Firearm mortality dropped nearly 3 percent between 2002 and 2003.

- The preliminary age-adjusted death rate for human immunode-ficiency virus (HIV) declined 4.1 percent between 2002 and 2003, continuing a downward trend observed since 1994.

- Age-adjusted death rates from alcohol dropped 4.3 percent and the rate for drug-related deaths fell 3.3 percent in 2003.

- Mortality increased for the following leading causes of death: Alzheimer disease, kidney disease, hypertension, and Parkinson disease.

The report is based on data recorded from approximately 93 percent of state death certificates issued in 2003.

Life Expectancy in the United States

Table 64.1 summarizes life expectancy and survival by age, race, and sex. Life expectancy at birth for 2002 represents the average number of years that a group of infants would live if the infants were to experience throughout life the age-specific death rates prevailing in 2002. In 2002 life expectancy at birth was 77.3 years, increasing by 0.1 year from 77.2 years in 2001. This increase is typical of the average yearly changes that occurred during the last 30 years in the United States. Throughout the past century, the trend in U.S. life expectancy was one of gradual improvement that has continued into the new century.

Life expectancy was 74.5 years for males, increasing by 0.1 year from 74.4 years in 2001. Life expectancy for females in 2002 was 79.9 years, increasing by 0.1 year from 79.8 years in 2001. The increase in life expectancy between 2001 and 2002 for females was primarily the result of decreases in mortality from heart disease, cancer, homicide,

Table 64.1. Expectation of Life by Age, Race[1], and Sex: United States, 2002.

Age	All races			White			Black		
	Total	Male	Female	Total	Male	Female	Total	Male	Female
0	77.3	74.5	79.9	77.7	75.1	80.3	72.3	68.8	75.6
1	76.8	74.1	79.4	77.2	74.6	79.7	72.4	68.8	75.6
5	72.9	70.2	75.4	73.3	70.7	75.8	68.5	65.0	71.7
10	67.9	65.3	70.5	68.3	65.7	70.8	63.6	60.1	66.8
15	63.0	60.3	65.5	63.4	60.8	65.9	58.7	55.2	61.8
20	58.2	55.6	60.7	58.6	56.1	61.0	53.9	50.5	57.0
25	53.5	51.0	55.8	53.8	51.4	56.1	49.3	46.0	52.1
30	48.7	46.3	51.0	49.0	46.7	51.2	44.7	41.6	47.4
35	44.0	41.6	46.1	44.3	42.0	46.4	40.1	37.1	42.7
40	39.3	37.0	41.4	39.6	37.4	41.6	35.6	32.8	38.1
45	34.8	32.6	36.7	35.0	32.9	36.9	31.3	28.5	33.7
50	30.3	28.3	32.2	30.5	28.5	32.4	27.3	24.6	29.5
55	26.1	24.1	27.7	26.2	24.3	27.9	23.4	21.0	25.4
60	22.0	20.2	23.5	22.1	20.3	23.6	19.9	17.6	21.6
65	18.2	16.6	19.5	18.2	16.6	19.5	16.6	14.6	18.0
70	14.7	13.2	15.8	14.7	13.3	15.8	13.5	11.8	14.7
75	11.5	10.3	12.4	11.5	10.3	12.3	10.9	9.5	11.7
80	8.8	7.8	9.4	8.7	7.7	9.3	8.6	7.5	9.2
85	6.5	5.7	6.9	6.4	5.7	6.8	6.6	5.8	7.0
90	4.8	4.2	5.0	4.7	4.1	4.9	5.1	4.5	5.3
95	3.6	3.2	3.7	3.4	3.0	3.5	3.9	3.6	4.0
100	2.7	2.5	2.8	2.4	2.3	2.5	3.0	2.9	3.0

[1]Race categories are consistent with the 1977 Office of Management and Budget guidelines.

Table 64.2. Life Expectancy at Birth, at 65 Years of Age, and at 75 Years of Age, According to Race and Sex: United States, Selected Years 1900–2002.

Specified age and year	All races Both sexes	All races Male	All races Female	White Both sexes	White Male	White Female	Black or African American[1] Both sexes	Black or African American[1] Male	Black or African American[1] Female
				Remaining life expectancy in years					
At birth									
1900[2,3]	47.3	46.3	48.3	47.6	46.6	48.7	33.0	32.5	33.5
1950[3]	68.2	65.6	71.1	69.1	66.5	72.2	60.8	59.1	62.9
1960[3]	69.7	66.6	73.1	70.6	67.4	74.1	63.6	61.1	66.3
1970	70.8	67.1	74.7	71.7	68.0	75.6	64.1	60.0	68.3
1980	73.7	70.0	77.4	74.4	70.7	78.1	68.1	63.8	72.5
1985	74.7	71.1	78.2	75.3	71.8	78.7	69.3	65.0	73.4
1990	75.4	71.8	78.8	76.1	72.7	79.4	69.1	64.5	73.6
1991	75.5	72.0	78.9	76.3	72.9	79.6	69.3	64.6	73.8
1992	75.8	72.3	79.1	76.5	73.2	79.8	69.6	65.0	73.9
1993	75.5	72.2	78.8	76.3	73.1	79.5	69.2	64.6	73.7
1994	75.7	72.4	79.0	76.5	73.3	79.6	69.5	64.9	73.9
1995	75.8	72.5	78.9	76.5	73.4	79.6	69.6	65.2	73.9
1996	76.1	73.1	79.1	76.8	73.9	79.7	70.2	66.1	74.2
1997	76.5	73.6	79.4	77.1	74.3	79.9	71.1	67.2	74.7
1998	76.7	73.8	79.5	77.3	74.5	80.0	71.3	67.6	74.8
1999	76.7	73.9	79.4	77.3	74.6	79.9	71.4	67.8	74.7
2000[4]	77.0	74.3	79.7	77.6	74.9	80.1	71.9	68.3	75.2
2001	77.2	74.4	79.8	77.7	75.0	80.2	72.2	68.6	75.5
2002	77.3	74.5	79.9	77.7	75.1	80.3	72.3	68.8	75.6
At 65 years									
1950[3]	13.9	12.8	15.0	**	12.8	15.1	13.9	12.9	14.9
1960[3]	14.3	12.8	15.8	14.4	12.9	15.9	13.9	12.7	15.1
1970	15.2	13.1	17.0	15.2	13.1	17.1	14.2	12.5	15.7
1980	16.4	14.1	18.3	16.5	14.2	18.4	15.1	13.0	16.8
1985	16.7	14.5	18.5	16.8	14.5	18.7	15.2	13.0	16.9
1990	17.2	15.1	18.9	17.3	15.2	19.1	15.4	13.2	17.2
1991	17.4	15.3	19.1	17.5	15.4	19.2	15.5	13.4	17.2
1992	17.5	15.4	19.2	17.6	15.5	19.3	15.7	13.5	17.4

1993	17.3	15.3	18.9	17.4	15.4	19.0	15.5	13.4	17.1
1994	17.4	15.5	19.0	17.5	15.6	19.1	15.7	13.6	17.2
1995	17.4	15.6	18.9	17.6	15.7	19.1	15.6	13.6	17.1
1996	17.5	15.7	19.0	17.6	15.8	19.1	15.8	13.9	17.2
1997	17.7	15.9	19.2	17.8	16.0	19.3	16.1	14.2	17.6
1998	17.8	16.0	19.2	17.8	16.1	19.3	16.1	14.3	17.4
1999	17.7	16.1	19.1	17.8	16.1	19.2	16.0	14.3	17.3
2000⁴	18.0	16.2	19.3	18.0	16.3	19.4	16.2	14.2	17.7
2001	18.1	16.4	19.4	18.2	16.5	19.5	16.4	14.4	17.9
2002	18.2	16.6	19.5	18.2	16.6	19.5	16.6	14.6	18.0

At 75 years

1980	10.4	8.8	11.5	10.4	8.8	11.5	9.7	8.3	**10.7
1985	10.6	9.0	11.7	10.6	9.0	11.7	10.1	8.7	11.1
1990	10.9	9.4	12.0	11.0	9.4	12.0	10.2	8.6	11.2
1991	11.1	9.5	12.1	11.1	9.5	12.1	10.2	8.7	11.2
1992	11.2	9.6	12.2	11.2	9.6	12.2	10.4	8.9	11.4
1993	10.9	9.5	11.9	11.0	9.5	12.0	10.2	8.7	11.1
1994	11.0	9.6	12.0	11.1	9.6	12.0	10.3	8.9	11.2
1995	11.0	9.7	11.9	11.1	9.7	12.0	10.2	8.8	11.1
1996	11.1	9.8	12.0	11.1	9.8	12.0	10.3	9.0	11.2
1997	11.2	9.9	12.1	11.2	9.9	12.1	10.7	9.3	11.5
1998	11.3	10.0	12.2	11.3	10.0	12.2	10.5	9.2	11.3
1999	11.2	10.0	12.1	11.2	10.1	12.1	10.4	9.2	11.1
2000⁴	11.4	10.1	12.3	11.4	10.1	12.3	10.7	9.2	11.6
2001	11.5	10.2	12.4	11.5	10.2	12.3	10.8	9.3	11.7
2002	11.5	10.3	12.4	11.5	10.3	12.3	10.9	9.5	11.7

**Data not available.

¹Data shown for 1900–60 are for the nonwhite population.

²Death registration area only. The death registration area increased from 10 States and the District of Columbia in 1900 to the coterminous United States in 1933.

³Includes deaths of persons who were not residents of the 50 States and the District of Columbia.

⁴Life expectancies (LEs) for 2000 were revised and may differ from those shown previously. LEs for 2000 were computed using population counts from census 2000 and replace LEs for 2000 using 1990-based post-census estimates.

cerebrovascular disease, and chronic lower respiratory disease. The increase in life expectancy for females could have been greater were it not for the offsetting effect of increases in mortality from accidents, Alzheimer disease, pneumonia, perinatal conditions, and septicemia. For males, life expectancy increased primarily because of decreases in mortality from heart disease, homicide, cancer, cerebrovascular disease, and HIV disease. The increase in life expectancy for males could have been greater were it not for the offsetting increases in mortality from accidents, diabetes, septicemia, perinatal conditions, and Alzheimer disease.

The difference in life expectancy between the sexes was 5.4 years in 2002, unchanged from the previous year. From 1900 to 1975, the difference in life expectancy between the sexes increased from 2.0 years to 7.8 years. The increasing gap during these years is attributed to increases in male mortality due to ischemic heart disease and lung cancer, both of which increased largely as the result of men's early and widespread adoption of cigarette smoking. Since 1979 the difference in life expectancy between the sexes has narrowed from 7.8 years to 5.4 years, reflecting proportionately greater increases in lung cancer mortality for women than for men and proportionately larger decreases in heart disease mortality among men.

Between 2001 and 2002, life expectancy for the black population rose 0.1 year to 72.3 years. For the total white population, life expectancy remained at 77.7 years. The difference in life expectancy between the white and black populations was 5.4 years in 2002, a historically record low level. The white-black difference in life expectancy narrowed from 14.6 years in 1900 to 5.7 years in 1982, but increased to 7.1 years in 1993 before beginning to decline again in 1994 (7.0 years). The increase in the gap from 1983 to 1993 was largely the result of increases in mortality among the black male population due to HIV infection and homicide.

Among the four race-sex groups, white females continued to have the highest life expectancy at birth (80.3 years), followed by black females (75.6 years), white males (75.1 years), and black males (68.8 years). Between 2001 and 2002, life expectancy increased one year for black males (from 68.6 in 2001 to 68.8 in 2002). Black males experienced an unprecedented decline in life expectancy every year for 1984–89, but annual increases in 1990–92 and 1994–2002. From 2001 to 2002, life expectancy for black females increased from 75.5 years to 75.6 years, an increase of 0.1 year. Life expectancy for white males rose 0.1 year, from 75.0 years in 2001 to two years in 2002. White female life expectancy increased during the same period by 0.1 year from 80.2 to 80.3 years. Overall, gains in life expectancy between 1980 and 2002 were 5.0 years for black males, 4.4 years for white males, 3.1 years for black females, and 2.2 years for white females.

The 2002 life table may be used to compare life expectancy at any age from birth onward. On the basis of mortality experienced in 2002, a person aged 65 years could expect to live an average of 18.2 more years for a total of 83.2 years, and a person age 100 years could expect to live an additional 2.7 years on average. Life expectancy at 100 years of age, particularly for the black population, should be interpreted with caution as these figures may be affected somewhat by inaccurate reporting of age.

Additional Information

National Center for Health Statistics
3311 Toledo Road
Hyattsville, MD 20782
Toll-Free: 866-441-NCHS (6247)
Phone: 301-458-4000
Website: http://www.cdc.gov/nchs
E-mail: nchsquery@cdc.gov

Chapter 65

Infant and Maternal Mortality Trends and Disparities

Preliminary data for 2002 show a significant increase in the infant mortality rate (IMR) to 7.0 infant deaths per 1,000 live births, the first rise in the U.S. IMR since 1958. The 2002 increase in infant mortality was concentrated in the neonatal period, particularly in deaths occurring within seven days of birth.

The rate of late fetal mortality (fetal deaths of 28 or more weeks of gestation per 1,000 live births plus fetal deaths) shows a three percent decline for 2002 (slightly greater than the average annual decline for 1990–2001). As a result, the perinatal mortality rate, which more fully describes the risk of death at late stages of pregnancy and shortly after birth, appears unchanged for 2002. The perinatal mortality rate had declined fairly consistently for more than half of a century.

Cause of Death

One way to better understand the increase in the IMR is to examine changes by cause using final 2001 and preliminary 2002 data. When examined by cause of infant death, three causes among the ten

This chapter includes: Excerpts from "Supplemental Analyses of Recent Trends in Infant Mortality," Centers for Disease Control and Prevention (CDC), February 8, 2005; and, "Disparities in Infant Mortality," © 2004 American Public Health Association. Reprinted with permission; "Maternal Mortality," U.S. Department of Health and Human Services (HHS), 2002; "African Americans Remain at Higher Risk," by Kauthan B. Umar, M.A., *Closing the Gap*, January/February 2004; also, Tables 23 and 43 from *Health, United States, 2005*, CDC.

leading causes of infant death appear to account for most of the current year increase:

- congenital malformations, deformations, and chromosomal abnormalities

- disorders related to short gestation and low birth weight, not elsewhere classified

- newborn affected by maternal complications of pregnancy

Historically, the majority of these deaths have been among infants born at low birthweight (weight at delivery of less than 2,500 grams or five and one-half pounds). Despite steady increases in preterm and low birthweight rates between 1990 and 2002, trends over this time period for these three causes do not indicate a consistent pattern of increase or decrease. However, the interpretation of the cause of death trends is complicated by the change in the international classification of diseases (ICD) revision in 1999 that created breaks in the comparability of cause of death statistics.

Historical Trends in Infant Mortality

The death registration area was completed in 1933 when all states were included in the collection of death statistics. Since then, with the exception of 1957–58, when a significant increase in the IMR was observed, the historical trend of the IMR has been one of steady, sometimes rapid decline. Through the 1930s and 1940s, the IMR declined by an average of four percent per year. The rate of decline slowed markedly to one percent per year for 1950 to 1964. Thereafter, until the early 1980s, infant mortality declined rapidly, by an average of almost five percent per year. From 1981 to 1989 the rate of decline again slowed to an average of two percent per year.

Recent Trends in Fetal and Infant Mortality

Over the more recent period, 1990 to 2001, the IMR declined 26 percent (from 9.2 to 6.8 per 1,000) for an average decrease of three percent per year. Between 1990 and 2001 the neonatal mortality rate declined from 5.8 to 4.5 per 1,000 (down 22 percent) and the postneonatal mortality rate from 3.4 to 2.3 (down 32 percent). Between 1990 and 2001, the late fetal mortality rate declined fairly steadily, by 23 percent, from 4.3 to 3.3 per 1,000. The perinatal mortality rate also declined steadily between 1990 and 2001, from 9.1 to 6.9 for a total of 24 percent. Although the pace of decline has slowed somewhat since the mid-1990s, significant declines in late fetal mortality and infant mortality have been observed through 2001 despite substantial increases in preterm and low birthweight risk, two important predictors of perinatal health.

As discussed, preliminary data for 2002 indicate a three percent rise in the IMR from 2001. The increase was observed for neonatal deaths only; a four percent increase in the neonatal mortality rate was reported, whereas the postneonatal rate remained constant. The increase in neonatal mortality was accompanied by a three percent decline in the late fetal mortality rate and, as a result, the perinatal mortality rate was unchanged for 2002.

Potential Explanatory Factors for the Changes in the Infant Mortality Rate

Changes in the characteristics of births and changes in birthweight and gestation-specific infant mortality rates (for example, the death rate for infants at a given weight or gestational age) may be related to changes in the IMR. Final birth data for 2002 indicate that the two key predictors of infant health, the percent of births born preterm (less than 37 completed weeks of gestation) and low birthweight, continued to climb, rising one to two percent for 2002. Increases in preterm and low birthweight rates of three and one percent respectively, were also noted between 2000 and 2001. Since 1990 preterm and low birthweight rates have risen fairly steadily, preterm by 14 percent (from 10.6 to 12.1 percent) and low birthweight by 11 percent (from 7.0 to 7.8 percent).

The bulk of the increase has been among moderately preterm (32–36 weeks of gestation) and moderately low birthweight (1,500–2,499 grams) infants. Between 1990 and 2002, the moderately preterm rate rose from 8.7 to 10.1 percent and the moderately low birthweight rate from 5.7 to 6.4 percent, whereas the very preterm rate (less than 32 weeks of gestation) rose from 1.92 to 1.96 percent and the very low birthweight rate (less than 1,500 grams) from 1.27 to 1.46 percent. Although still at increased risk compared with term or normal birthweight infants, infants born moderately preterm and moderately low birthweight, are at substantially lower risk than their very preterm and very low birthweight counterparts for early death. For 2001, 18 percent of infants born very preterm did not survive the first year of life compared with less than one percent of infants born moderately preterm.

Multiple births, more than half of which are born preterm and/or low birthweight, have contributed importantly to recent increases in preterm and low birthweight rates. Between 1990 and 2002 the multiple birth rate climbed 42 percent (a three percent rise was reported between 2001 and 2002); in 2002 nearly one-fourth of all low birthweight infants were born in a multiple delivery. Multiple births do not account for all of the preterm/low birthweight rise; however, the preterm rate for singletons alone increased seven percent over this period. (While the rate of moderately preterm singleton births rose from 8.01 to 8.87 percent between 1990 and 2002, the very preterm rate for singletons declined slightly, from 1.69 to 1.57 percent.)

The increased use of assisted reproductive therapies such as in-vitro fertilization has been strongly associated with the growth in multiple gestation pregnancies and may also be associated with an increased risk of low birthweight among singletons. One percent of all 2001 births were the result of assisted reproductive therapy procedures.

Changes in the management of labor and delivery influenced at least in part by the increased use of medical technologies (e.g., ultrasound), and more aggressive management of premature rupture of the membranes may also be related to the trends in preterm/low birthweight births as induction of labor and cesarean delivery occur more often at earlier gestational ages; the use of induction of labor and of cesarean delivery among births delivered preterm has risen substantially in recent years.

Recent declines in infant mortality have been attributed to improvement in birthweight and gestation-specific infant mortality rates, not to the prevention of preterm or low birthweight. The decline in birthweight and gestation-specific mortality has been attributed primarily to improvements in obstetric and neonatal care such as pulmonary surfactants for preterm infants.

Definition of Terms

Infant Mortality Rate: Deaths of infants aged less than one year per 1,000 or 100,000 live births. The infant mortality rate is the sum of the neonatal and postneonatal mortality rates.

Neonatal Mortality Rate: Deaths of infants aged 0–27 days per 1,000 live births. The neonatal mortality rate is the sum of the early neonatal and late neonatal mortality rates.

Early Neonatal Mortality Rate: Deaths of infants aged 0–6 days per 1,000 live births.

Late Neonatal Mortality Rate: Deaths of infants aged 7–27 days per 1,000 live births.

Postneonatal Mortality Rate: Deaths to infants aged 28 days–1 year per 1,000 live births.

Late Fetal Mortality Rate: Fetal deaths of 28 or more weeks of gestation per 1,000 live births plus fetal deaths.

Perinatal Mortality Rate: Late fetal deaths plus early neonatal deaths per 1,000 live births plus fetal deaths.

Table 65.1. Infant deaths and infant, neonatal, and postneonatal mortality rates: United States, 1933, 1940, 1950, 1960, 1970, 1975, 1980, 1985, and 1990–2001 final, and 2002 (preliminary and latest processed) [Rates per 1,000 live births].

| | | Infant mortality rate | | | | |
| | | | Neonatal (under 28 days) | | | Postneonatal |
Year	Infant deaths	Total	Total	Under 7 days	7–27 days	(28 days–11 months)
2002[1]	28,042	7.0	4.7	3.7	0.9	2.3
2001	27,568	6.8	4.5	3.6	0.9	2.3
2000	28,035	6.9	4.6	3.7	1.0	2.3
1999	27,937	7.1	4.7	3.8	1.0	2.3
1998	28,371	7.2	4.8	3.8	1.0	2.4
1997	28,045	7.2	4.8	3.8	0.9	2.5
1996	28,487	7.3	4.8	3.8	0.9	2.5
1995	29,583	7.6	4.9	4.0	0.9	2.7
1994	31,710	8.0	5.1	4.2	0.9	2.9
1993	33,466	8.4	5.3	4.3	0.9	3.1
1992	34,628	8.5	5.4	4.4	1.0	3.1
1991	36,766	8.9	5.6	4.6	1.0	3.4
1990	38,351	9.2	5.8	4.8	1.0	3.4
1985	40,030	10.6	7.0	5.8	1.2	3.7
1980	45,526	12.6	8.5	7.1	1.4	4.1
1975	50,525	16.1	11.6	10.0	1.6	4.5
1970	74,667	20.0	15.1	13.6	1.5	4.9
1960	110,873	26.0	18.7	16.7	2.0	7.3
1950	103,825	29.2	20.5	17.8	2.7	8.7
1940	110,984	47.0	28.8	23.3	5.5	18.3
1933[2]	120,887	58.1	34.0	26.3	7.7	24.1

[1] Partially edited data processed through January 2004.

[2] First year in which all states were included in the collection of death statistics.

Source: Various CDC/NCHS publications.

Table 65.2. Infant deaths and infant mortality rates for all causes and infant mortality rates by leading causes: United States, preliminary 2002, and final 1990–2001 [Rates per 100,000 live births].

Cause of death (Based on the *International Classification of Diseases, Tenth Revision*, 1992)	ICD-10[1]				ICD-9[2,3]								
	2002[4]	2001	2000	1999	1998	1997	1996	1995	1994	1993	1992	1991	1990
All causes (deaths)	27,977	27,568	28,035	27,937	28,371	28,045	28,487	29,583	31,710	33,466	34,628	36,766	38,351
All causes (rates)	696.1	684.8	690.7	705.6	719.8	722.6	732.0	758.6	802.2	836.6	851.9	894.4	922.3
Congenital malformations, deformations, and chromosomal abnormalities (Q00–Q99)	140.7	136.9	141.5	138.2	157.6	159.2	164.0	168.1	173.4	178.2	183.2	186.9	198.1
Disorders relating to short gestation and low birthweight, not elsewhere classified (P07)	114.4	109.5	108.3	110.9	104.0	101.1	100.3	100.9	107.6	107.7	99.3	100.7	96.5
Sudden infant death syndrome (R95)	50.6	55.5	62.2	66.9	71.6	77.1	78.4	87.1	103.0	116.7	120.3	130.1	13C.3
Newborn affected by maternal complications of pregnancy (P01)	42.9	37.2	34.6	35.3	34.1	32.1	32.1	33.6	32.8	33.6	35.9	37.4	39.8
Newborn affected by complications of placenta, cord and membranes (P02)	25.3	25.3	26.2	25.9	24.4	24.7	24.4	24.7	24.0	24.8	24.4	23.4	23 4

Respiratory distress of newborn (P22)	23.8	25.1	24.6	28.0	32.9	33.5	35.0	37.3	39.6	45.4	50.8	62.5	68.5
Accidents (unintentional injuries) (V01–X59)	22.2	24.2	21.7	21.3	18.3	19.0	20.0	19.5	21.7	21.6	19.2	22.3	21.8
Bacterial sepsis of newborn (P36)	18.3	17.3	18.9	17.5	18.7	18.4	17.6	18.4	18.7	17.2	19.8	19.3	19.2
Diseases of the circulatory system (I00–I99)	16.1	15.4	16.3	16.8	25.2	24.7	24.3	24.8	24.1	23.6	23.2	22.8	24.5
Intrauterine hypoxia and birth asphyxia (P20–P21)	14.4	13.3	15.5	15.5	11.7	11.6	11.0	12.2	13.6	13.7	15.1	14.6	18.3

[1] World Health Organization. *International Statistical Classification of Diseases and Related Health Problems, Tenth Revision.* Geneva: World Health Organization. 1992.

[2] World Health Organization. *Manual of the International Statistical Classification of Diseases, Injuries, and Causes of Death, based on the recommendations of the Ninth Revision Conference, 1975.* Geneva: World Health Organization. 1977.

[3] Cause of death titles in ICD-9 differ in some cases from those in ICD-10. Breaks in the comparability of some causes listed have resulted in changes in category titles and from coding rules used to select the underlying cause of death. Comparisons between 1998 and 1999 infant mortality rates by cause of death in this table should not be made. The trends displayed should be interpreted separately as trends from 1990–1998 and 1999–2002.

[4] Preliminary data for 2002 processed through July 10, 2003.
Source: Various CDC/NCHS publications.

Low Birthweight Rate: Births with weight at delivery of less than 2,500 grams per 100 live births. The low birthweight rate is the sum of the moderately low and very low birthweight rates.

Moderately Low Birthweight Rate: Births with weight at delivery of 1,500–2,499 grams per 100 live births.

Very Low Birthweight Rate: Births with weight at delivery of less than 1,500 grams per 100 live births.

Term: Births at 37–41 weeks of gestation.

Preterm Rate: Births at less than 37 completed weeks of gestation per 100 live births. The preterm rate is the sum of the moderately and very preterm rates.

Moderately Preterm Rate: Births at 32–36 weeks of gestation per 100 live births.

Very Preterm Rate: Births at less than 32 weeks of gestation per 100 live births.

Disparities in Infant Mortality

Nearly 28,000 infants died before their first birthday in 2000—an infant mortality rate of 6.9 per 1000 live births. The U.S. infant mortality rate is higher than that in 27 other nations—more than twice the rate of Hong Kong or Sweden.[1]

Infant Mortality Rates Vary Based on Race and Ethnicity

The 2000 infant mortality rate per 1000 live births for babies born to:[1]

- African Americans was 13.6.
- Native Americans was 8.2.
- Hispanics was 5.6.
- Asian/Pacific Islanders was 4.8.
- Whites was 5.7.

African Americans. African American infants are more than twice as likely to die before their first birthday as white infants.[1] In addition, African American infant mortality rates are increasing.[4] The rate of sudden infant death syndrome (SIDS) among African Americans is twice that of whites.[3]

Hispanics. Overall, Hispanic infants do not have higher mortality rates than other groups.[6] But this rate does not reflect the diversity within this group—the Puerto Rican infant mortality rate was 7.8 per 1,000 live births in 1998.[4]

American Indians/Alaska Natives. American Indians and Alaska Natives have an infant death rate almost double that for whites.[2] American Indians and Alaska Natives experience high rates of SIDS and fetal alcohol syndrome (FAS).[4]

Native Hawaiian/Pacific Islander. Native Hawaiian and other Pacific Islander infant mortality rate is 31 percent greater than that of whites.[3]

Asians. Asians have a lower infant mortality rate than whites, but the highest rate of infant deaths from birth defects.[3]

Causes of Infant Mortality Vary Based on Race and Ethnicity

Prematurity/low birthweight is the leading cause of death in the first month of life. Birth defects are the leading cause of death in the first year of life.[1]

African Americans. The rate of deaths due to prematurity/low birthweight for black infants was nearly four times that for white ones.[1]

Hispanics. Hispanics/Latinos, in particular Puerto Ricans, exhibit a high rate of central nervous system anomalies, which include spina bifida, anencephaly, and congenital hydrocephalus.[4]

Some Potential Reasons for Disparities in Infant Mortality

Age. Younger and older mothers have higher preterm birth rates.[1]

Cigarette smoking. Smoking is a potential factor for low birthweight and growth retardation. Asian/Pacific Islanders smoke the least and American Indian/Alaska Natives smoke the most.[4]

Alcohol consumption. Alcohol consumption is a potential factor in poor pregnancy outcomes. Whites and American Indian/Alaska Natives have the highest alcohol consumption and Asian/Pacific Islanders have the lowest.[4]

Unintended pregnancy. Births resulting from unwanted conceptions may suffer from elevated risks of infant mortality and low birthweight. In one study, African American women indicated 29 percent of their births in the previous five years were unintended as opposed to 9.2 percent of white women.[4]

Cultural. Mexican Americans reported more prenatal stress, less support from the baby's father, and more drug/alcohol use.

Obesity. Asian/Pacific Islanders have the lowest obesity rate and African Americans have the highest.[4]

Unequal Care. Rates of prenatal care in the first trimester:[6]

- 85 percent for whites
- 77 percent for Native Hawaiians/Pacific Islanders
- 75 percent for Hispanics
- 74 percent for African Americans
- 69 percent for American Indians/Alaska Natives

Education. More educated pregnant women have greater rates of prenatal care during the first trimester than less educated pregnant women.[6]

References

1. March of Dimes 2003 Data Book for Policy Makers, "Maternal, Infant, and Child Health in the United States."

2. "Healthy People 2010: An Overview," http://www.healthypeople .gov.

3. http://www.epi.umn.edu/let/nfntmort.html

4. http://raceandhealth.hhs.gov/3rdpgblue/infant/ red.htm

5. http://healthdisparities.nih.gov/whatare.html

6. "National Healthcare Disparities Report," U.S. Dept. Health and Human Services, December 2003, Prepublication Copy.

Maternal Mortality

During the past several decades, there was a dramatic decrease in maternal mortality. Between 1970 and 1980, maternal mortality decreased from 21.5 to 9.4 deaths per 100,000 live births, a 56 percent drop. However, from 1980–1998, the rate remained between 6 and 7 maternal deaths per 100,000 live births. In 1999, there were 001 maternal deaths related to complications of pregnancy, childbirth, and the postpartum period, a rate of 8.3 per 100,000 live births. Though an increase from the 1998 rate of 6.1, this difference is attributable to changes made in the classification and coding of maternal deaths starting with 1999 data.

In 1999, the maternal mortality rate for Black women (23.3 per 100,000 live births) was more than four times the rate for White women (5.5 per 100,000 live births) and three times the rate for Hispanic women (7.9 per 100,000 live births).

The risk of maternal death increases with age. In 1999, women aged 35 years and older had nearly three times the risk of death (23.0 per 100,000 live births) as women aged 25–29 (8.2 per 100,000 live births). Black women aged 35 years and older had the highest rate of maternal mortality of nearly 70 deaths per 100,000 live births.

African Americans Remain at Higher Risk

In a decade-long study, the Centers for Disease Control and Prevention (CDC) found that African American women die three times more often from pregnancy-related complications than non-Hispanic White women. This gap, which has persisted for more than 60 years, is the largest and most difficult disparity to understand in the area of maternal and child health.

"Any pregnancy-related death is one too many," said Secretary of the Department of Health and Human Services (HHS) Tommy G. Thompson, in a February 20, 2003, press release. "We must focus our research on finding ways to reduce these deaths."

Data from CDC's Pregnancy Mortality Surveillance System (PMSS) from 1991 to 1999 indicate that although maternal mortality is rare, on average 12 women die each year for every 100,000 live births. For African American women, though, the rate is 30.0 deaths per 100,000 live births compared with 8.1 deaths for White women.

African American women are three times more likely to die from ectopic pregnancies, (when the placenta and fetus develop outside of

Table 65.3. Infant mortality rates, according to race, Hispanic origin, geographic division, and state: United States, average annual 1989–91, 1997–99, and 2000–2002.[t]

Geographic division and state	All races			Not Hispanic or Latino					
				White			Black or African American		
	1989–91[1]	1997–99[2]	2000–2002[2]	1989–91[1]	1997–99[2]	2000–2002[2]	1989–91[1]	1997–99[2]	2000–2002[2]
	Infant (under one year of age) deaths per 1,000 live births								
United States	9.0	7.1	6.9	7.3	5.9	5.7	17.2	13.9	13.6
New England[4]	7.3	5.7	5.4	6.2	4.7	4.5	15.1	11.8	12.1
Connecticut	7.9	6.7	6.4	5.9	4.8	4.9	17.0	13.4	14.3
Maine	6.6	5.5	5.1	6.2	5.6	5.0	*	*	*
Massachusetts	7.0	5.2	4.8	5.9	4.4	4.0	14.2	10.8	10.5
New Hampshire[4]	7.1	4.8	4.9	7.2	4.4	4.5	*	*	*
Rhode Island	8.7	6.7	6.7	7.5	4.8	5.3	*13.6	*12.4	*12.6
Vermont	6.6	6.2	5.5	6.3	6.0	5.5	*	*	*
Middle Atlantic	9.2	6.7	6.4	6.6	5.0	5.0	18.5	13.3	12.5
New Jersey	8.4	6.5	6.1	6.1	4.3	4.0	17.8	13.9	13.6
New York	9.5	6.4	6.1	6.3	4.6	4.8	18.4	11.9	11.2
Pennsylvania	9.2	7.4	7.3	7.2	5.8	5.9	19.1	16.0	14.4
East North Central	9.8	8.0	7.7	7.7	6.4	6.2	19.1	16.0	15.9
Illinois	10.7	8.5	7.8	7.6	6.2	5.9	20.5	17.1	15.8
Indiana	9.4	7.9	7.7	8.4	7.0	7.0	17.3	15.2	13.9
Michigan	10.5	8.1	8.1	7.7	6.1	6.0	20.7	16.1	16.9
Ohio	9.0	8.0	7.7	7.7	6.8	6.3	16.2	14.5	15.3
Wisconsin	8.4	6.8	6.9	7.4	5.6	5.6	17.0	15.7	17.9
West North Central	8.5	6.9	6.6	7.4	6.1	5.8	17.5	15.2	14.1
Iowa	8.2	6.1	5.8	7.8	5.7	5.5	15.8	17.2	*11.4
Kansas	8.5	7.3	7.0	7.8	7.1	6.4	15.4	12.0	14.7
Minnesota	7.3	6.0	5.5	6.4	5.4	4.7	18.5	12.5	10.8
Missouri	9.7	7.6	7.7	8.0	6.1	6.3	18.0	16.4	15.6
Nebraska	8.1	7.2	7.0	7.2	6.3	6.2	18.3	17.0	15.0
North Dakota	8.0	7.3	7.8	7.3	6.7	6.8	*	*	*
South Dakota	9.5	8.5	6.4	7.5	7.1	5.4	*	*	*

South Atlantic	10.4	8.3	8.0	7.6	6.2	6.0	17.2	1.1	13.7
Delaware	11.2	8.3	9.6	8.2	6.0	7.9	20.1	1.1	14.9
District of Columbia	20.3	14.1	11.4	*8.2	*	*	23.9	1.4	15.3
Florida	9.4	7.2	7.2	7.2	6.0	5.7	16.2	1.5	13.0
Georgia	11.9	8.4	8.7	8.4	6.0	6.3	17.9	1.3	13.4
Maryland	9.1	8.6	7.7	6.3	5.5	5.3	15.0	1.8	12.7
North Carolina	10.7	9.2	8.4	8.0	6.9	6.4	16.9	1.9	15.1
South Carolina	11.8	9.8	9.0	8.4	6.5	6.0	17.2	1.8	14.9
Virginia	9.9	7.5	7.2	7.4	5.8	5.5	18.0	1.3	13.6
West Virginia	9.1	8.3	7.9	8.8	8.2	7.7	*15.7	*12.7	*11.7
East South Central	10.4	8.8	8.8	8.1	6.8	6.8	16.5	1.6	15.0
Alabama	11.4	9.8	9.3	8.6	7.3	6.8	16.8	1.8	14.7
Kentucky	8.7	7.4	6.7	8.1	6.9	6.4	14.4	2.2	10.8
Mississippi	11.5	10.3	10.5	7.9	6.7	7.0	15.2	1.5	14.7
Tennessee	10.2	8.2	9.0	7.8	6.2	7.0	18.2	5.0	17.0
West South Central[4]	8.4	7.0	6.8	7.2	6.4	6.2	14.2	2.3	12.3
Arkansas	9.8	8.5	8.3	8.1	7.5	7.5	15.2	2.8	12.8
Louisiana[4]	10.2	9.3	9.8	7.5	6.4	6.9	14.3	3.7	13.7
Oklahoma[4]	8.0	8.2	8.0	7.3	7.9	7.4	12.7	3.4	14.5
Texas	7.9	6.3	5.9	6.9	5.8	5.5	14.1	1.1	11.1
Mountain	8.4	6.7	6.2	7.9	6.2	5.7	16.9	2.7	13.5
Arizona	8.8	7.1	6.7	8.2	6.5	6.5	17.3	3.7	14.4
Colorado	8.7	6.8	6.0	8.0	6.3	5.2	16.7	3.7	13.7
Idaho	8.9	6.8	6.6	8.9	6.6	6.2	*	*	*
Montana	9.0	7.0	6.9	8.0	6.2	6.4	*	*	*
Nevada	8.6	6.8	6.0	7.8	6.8	5.1	16.9	1.8	13.7
New Mexico	8.4	6.7	6.4	8.1	6.7	6.0	*17.2	*	*15.8
Utah	7.0	5.4	5.3	6.8	5.3	5.0	*	*	*
Wyoming	8.4	6.7	6.5	8.0	6.3	6.3	*	*	*
Pacific	7.7	5.7	5.5	7.0	5.1	4.9	15.4	2.0	11.2
Alaska	9.2	6.5	6.8	7.2	5.5	5.1	*	*	*
California	7.6	5.7	5.4	6.9	5.0	4.7	15.4	2.2	11.4
Hawaii	7.0	6.9	7.2	5.5	5.8	6.3	*13.6	*	*
Oregon	8.0	5.6	5.5	7.4	5.4	5.6	21.3	*8.8	*10.4
Washington	8.0	5.4	5.5	7.4	4.9	5.2	15.1	11.4	9.5

Table 65.3. Part II

Infant[3] deaths per 1,000 live births

	Hispanic or Latino[5]			American Indian or Alaska Native[6]			Asian or Pacific Islander[6]		
	1989–91[1]	1997–99[2]	2000–2002[2]	1989–91[1]	1997–99[2]	2000–2002[2]	1989–91[1]	1997–99[2]	2000–2002[2]
United States	7.5	5.8	5.5	12.6	9.1	8.9	6.6	5.1	4.8
New England[7]	8.1	7.6	6.5	*	*	*	5.8	3.8	3.9
Connecticut	7.9	8.9	7.1	*	*	*	*	*	*3.7
Maine	*	*	*	*	*	*	*	*	*
Massachusetts	8.3	6.3	6.0	*	*	*	5.7	*3.5	3.7
New Hampshire[7]	N/A	*	*	*	*	*	*	*	*
Rhode Island	*7.2	*8.3	8.0	*	*	*	*	*	*
Vermont	*	*	*	*	*	*	*	*	*
Middle Atlantic	9.1	6.3	6.0	*11.6	*	*7.9	6.4	4.2	3.4
New Jersey	7.5	6.4	6.3	*	*	*	5.6	4.4	3.3
New York	9.4	5.9	5.5	*15.2	*	*	6.4	4.0	3.4
Pennsylvania	10.9	8.2	8.6	*	*	*	7.8	*4.7	*4.0
East North Central	8.7	7.2	6.5	11.6	8.4	9.7	6.1	6.0	5.6
Illinois	9.2	6.9	6.4	*	*	*	6.0	6.3	6.5
Indiana	*7.2	7.4	6.4	*	*	*	*	*6.4	*
Michigan	7.9	7.0	6.7	*10.7	*	*	*6.1	6.0	4.9
Ohio	8.0	8.8	7.6	*	*	*	*4.8	*4.9	*4.8
Wisconsin	*7.3	9.2	6.2	*11.9	*9.2	*11.5	*6.7	*5.7	*5.2
West North Central	9.3	6.5	7.0	17.1	12.3	10.9	7.4	6.6	5.6
Iowa	*11.9	*5.6	*6.7	*	*	*	*	*	*
Kansas	8.7	5.8	7.1	*	*	*	*	*	*
Minnesota	*8.4	7.0	6.5	17.3	*10.9	*10.3	*5.1	7.0	6.1
Missouri	*9.1	*5.6	7.2	*	*	*	*9.1	*5.7	*4.5
Nebraska	*8.8	8.7	7.2	*18.2	*	*15.8	*	*	*
North Dakota	*	*	*	*13.8	*13.4	*13.4	*	*	*
South Dakota	*	*	*	19.9	15.2	11.6	*	*	*

South Atlantic	7.4	5.1	5.4	12.7	10.7	8.5	6.8	5.2	5.3
Delaware	*	*	*7.9	*	*	*	*	*	*
District of Columbia	*8.8	*	*7.5	*	*	*	*	*	*
Florida	7.1	4.7	5.2	*	*8.5	*5.8	*6.2	4.5	6.1
Georgia	9.0	4.9	6.0	*	*	*	*8.2	5.0	6.8
Maryland	7.2	5.4	5.7	*	*	*	7.5	5.2	*4.5
North Carolina	*7.5	6.7	5.6	12.2	13.7	10.6	*6.3	5.8	6.9
South Carolina	*	*7.5	*4.6	*	*	*	*	*	*
Virginia	7.6	5.0	4.8	*	*	*	6.0	5.2	4.6
West Virginia	*	*	*	*	*	*	*	*	*
East South Central	*5.9	6.7	6.2	*	*	*10.1	*7.7	6.2	*5.4
Alabama	*	*7.5	7.0	*	*	*	*	*	*
Kentucky	*	*	*4.8	*	*	*	*	*	*
Mississippi	*	*	*	*	*	*	*	*	*
Tennessee	*	*7.0	6.2	*	*	*	*	*	*
West South Central[7]	7.0	5.5	5.1	8.4	7.9	7.5	6.7	4.4	4.4
Arkansas	*	*6.2	*4.5	*	*	*	*	*	*
Louisiana[7]	N/A	*	*6.0	*	*	*	*	*	*3.1
Oklahoma[7]	N/A	5.1	5.7	7.8	8.0	7.6	*	*	*
Texas	7.0	5.5	5.1	*	*8.6	*	6.8	4.4	4.0
Mountain	7.9	6.7	6.2	11.6	8.8	8.6	8.1	5.7	5.9
Arizona	8.0	7.1	6.0	11.4	8.6	9.4	*8.5	*6.1	*5.3
Colorado	8.5	7.0	6.2	*16.5	*	*11.8	*7.8	*5.9	*6.2
Idaho	*7.2	7.0	8.8	*	*	*	*	*	*
Montana	7.0	*	*	16.7	*12.0	*9.9	*	*	*
Nevada	7.8	5.6	5.1	*	*	*	*	*4.7	*4.7
New Mexico	*7.0	6.5	6.3	9.8	7.7	6.8	*	*	*8.4
Utah	*	5.9	6.5	*10.0	*	*	*10.7	*6.5	*
Wyoming	*	*	*	*	*	*	*	*	*
Pacific	7.1	5.3	5.1	14.6	8.9	9.3	6.5	5.3	4.9
Alaska	*	*	*	15.7	9.1	11.2	*	*	*
California	7.0	5.3	5.1	11.0	8.9	7.6	6.4	4.9	4.5
Hawaii	10.7	*7.0	*6.0	*	*	*	7.1	7.4	7.3
Oregon	8.5	6.2	5.1	*15.7	*	*	*8.4	*5.2	*3.7
Washington	7.6	5.0	5.1	19.6	9.6	10.6	6.2	4.9	4.8

Table 65.3. Part III Notes

t Data are based on linked birth and death certificates for infants.

* Estimates are considered unreliable. Rates preceded by an asterisk are based on fewer than 50 deaths. Rates not shown are based on fewer than 20 deaths.

N/A Data not available.

[1] Rates based on unweighted birth cohort data.

[2] Rates based on period file using weighted data. In Appendix I, National Vital Statistics System, Linked Birth/Infant Death Data Set.

[3] Under one year of age.

[4] Rates for white and black are substituted for non-Hispanic white and non-Hispanic black for Louisiana 1989, Oklahoma 1989–90, and New Hampshire 1989–91.

[5] Persons of Hispanic origin may be of any race.

[6] Includes persons of Hispanic origin.

[7] Rates for Hispanic origin exclude data from States not reporting Hispanic origin on the birth certificate for one or more years in a three year period. Note: National linked files do not exist for 1992–94.
Source: Centers for Disease Control and Prevention, National Center for Health Statistics, National Vital Statistics System, Linked Birth/Infant Death Data Set.

the uterus) and preeclampsia (a combination of hypertension, fluid retention, and protein loss in the urine). African American women are also two times more likely to leak amniotic fluids during pregnancy, which leads to infection, according to the *Almanac*, the University of Pennsylvania's faculty news journal. These three conditions account for 59 percent of all maternal deaths in the United States.

According to a 2002 CDC study, it is the limited access that minority communities have to health care that possibly leads to higher maternal mortality rates. The study revealed that African American women were more than twice as likely as White women to receive delayed or no prenatal care. Moreover, the majority of women in the study said they wanted earlier prenatal care but were hindered by outside barriers like a lack of money or insurance and the inability to obtain an appointment.

Removing barriers to and actively promoting the use of prenatal services is key to reducing maternal mortality according to Dr. Audrey Saftlas, professor of epidemiology at the University of Iowa College of Public Health. In a study published in the *American Journal of Epidemiology*, Saftlas argued that the health care system should make comprehensive reproductive health services more available to African American women while ensuring that women are able and willing to use services.

"With current medical knowledge and technology, more than half of maternal deaths can be prevented," Saftlas said. "We need to develop strategies to improve the content of and access to prenatal care for all Black women—not just Black women at high risk, but also those considered at low risk."

Indeed, there is a misconception that by focusing on high-risk women, incidents of pregnancy-related deaths will be easier to prevent, according to Dr. Margaret A. Harper, primary author of "Pregnancy-Related Death and Health Care Services."

But she said that about 10 to 15 percent of women who are thought to be at risk for a complication actually go on to have a problem. As a result, focusing on risk factors can give patients and providers a false sense of security, leaving them ill-prepared if complications arise, Harper said. If lack of prenatal care and known risk factors do not fully explain the causes of maternal mortality, then what needs to be done?

Dr. Luigi Mastroianni, Jr., professor of Obstetrics and Gynecology at the University of Pennsylvania School of Medicine, argues for a "need to speed up the development of superior methods to predict risk, achieve timely intervention, and develop effective therapies."

Table 65.4. Maternal mortality for complications of pregnancy, childbirth, and the puerperium, according to race, Hispanic origin, and age: United States, selected years 1950–2002. (Data are based on death certificates.)

Race, Hispanic origin, and age	1950[1]	1960[1]	1970	1980	1990	1995	1999[2]	2000	2001	2002
					Number of deaths					
All persons	2,960	1,579	803	334	343	277	391	396	399	357
White	1,873	936	445	193	177	129	214	240	228	190
Black or African American	1,041	624	342	127	153	133	154	137	150	148
American Indian or Alaska Native				3	4	1	5	6	5	0
Asian or Pacific Islander				11	9	14	18	13	16	19
Hispanic or Latino[3]					47	43	67	81	81	62
White, not Hispanic or Latino[3]					125	84	149	160	151	128
					Deaths per 100,000 live births					
All persons										
All ages, age adjusted[4]	73.7	32.1	21.5	9.4	7.6	6.3	8.3	8.2	8.8	7.6
All ages, crude	83.3	37.1	21.5	9.2	8.2	7.1	9.9	9.8	9.9	8.9
Under 20 years	70.7	22.7	18.9	7.6	7.5	3.9	6.6	*	8.8	6.7
20–24 years	47.6	20.7	13.0	5.8	6.1	5.7	6.2	7.4	6.9	5.8
25–29 years	63.5	29.8	17.0	7.7	6.0	6.0	8.2	7.9	8.5	7.5
30–34 years	107.7	50.3	31.6	13.6	9.5	7.3	10.1	10.0	10.1	9.3
35 years and over 5	222.0	104.3	81.9	36.3	20.7	15.9	23.0	22.7	18.9	18.4
White										
All ages, age adjusted[4]	53.1	22.4	14.4	6.7	5.1	3.6	5.5	6.2	6.5	4.8
All ages, crude	61.1	26.0	14.3	6.6	5.4	4.2	6.8	7.5	7.2	6.0
Under 20 years	44.9	14.8	13.8	5.8	*	*	*	*	7.4	*
20–24 years	35.7	15.3	8.4	4.2	3.9	3.5	4.0	5.6	5.3	3.4
25–29 years	45.0	20.3	11.1	5.4	4.8	4.0	5.4	5.9	5.8	4.6
30–34 years	75.9	34.3	18.7	9.3	5.0	4.0	7.0	7.1	8.1	6.7
35 years and over[5]	174.1	73.9	59.3	25.5	12.6	9.1	16.6	18.0	11.4	13.3

Black or African American									
All ages, age adjusted[4]	92.0	65.5	24.9	21.7	20.9	23.3	20.1	22.4	22.9
All ages, crude	103.6	60.9	22.4	22.4	22.1	25.4	22.0	24.7	24.9
Under 20 years	54.8	32.3	13.1	*	*	*	*	*	*
20–24 years	56.9	41.9	13.9	14.7	15.3	14.0	15.3	14.6	14.9
25–29 years	92.8	65.2	22.4	14.9	21.0	26.6	21.8	24.7	27.1
30–34 years	150.6	117.8	44.0	44.2	31.2	36.1	34.8	30.6	28.4
35 years and over[5]	299.5	207.5	100.6	79.7	61.4	69.9	62.8	71.0	62.9
Hispanic or Latino[3, 6]									
All ages, age adjusted[4]				7.4	5.4	7.9	9.0	8.8	6.0
All ages, crude				7.9	6.3	8.8	9.9	9.5	7.1
White, not Hispanic or Latino[3]									
All ages, age adjusted[4]				4.4	3.3	4.9	5.5	5.8	4.4
All ages, crude				4.8	3.5	6.4	6.8	6.5	5.6

Blank spaces indicate that data were not available.

* Rates based on fewer than 20 deaths are considered unreliable and are not shown.

[1] Includes deaths of persons who were not residents of the 50 States and the District of Columbia.

[2] Starting with 1999 data, changes were made in the classification and coding of maternal deaths under ICD-10. The large increase in the number of maternal deaths between 1998 and 1999 is due to changes associated with ICD-10.

[3] Prior to 1997, excludes data from states lacking an Hispanic-origin item on the death certificate.

[4] Rates are age adjusted to the 1970 distribution of live births by mother's age in the United States.

[5] Rates computed by relating deaths of women 35 years and over to live births to women 35–49 years.

[6] Age-specific maternal mortality rates are not calculated because rates based on fewer than 20 deaths are considered unreliable.

Notes: Underlying cause of death code numbers are based on the applicable revision of the International Classification of Diseases (ICD) for data years shown.

Sources: Centers for Disease Control and Prevention, National Center for Health Statistics, National Vital Statistics System; numerator data from annual mortality files; denominator data from annual natality files; Kochanek KD, Murphy SL, Anderson RN, Scott C. Deaths: Final data for 2002. *National vital statistics reports*. Vol. 53 No. 5. Hyattsville, Maryland: National Center for Health Statistics. 2004.

Chapter 66

Childhood Risk of Injury-Related Death

Children at Risk

Children are at significant risk from unintentional injury-related death and disability. Injury rates vary with a child's age, gender, race, and socioeconomic status. Younger children, males, minorities, and poor children suffer disproportionately. Poverty is the primary predictor of injury. Racial disparities in unintentional injury rates appear to have more to do with living in impoverished environments than with ethnicity. Strategies that reduce financial barriers to safety devices, increase education efforts, and improve the safety of the environment are effective at reducing death and injury among populations at risk.

Low-Income Children

- Unintentional injuries disproportionately affect poor children. Injuries to poor children also result in more fatalities than injuries to children with greater economic resources. Children from low-income families are twice as likely to die in a motor vehicle crash, four times more likely to drown, and five times more likely to die in a fire.

- Children ages five and under are more likely to live in poverty than any other age group. More than 3.9 million children ages five and under in the United States live in poverty.

This chapter includes: "Children at Risk Fact Sheet," and "Airway Obstruction Injury Fact Sheet," © 2004 Safe Kids Worldwide. Reprinted with permission.

535

- Several factors common to low-income families may increase a child's risk of injury, including single-parent households, lack of education, young maternal age, and multiple siblings.

- Children from low-income families live in more hazardous environments that may increase their risk of injury. Risk factors include substandard and overcrowded housing, lack of safe recreational facilities, proximity of housing to busy streets, inadequate childcare or supervision, increased exposure to physical hazards, and limited access to health care.

- Low-income families are less likely to use safety devices due to lack of money, lack of transportation to obtain safety devices, lack of control over housing conditions, or all of these.

- Despite an overall decline in injury-related death, death rates for children of low-income families continue to increase. This phenomenon may be explained by the higher incidence of the most severe types of injuries, such as firearm and pedestrian injuries, among low-income children.

Native American and Black Children

- Black and Native American children have disproportionate death and injury rates due to higher levels of poverty and lower levels of education, employment, and income. These children are more likely to lack health insurance, have difficulty obtaining appropriate and necessary medical care, have lower incomes creating significant financial barriers to care, receive care in hospital emergency rooms, and practice fewer safety behaviors. They are less likely to receive lifesaving preventive services.

- Among children ages 14 and under, Native American children have the highest unintentional injury death rate in the United States and are nearly two times more likely to die from unintentional injury than white children.

- More than 40 percent of Native American children are poor, which is more than three times the poverty rate of white children. Factors that contribute to higher death and injury rates among Native American children are more strongly associated with economic conditions than culturally based parenting differences.

- Among children ages 14 and under, black children have the second highest unintentional child injury death rate in the United States, a rate one and a half times that of white children.

- More than 30 percent of black children live below poverty level, a percentage twice that of white children.

Rural and Urban Children

- Children living in rural areas are at significantly greater risk from unintentional injury-related death than children living in urban areas. These children are especially at risk from drowning, motor vehicle crashes, unintentional firearm injury, residential fires, and agricultural work-related injury.

- Injuries in rural settings occur in remote, sparsely populated areas that tend to lack organized systems of trauma care resulting in prolonged response and transport times. A short supply of medical facilities, equipment, and personnel to treat injuries in rural areas also contributes to increased risk.

- Minority children living in rural areas are especially at risk from unintentional injury-related death. These children represent a smaller percentage of the rural population, and their specific needs are unlikely to be met.

- Higher death rates from unintentional injury in southern and mountain states reflect the high number of people living in rural and impoverished communities.

- Higher injury fatality rates in rural communities are due in part to the high number of farm-related injuries. Children account for 20 percent of all injury-related farm fatalities and represent an even larger portion of nonfatal injuries.

- Inner-city children are at greater risk from sustaining severe nonfatal injuries than suburban and rural children. However, their mortality rates from injury are lower, possibly due to proximity to hospitals and trauma centers.

Male Children

- At virtually all ages, for the majority of causes of injury, males have significantly higher risk of death and injury than females primarily due to greater exposure to activities that result in injury and patterns of risk-taking and rougher play.

Young Children

- Children ages four and under are at greater risk from unintentional injury-related death and disability and account for 49 percent of these deaths among children ages 14 and under.

- Infants have higher rates of unintentional injury-related death than older children, particularly from suffocation, falls, and motor vehicle occupant injury.

- Preschoolers are developing motor skills but have poor impulse control and judgment. Their natural curiosity and lack of fear lead them into potentially dangerous situations. These children are more likely to die from drowning, residential fire and burn injury, poisoning, motor vehicle occupant injury, pedestrian injury, and airway obstruction injury.

- Leading causes of unintentional injury-related death vary throughout childhood and are dependent upon a child's developmental abilities and exposure to potential hazards. Injuries tend to occur when a task's demands exceed the child's abilities to complete the task safely.

Children with Special Needs

- Children with developmental disabilities, both physical and psychological, have higher rates of injury. Sensory neural deficits, such as blindness or deafness, may also increase the risk of certain types of injury.

- Children with cognitive, emotional, or social limitations have significantly higher rates of injury which may be due in part to a lack of appropriate prevention education.

- Children with attention deficit hyperactivity disorder (ADHD) are more likely to suffer from bicycle- and pedestrian-related injuries, head injuries, and multiple injuries than children without ADHD. Children with ADHD are also more likely to suffer more severe injuries and develop functional limitations as a result of their injuries.

Airway Obstruction

Airway obstruction injury is the leading cause of unintentional injury-related death among infants under age one. These injuries occur when children are unable to breathe normally because food or objects block their internal airways (choking), materials block or cover their external airways (suffocation), or items become wrapped around their necks and interfere with breathing (strangulation). Children, especially those under age three, are particularly vulnerable to airway obstruction death and injury due to their small upper airways, their relative inexperience with chewing, and their natural tendency to put objects in their mouths. Additionally, infants' inability to lift their heads or extricate themselves from tight places puts them at greater risk.

Airway Obstruction Deaths and Injuries

- In 2001, 864 children ages 14 and under died from unintentional airway obstruction injuries. Of these children, 87 percent were ages four and under.

- In 2001, 695 children ages 14 and under died from unintentional suffocation, strangulation, and entrapment.

- In 2001, 169 children ages 14 and under died from choking (30 percent food and 70 percent nonfood) and more than 17,500 children were treated in hospital emergency departments for choking-related episodes.

- In 2002, eight children ages two to eleven died from choking on or aspiration of a toy; three of these deaths involved balloons. Choking and suffocation/asphyxia deaths account for 62 percent of all toy-related fatalities.

- In 2002, more than 80 percent of children treated in hospital emergency rooms for airway obstruction injuries were ages four and under.

When and Where Airway Obstruction Deaths and Injuries Occur

The majority of childhood suffocations, strangulations, and choking deaths occur in the home.

Suffocation

- Sixty percent of infant suffocation occurs in the sleeping environment. Infants can suffocate when their faces become wedged against or buried in a mattress, pillow, infant cushion, other soft bedding, or when someone in the same bed rolls over onto them. Infants can also suffocate when their mouths and noses are covered by or pressed against a plastic bag.

- It is estimated that as many as 900 infants whose deaths are attributed to Sudden Infant Death Syndrome (SIDS) each year are found in potentially suffocating environments, frequently on their stomachs, with their noses and mouths covered by soft bedding. Soft bedding may also be a factor in the deaths of children in playpens. Since 1988, at least 100 babies have died of suffocation or SIDS while in playpens with soft bedding or improper or extra mattresses.

- Children can suffocate when they become trapped in household appliances, such as refrigerators or dryers, and toy chests.

- Each year, cribs and play yards are involved in nearly 53 percent of all nursery product-related deaths among children ages five and under. Cribs (primarily older, used cribs) are responsible for about 26 strangulation and suffocation deaths each year.

Choking

- The majority of childhood choking injuries are associated with food items. Children are at risk from choking on small, round foods such as hot dogs, candies, nuts, grapes, carrots, and popcorn.

- Non-food choking hazards tend to be round or conforming objects such as coins, small balls, and balloons. More than 110 children, most of them ages five and under, have died from balloon-related suffocation since 1973.

Strangulation

- Strangulation occurs among children when consumer products become wrapped around their necks. Common items include clothing drawstrings, ribbons or other decorations, necklaces, pacifier strings, and window blind or drapery cords.

- Since 1991, at least 130 children have strangled on window covering cords. The majority of deaths involved outer blind cords and occurred when the cord was hanging near the floor or crib, or when furniture was placed near the cord. Other deaths occurred when children, ages nine months to seventeen months, strangled in loops formed by inner blind cords.

- Since 1985, at least 22 children have died from entanglement of clothing drawstrings, most often hood or neck drawstrings. In addition, more than half of drawstring entanglement incidents involved playground slides.

- Children strangle in openings that permit the passage of their bodies, yet are too small for and entrap their heads. These include

spaces in bunk beds, cribs, playground equipment, baby stroll-
ers, carriages, and high chairs. Since 1990, at least 57 children,
nearly all ages three and under, have died due to entrapment in
bunk beds alone.

Who Is at Risk?

- Children ages four and under, especially under age one, are at
  greatest risk for all forms of airway obstruction injury.

- Male, low-income and nonwhite children are at increased risk
  from suffocation, choking, and strangulation.

- Black infants are more likely than white infants to be placed to
  sleep on their stomachs and on softer bedding.

- Children placed in adult beds are at increased risk for airway
  obstruction injury. Since 1990, at least 296 children ages two and
  under have died in adult beds as a result of entrapment in the
  bed structure. Additionally, 209 children in this age group died
  in adult beds from smothering as a result of being covered by
  another person's body.

Airway Obstruction Prevention Laws and Regulations

- The Child Safety Protection Act bans any toy intended for use
  by children under age three that may pose a choking, aspiration,
  or ingestion hazard and requires choking hazard warning labels
  on packaging for these items when intended for use by children
  ages three to six.

- The U.S. Consumer Product Safety Commission (CPSC) has issued
  voluntary guidelines for drawstrings on children's clothing to prevent children from strangling in the neck and waist drawstrings
  of upper outerwear garments, such as jackets and sweatshirts.

- In 1999, the CPSC voted to issue a mandatory standard for bunk
  beds to address entrapment hazards. The standard restricts opening sizes, requires guardrails and specifies company identification
  and age-specific warning labels to be present on all new bunk beds.

Health Care Costs and Savings

- The total annual cost of airway obstruction injury among children ages 14 and under is nearly $3.7 billion. Children ages four
  and under account for more than 78 percent of these costs.

Prevention Tips

- Place an infant on her back on a firm, flat crib mattress in a crib that meets national safety standards. Remove pillows, comforters, toys, and other soft products from the crib. Never hang anything on or above a crib with string or ribbon longer than seven inches.

- Always supervise young children while they are eating and playing. Do not allow children under age six to eat small, round, or hard foods including hot dogs. Keep small items such as safety pins, jewelry, and buttons out of children's reach. Learn first aid and CPR.

- Ensure that children play with age-appropriate toys, as indicated by safety labels. Inspect old and new toys regularly for damage. Consider purchasing a small parts tester to determine whether or not small toys and objects in your home may present a choking hazard to young children.

- Remove hood and neck drawstrings from all children's outerwear. To prevent strangulation, never allow children to wear necklaces, purses, scarves, or clothing with drawstrings while on playgrounds.

- Tie up all window blind and drapery cords, or cut the ends and retrofit with safety tassels. The inner cords of blinds should be fitted with cord stops. Never place a crib near a window.

- Do not allow a child under age six to sleep on the top bunk of a bunk bed. Ensure that all spaces between the guardrail and bed frame, and all spaces in the head and foot boards, are less than 3.5 inches.

Additional Information

Safe Kids USA
1301 Pennsylvania Ave., N.W., Suite 1000
Washington, DC 20004
Phone: 202-662-0600
Fax: 202-393-2072
Website: http://www.usa.safekids.org

Chapter 67

Work-Related Fatalities

Fatal Injuries

Data for the figures in this chapter come from two sources: NIOSH National Traumatic Occupational Fatalities (NTOF) Surveillance System, which is a death-certificate-based census of occupational deaths for U.S. workers aged 16 or older; and the Bureau of Labor Statistics' (BLS) Census of Fatal Occupational Injuries (CFOI) Surveillance System.

BLS reported 5,524 fatal occupational injuries in 2002. Rates of these injuries declined 23.1% during 1992–2002, from 5.2 per 100,000 full-time workers in 1992 to 4.0 in 2002. During 1980–2000, the states with the highest rates of occupational injury death were Alaska, Wyoming, Montana, Idaho, West Virginia, and Mississippi. Most fatal injuries occurred among workers who were aged 25–54 (66.6%), male (92.0%), and white, non-Hispanic (71.0%). The majority of fatal injuries (55.2% or 2,999 cases) occurred among two occupational groups: operators, fabricators, and laborers (34.9% or 1,895 cases); and precision production, craft, and repair workers (20.3% or 1,104 cases). Two industry sectors accounted for more than 40% of fatal occupational

This chapter includes: Excerpts from "Chapter 2: Fatal and Nonfatal Injuries, and Selected Illnesses and Conditions," from *Worker Health Chartbook 2004*, Centers for Disease Control and Prevention (CDC), 2004; and "Work-Related Roadway Crashes: Who's at Risk," National Institute for Occupational Safety and Health (NIOSH), NIOSH Publication No. 2004-137, March 2004.

injuries: construction (22.6% or 1,121 cases) and transportation and public utilities (18.3% or 910 cases). Deaths due to motor vehicle incidents had the highest rates from 1980 through 1998. During 1992–2000, the number of fatal occupational injuries associated with highway incidents increased 18.5%.

How did annual rates of fatal occupational injuries differ by cause of death during 1980–1998?

During 1980–1998, fatal occupational injury rates declined for the six leading causes of death, though not always consistently. During this period, deaths due to motor vehicle incidents had the highest rates.

Deaths due to machines had the second highest rate until 1990, when they were surpassed by deaths due to homicides. For 1998, the rates of death for homicides and falls were second highest, followed closely by the rate for machine-related deaths. (Source: NIOSH [2001].)

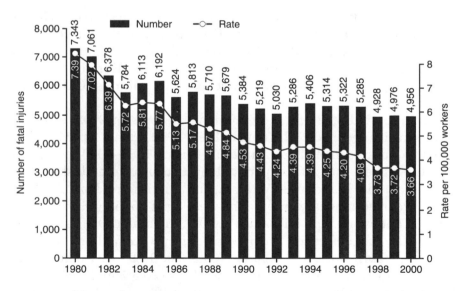

Figure 67.1. Numbers and rates of traumatic occupational fatalities, 1980–2000. (All data for 1980–2000 exclude New York City.) The numbers of traumatic occupational fatalities decreased 33% during 1980–2000, from 7,343 fatalities in 1980 to 4,956 in 2000. During this period, the average annual rate for traumatic occupational fatalities decreased 50%—from 7.4 per 100,000 civilian workers in 1980 to 3.7 in 2000. (Source: NIOSH [2003].)

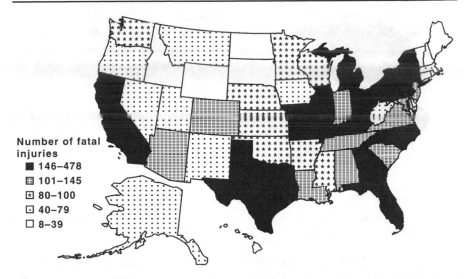

Figure 67.2. *Number of fatal occupational injuries by State, 2002. BLS reported a low of 8 fatal occupational injuries in Rhode Island and a high of 478 in California for 2002. High fatality counts were also reported for Texas (417), Florida (354), New York (238), and Ohio (202). (Source: BLS [2003c].)* [a]

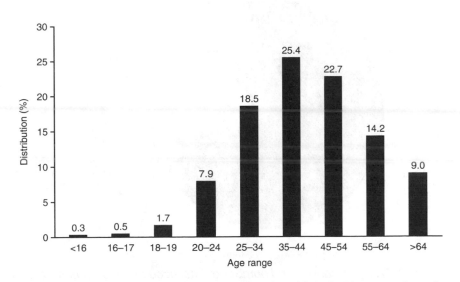

Figure 67.3. *Distribution of fatal occupational injuries by age of worker, 2002. In 2002, two-thirds of all fatally injured workers were aged 25–54. The highest percentage and number of fatalities (25.4% or 1,402 cases) were reported for workers aged 35–44. (Source: BLS [2003c].)* [a]

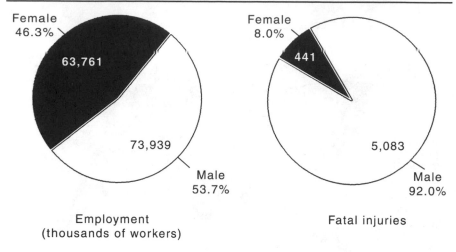

Figure 67.4. *Employment and fatality profiles by sex, 2002. Male workers held 53.7% of the estimated 137.7 million jobs for employed workers in 2002, and they incurred 92.0% of the 5,524 fatal occupational injuries. (Source: BLS [2003c].)* [a]

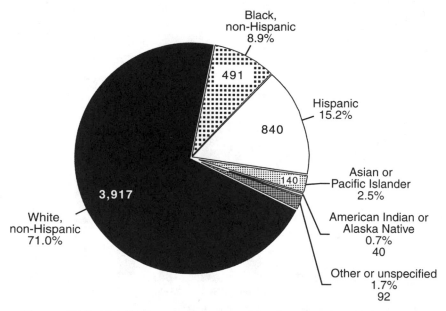

Figure 67.5. *Distribution and number of fatal occupational injuries by race, 2002. The 3,917 fatal injuries among white, non-Hispanic workers represented 71.0% of all fatal occupational injuries in 2002. Hispanic workers accounted for 840 cases or 15.2% of fatal occupational injuries in 2002. (Source: BLS [2003c].)* [a]

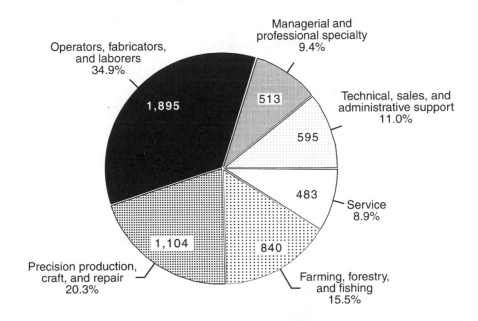

Figure 67.6. Distribution and number of fatal occupational injuries by occupation, 2002. In 2002, the majority of fatal injuries (55.2% or 2,999 cases) occurred among two occupational groups: operators, fabricators, and laborers (34.9% or 1,895 cases) and precision production, craft, and repair workers (20.3% or 1,104 cases). (Source: BLS [2003c].) [a]

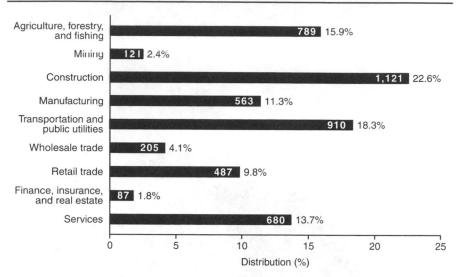

Figure 67.7. *Distribution and number of fatal occupational injuries by private industry sector, 2002. In 2002, two industry sectors accounted for more than 40% of fatal occupational injuries: construction (22.6% or 1,121 cases) and transportation and public utilities (18.3% or 910 cases). (Source: BLS [2003c].)* [a]

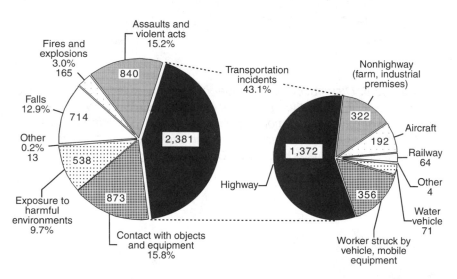

Figure 67.8. *Distribution and number of fatal occupational injuries by event or exposure, 2002. Transportation-related incidents caused 43.1% of the fatal occupational injuries in 2002, including 1,372 highway fatalities (which accounted for 24.9% of all occupational fatalities). (Source: BLS [2003c].)* [a]

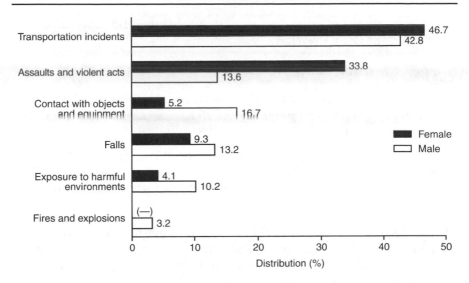

Figure 67.9. *Distribution of fatal occupational injuries by sex of worker and event or exposure, 2002. Fatal injuries to male and female workers were not distributed consistently by type of event or exposure in 2002 because of differences in the types of jobs held by men and women. Fatal injuries in female workers were most frequently associated with transportation incidents (46.7%) and assaults and violent acts (33.8%). Transportation incidents also accounted for the most fatalities in male workers (42.8%), and contact with objects and equipment accounted for an additional 16.7% of male fatalities. (Note: A dash in parentheses indicates that no data were reported or that data do not meet BLS publication criteria.) (Source: BLS [2003c].)* [a]

Reference

[a] BLS [2003c]. Census of fatal occupational injuries. Fatal injuries. Washington, DC: U.S. Department of Labor, Bureau of Labor Statistics, Safety and Health Statistics Program.

Roadway Crashes Are the Leading Cause of Occupational Fatalities in the U.S.

- From 1992 through 2001, roadway crashes were the leading cause of occupational fatalities in the U.S., accounting for 13,337 civilian worker deaths (22% of all injury-related deaths).

- The annual numbers of work-related roadway deaths increased over the decade, despite overall declines in the number and rate of occupational fatalities from all causes. Fatality rates showed little change, hovering around one fatality per 100,000 full-time equivalent (FTE) workers.

Worker Characteristics

- Eighty-nine percent of the victims were male; the fatality rate for males (1.7 deaths per 100,000 FTE) was almost six times higher than the rate for females (0.3).

- The age group with the largest number of roadway crash fatalities was 35–44 year olds (3,275, 25% of crash fatalities) followed closely by 45–54 year olds (2,904, 22%) and 25–34 year olds (2,899, 22%).

- After age 64, crash-related fatality rates increased substantially. Workers 75 years and older had the highest fatality rate of all age groups (6.4 deaths per 100,000 FTE), followed by workers 65–74 years old (3.8).

Data source: Census of Fatal Occupational Injuries (CFOI).[1]

Industry and Occupation Characteristics

- The industry divisions with the highest number of fatalities were transportation/communications/public utilities (TCPU) (4,358, 33% of the total), services (1,884, 14%), construction (1,403, 11%), and manufacturing (1,093, 8%).

- The highest fatality rates by industry were in TCPU (4.6 deaths per 100,000 FTE), mining (3.4), and agriculture/forestry/fishing (2.6).

- The occupation divisions with the greatest proportion of fatalities were transportation/material movers (6,212, 47%), precision production/craft/repairers (1,178, 9%), sales (975, 7%), and service (961, 7%).

- The highest fatality rates by occupation were among transportation/material movers (11.1 deaths per 100,000 FTE), farmers/foresters/fishers (2.5), and laborers (1.4).

- Truck drivers, who are included among transportation/material mover occupations, had a rate of 17.6 deaths per 100,000 FTE, a rate considerably higher than that for this occupation group as a whole.

Data source: CFOI.[1]

Crash Characteristics

- Work related crash fatalities most often resulted from collisions between vehicles (49%). Other prominent crash types were single-vehicle incidents that did not involve a collision with another vehicle or with a pedestrian (non-collisions) (26%) and collisions between a vehicle and a stationary object on the roadside (18%).

- Sixty-two percent of fatalities occurred between 7 a.m. and 4 p.m.; 38% occurred on U.S. or state-designated highways, 26% on interstate highways, and 24% on a local road or street.

Data source: CFOI.[1]

Vehicles

- Vehicles occupied by fatally injured workers were most often semi-trucks (3,780, 28%), cars (3,140, 24%), other and unspecified trucks (2,359, 18%), and pick-up trucks (1,607, 12%). [Data source: CFOI.[1]]

- Between 1992 and 2001, truck occupant deaths increased, as car occupant deaths decreased. [Data source: CFOI.[1]]

- Sixty-two percent of vehicles occupied by a fatally injured worker were registered to a business or government, 17% were registered to the driver, and 12% to an individual other than the driver. [Data source: FARS.[2]]

- Crashes involving large trucks (more than 10,000 lb. gross vehicle weight rating) were seven times as likely to be fatal to other motorists as to truck occupants. An average of 4,425 motorists involved in collisions with large trucks died each year from 1992 through 2001, compared to 681 large-truck occupants. [Data source: Traffic Safety Facts 2001.[3]]

Vehicle Occupants and Drivers

- Between 1997 and 2002, 28% of fatally injured workers were wearing a seat belt; 56% were unbelted or had no seat belt available. Belt use was unknown for the remaining 16%.

- Factors associated with the worker's vehicle that contributed to the crash included: running off the road or failing to stay in the proper lane (46%); driving over the speed limit or too fast for conditions (23%); driver inattention (11%); and the driver being drowsy or asleep (7%). Note: Up to four factors may be reported for each vehicle.

- In 8% of crashes fatal to a worker, the driver of the worker's vehicle was determined to have been drinking. Data source: FARS.[2]

Data Sources

[1] Census of Fatal Occupational Injuries (CFOI), 1992-2001 (special research file prepared for NIOSH by the Bureau of Labor Statistics; excludes New York City).

[2] Fatality Analysis Reporting System (FARS), 1997-2002; National Highway Traffic Safety Administration (NHTSA) (public-use microdata files).

[3] Traffic Safety Facts 2001 [NHTSA]. Publication DOT HS 809 484 (December 2002).

Employment data used to calculate fatality rates: Current Population Survey, 1992-2001 (microdata files).

Chapter 68

Suicide Facts and Statistics

Suicide Facts

- Most popular press articles suggest a link between the winter holidays and suicides (Annenberg Public Policy Center of the University of Pennsylvania 2003). However, this claim is just a myth. In fact, suicide rates in the United States are lowest in the winter and highest in the spring (CDC 1985, McCleary et al. 1991, Warren et al. 1983).

- Suicide took the lives of 30,622 people in 2001 (CDC 2004).

- Suicide rates are generally higher than the national average in the western states and lower in the eastern and midwestern states (CDC 1997).

- In 2002, 132,353 individuals were hospitalized following suicide attempts; 116,639 were treated in emergency departments and released (CDC 2004).

- In 2001, 55% of suicides were committed with a firearm (Anderson and Smith 2003).

This chapter includes: "Suicide Facts," Centers for Disease Control and Prevention (CDC), reviewed December 2, 2005; and "CDC Reports Latest Data on Suicide Behaviors, Risk Factors, and Prevention," listed under "Youth-Related Suicide Findings," CDC, June 10, 2004; also, "Suicide–Some Answers," under the heading "Mental Illness and Suicide," from Substance Abuse and Mental Health Services Administration, (SAMHSA), 2000.

Groups At Risk

Males

- Suicide is the eighth leading cause of death for all U.S. men (Anderson and Smith 2003).

- Males are four times more likely to die from suicide than females (CDC 2004).

- Suicide rates are highest among Whites and second highest among American Indian and Native Alaskan men (CDC 2004).

- Of the 24,672 suicide deaths reported among men in 2001, 60% involved the use of a firearm (Anderson and Smith 2003).

Females

- Women report attempting suicide during their lifetime about three times as often as men (Krug et al. 2002).

Youth

The overall rate of suicide among youth has declined slowly since 1992 (Lubell, Swahn, Crosby, and Kegler 2004). However, rates remain unacceptably high. Adolescents and young adults often experience stress, confusion, and depression from situations occurring in their families, schools, and communities. Such feelings can overwhelm young people and lead them to consider suicide as a solution. Few schools and communities have suicide prevention plans that include screening, referral, and crisis intervention programs for youth.

- Suicide is the third leading cause of death among young people ages 15 to 24. In 2001, 3,971 suicides were reported in this group (Anderson and Smith 2003).

- Of the total number of suicides among ages 15 to 24 in 2001, 86% (n=3,409) were male and 14% (n=562) were female (Anderson and Smith 2003).

- American Indian and Alaskan Natives have the highest rate of suicide in the 15 to 24 age group (CDC 2004).

- In 2001, firearms were used in 54% of youth suicides (Anderson and Smith 2003).

The Elderly

Suicide rates increase with age and are very high among those 65 years and older. Most elderly suicide victims are seen by their primary care provider a few weeks prior to their suicide attempt and diagnosed with their first episode of mild to moderate depression (DHHS 1999). Older adults who are suicidal are also more likely to be suffering from physical illnesses and be divorced or widowed (DHHS 1999; Carney et al. 1994; Dorpat et al. 1968).

- In 2001, 5,393 Americans over age 65 committed suicide. Of those, 85% (n=4,589) were men and 15% (n=804) were women (CDC 2004).

- Firearms were used in 73% of suicides committed by adults over the age of 65 in 2001 (CDC 2004).

Risk Factors

The first step in preventing suicide is to identify and understand the risk factors. A risk factor is anything that increases the likelihood that persons will harm themselves. However, risk factors are not necessarily causes. Research has identified the following risk factors for suicide (DHHS 1999):

- previous suicide attempt(s)
- history of mental disorders, particularly depression
- history of alcohol and substance abuse
- family history of suicide
- family history of child maltreatment
- feelings of hopelessness
- impulsive or aggressive tendencies
- barriers to accessing mental health treatment
- loss (relational, social, work, or financial)
- physical illness
- easy access to lethal methods
- unwillingness to seek help because of the stigma attached to mental health and substance abuse disorders or suicidal thoughts

- cultural and religious beliefs—for instance, the belief that suicide is a noble resolution of a personal dilemma

- local epidemics of suicide

- isolation, a feeling of being cut off from other people

Protective Factors

Protective factors buffer people from the risks associated with suicide. A number of protective factors have been identified (DHHS 1999):

- effective clinical care for mental, physical, and substance abuse disorders

- easy access to a variety of clinical interventions and support for help seeking

- family and community support

- support from ongoing medical and mental health care relationships

- skills in problem solving, conflict resolution, and nonviolent handling of disputes

- cultural and religious beliefs that discourage suicide and support self-preservation instincts

References

Anderson RN, Smith BL. Deaths: leading causes for 2001. *National Vital Statistics Report 2003*; 52(9):1–86.

Annenberg Public Policy Center of the University of Pennsylvania. *Suicide and the Media*. Available online from: URL: http://www .annenbergpublicpolicycenter.org/07_adolescent_risk/suicide/ dec14%20suicide%20report.htm.

Carney SS, Rich CL, Burke PA, Fowler RC. Suicide over 60: the San Diego study. *Journal of American Geriatric Society* 1994; 42:174–80.

Centers for Disease Control and Prevention, National Center for Injury Prevention and Control. *Suicide Surveillance*, 1970–1980. (1985).

Centers for Disease Control and Prevention. Regional variations in suicide rates—United States 1990–1994, August 29, 1997. *MMWR* 1997; 46(34):789–92. Available online from: URL: http://www.cdc.gov/ mmwr/preview/mmwrhtml/00049117.htm.

Centers for Disease Control and Prevention, National Center for Injury Prevention and Control (producer). Web-based Injury Statistics Query and Reporting System (WISQARS) [Online]. (2004). Available online from: URL: http://www.cdc.gov/ncipc/wisqars/default.htm. [2004 June 21 accessed].

Department of Health and Human Services. *The Surgeon General's call to action to prevent suicide*. Washington (DC): Department of Health and Human Services; 1999. Available online from: URL: http://www.surgeongeneral.gov/library/calltoaction/default.htm.

Dorpat TL, Anderson WF, Ripley HS. The relationship of physical illness to suicide. In: Resnik HP, editor. *Suicide behaviors: diagnosis and management*. Boston (MA): Little, Brown, and Co.; 1968:209–19.

Krug EG, Dahlberg LL, Mercy JA, Zwi AB, Lozano R, editors. *World report on violence and health* [serial online]. 2004 May. Available online from: URL: http://www.who.int/violence_injury_prevention/violence/world_report/wrvh1/en.

Lubell KM, Swahn MH, Crosby AE, Kegler SR. Methods of suicide among persons aged 10–19 years—United States, 1992–2001. *MMWR* 2004; 53:471–473. Available online from: URL: http://www.cdc.gov/mmwr/PDF/wk/mm5322.pdf.

McCleary R, Chew K, Hellsten JJ, Flunn-Bransford M. Age-and Sec-Specific Cycles in United States Suicides, 1973–1985. *American Journal of Public Health* 1991; 81:1494–7.

Warren CW, Smith JC, Tyler CW. Seasonal Variation in Suicide and Homicide: A Question of Consistency. *Journal of Biosocial Sciences* 1983; 15:349–356.

Youth-Related Suicide Findings

Analysis of data on suicide methods by the Centers for Disease Control and Prevention (CDC) found that among youth aged 10–14 years, suffocation (mostly hangings) has replaced firearms as the most common method of suicide. In 2001, suffocation suicides in this age group occurred nearly twice as often as firearms suicides, the most frequently used method before 1997. The findings were released in the June 10, 2004 *Morbidity and Mortality Weekly Report* along with data on the relationship between suicide attempts and physical fighting in high school students, school-associated suicides, suicide trends in Hispanic populations, and suicide trends in China.

"Suicide remains the third leading cause of death among young people in this country," said Dr. Ileana Arias, acting director of CDC's Injury Center. "We must focus on the underlying reasons for suicide and a comprehensive strategy to prevent them."

Other Youth-Related Findings

- One in 20 high school students reported both suicide attempts and involvement in physical fights in the past year. Students who reported attempting suicide in the past 12 months were nearly four times as likely to report involvement in physical fights.

- Of the lethal acts of school violence carried out by students between July 1, 1994, and June 30, 1999, more than 20 percent were suicides. One in four suicide victims injured or killed someone else before their suicide.

- Hispanic males were almost six times as likely to die by suicide as Hispanic females, representing 85 percent of the 8,744 Hispanic suicides between 1997 and 2001. Hispanic youth are the fastest growing segment of the U.S. population and account for one-fourth of all Hispanic suicide deaths.

- Suicide is the fifth leading cause of death in China, where more than 287,000 people were victims of suicide annually between 1995 and 1999. In most countries suicides are most common among males, but in China, suicides and suicide attempts were most common among young Chinese women between the ages of 15 and 34.

Suicide is a major public health problem for youth in the United States and abroad. Several of the studies identified a connection between interpersonal violence and suicide. CDC researchers believe a promising approach for future suicide prevention efforts is to determine if effective strategies for preventing youth violence, such as school-based curricula, are also effective for preventing youth suicide. In addition, the findings highlight the need for parents, teachers, and other youth influencers to be aware of potential signs of suicidal behavior, such as fighting and expressions of suicidal thoughts.

CDC's suicide prevention efforts include describing and tracking the problem of self-directed violence; using research to increase knowledge of the risk and protective factors related to suicidal behavior; evaluating and demonstrating ways to prevent suicidal behavior; effectively communicating scientific information about suicide prevention; and integrating proven suicide prevention efforts.

Mental Illness and Suicide

Although the great majority of people who suffer from a mental illness do not die by suicide, having a mental illness does increase the likelihood of suicide compared to people who do not have one. An estimated 2–15 % of persons who have been diagnosed with major depression die by suicide. Suicide risk is highest in depressed individuals who feel hopeless about the future, those who have just been discharged from the hospital, those who have a family history of suicide, and those who have made a suicide attempt in the past.

An estimated 3–20% of persons who have been diagnosed with bipolar disorder die by suicide. Hopelessness, recent hospital discharge, family history, and prior suicide attempts all raise the risk of suicide in these individuals. An estimated 6–15% of persons diagnosed with schizophrenia die by suicide. Suicide is the leading cause of premature death in those diagnosed with schizophrenia. Between 75 and 95% of these individuals are male. Also at high risk are individuals who suffer from depression at the same time as another mental illness. Specifically, the presence of substance abuse, anxiety disorders, schizophrenia, and bipolar disorder put those with depression at greater risk for suicide.

People with personality disorders are approximately three times as likely to die by suicide than those without. Between 25 and 50% of these individuals also have a substance abuse disorder or a major depressive disorder. People who die by suicide are frequently suffering from undiagnosed, undertreated, or untreated depression.

Substance Use Disorders

Suicide risk is increased by both legal and illicit substance use. Research has addressed the increased risk for particular substance use (for example, alcohol), as well as multiple drug use. Substance use disorders as it is used here include intoxication, binge drinking, withdrawal, substance dependence, and substance abuse. Substance use disorders and suicide occur more frequently among youth and adults, compared to older persons. For particular groups at risk, such as American Indians and Alaskan Natives, depression and alcohol use and abuse are the most common risk factors for completed suicide. Alcohol and substance abuse problems contribute to suicidal behavior in several ways. Persons who are dependent on substances often have a number of other risk factors for suicide (runaway and homeless youth). In addition to being depressed, they are also likely to have social and financial problems. Substance use disorders can be common among persons prone to be impulsive, and among persons who engage in many types of high-risk behaviors that result in self-harm.

Alcohol-Related Suicides

- Between 40 and 60% of those who die by suicide are intoxicated at the time of death. An estimated 18–66% of those who die by suicide have some alcohol in their blood at the time of death.

- An estimated 1–6% of individuals with alcohol dependency will die by suicide. People who are addicted to alcohol are at higher risk if they also suffer from depression. At the time of death by suicide, 50–75% of alcohol-dependent individuals are suffering from depression.

- Adolescents who die by suicide are more likely to use a firearm than another method if they have alcohol in their blood at the time of death.

- Suicide rates among 18–20 year-olds were found to decrease among several states where the minimum legal drinking age was raised to 21.

Other Substance Use Disorders

- Intoxication by drugs or alcohol may increase suicide risk by decreasing inhibitions, increasing aggressiveness and impairing judgment. Additionally, substance use such as alcohol increases the lethality of some medications, making it more likely that a suicide attempt via overdose will be lethal.

- Research suggests that adolescents who use marijuana and/or cigarettes are at increased risk of suicide. Studies have also found that as many as 20% of those who die by suicide have used cocaine in the days prior to death.

Additional Information

Substance Abuse and Mental Health Services Administration
1 Choke Cherry Rd., Room 8-1036
Rockville, MD 20857
Toll-Free Suicide Prevention Hotline: 800-273-8255
Toll-Free TTY: 800-799-4889
Website: http://www.samhsa.gov

American Association of Suicidology
5221 Wisconsin Ave. N.W.
Washington, DC 20016
Phone: 202-237-2280
Website: http://www.suicidology.org
E-mail: info@suicidology.org

AAS provides an online listing by state of suicide survivors support groups.

Compassionate Friends
P.O. Box 3696
Oak Brook, IL 60522-3696
Toll-Free: 877-969-0010
Fax: 630-990-0246
Website: http://www.compassionatefriends.org
E-mail: nationaloffice@compassionatefriends.org

Offers support groups and resources for parents who have had a child die and children who have had a sibling die.

Suicide Prevention Resource Center
55 Chapel Street
Newton, MA 02458-1060
Toll-Free: 877-GET-SPRC (438-7772)
TTY: 617-964-5448
Website: http://www.sprc.org
E-mail: info@sprc.org

Offers Internet links to suicide survivor support groups and resources for survivors of suicide.

Yellow Ribbon
P.O. Box 644
Westminster, CO 80036-0644
Phone: 303-429-3530
Fax: 303-426-4496
Website: http://www.yellowribbon.org
E-mail: ask4help@yellowribbon.org

Yellow Ribbon has an online directory of support group information available at http://www.yellowribbon.org/SurvivorSupportGroups.html.

Chapter 69

Alcohol-Attributable Deaths

Excessive alcohol consumption is the third leading preventable cause of death in the United States[1] and is associated with multiple adverse health consequences, including liver cirrhosis, various cancers, unintentional injuries, and violence. To analyze alcohol-related health impacts, the Centers for Disease Control and Prevention (CDC) estimated the number of alcohol-attributable deaths (AADs) and years of potential life lost (YPLLs) in the United States during 2001. This report summarizes the results of that analysis, which indicated that approximately 75,766 AADs and 2.3 million YPLLs, or approximately 30 years of life lost on average per AAD, were attributable to excessive alcohol use in 2001. These results emphasize the importance of adopting effective strategies to reduce excessive drinking, including increasing alcohol excise taxes, and screening for alcohol misuse in clinical settings.

Alcohol-Related Disease Impact (ARDI) software was used to estimate the number of AADs and YPLLs. ARDI estimates AADs by multiplying the number of deaths from a particular alcohol-related condition by its alcohol-attributable fraction (AAF). Certain conditions (for example, alcoholic cirrhosis of the liver) are, by definition, 100% alcohol-attributable. For the majority of the chronic conditions profiled in ARDI, the system calculates AAFs by using relative risk

"Alcohol-Attributable Deaths and Years of Potential Life Lost—United States, 2001," *MMWR Weekly* 53(37); 866–870, Centers for Disease Control and Prevention (CDC), September 24, 2004.

estimates from meta-analyses [2, 3] and prevalence data on alcohol use from the Behavioral Risk Factor Surveillance System. For some conditions, especially those with an acute onset (injuries), ARDI includes direct estimates of AAFs. Direct estimates of AAFs are based on studies assessing the proportion of deaths from a particular condition that occurred at or above a specified blood alcohol concentration (BAC).[4, 5] For acute conditions, a death is alcohol-attributable if the decedent (or, as in the case of motor-vehicle traffic, a driver or non-occupant) had a BAC of greater than 0.10 g/dL. AAFs for motor-vehicle—traffic deaths are obtained from the Fatality Analysis Reporting System.[6] YPLLs, a commonly used measure of premature death, are then calculated by multiplying age- and sex-specific AAD estimates by the corresponding estimate of life expectancy. For chronic conditions, AADs and YPLLs were calculated for decedents aged 20 years and older; for the majority of acute conditions, they were calculated for decedents aged 15 years and older. However, ARDI also provides estimates of AADs and YPLLs for persons aged less than 15 years who died from motor-vehicle crashes, child maltreatment, or low birthweight. Consistent with World Health Organization recommendations,[7] the harmful and beneficial effects of alcohol use are reported separately.

In 2001, an estimated 75,766 AADs and 2.3 million YPLLs were attributable to the harmful effects of excessive alcohol use (Table 69.1). Of the 75,766 deaths, 34,833 (46%) resulted from chronic conditions, and 40,933 (54%) resulted from acute conditions. Overall, 54,847 (72%) of all AADs involved males, and 4,554 (6%) involved persons under 21 years. Of the deaths among males, 41,202 (75%) involved men aged 35 years and older; of those deaths, 41,202 (58%) were attributed to chronic conditions. For males and females combined, the leading chronic cause of AADs was alcoholic liver disease (12,201), and the leading acute cause of AADs was injury from motor-vehicle crashes (13,674). In addition, in 2001, an estimated 11 lives were saved because of the potential benefits of excessive alcohol use, all of which were attributable to a reduced risk for death from cholelithiasis (gall bladder disease).

Of the estimated 2,279,322 YPLLs, 788,005 (35%) resulted from chronic conditions, and 1,491,317 (65%) resulted from acute conditions. Overall, 1,679,414 (74%) of the total YPLLs were among males, and 271,392 (12%) involved persons under 21 years. Of all YPLLs among males, 973,214 (58%) involved men 35 years and older, of which 53% were attributed to chronic conditions. Deaths from alcoholic liver disease resulted in 316,321 YPLLs, and deaths from motor-vehicle— traffic crashes resulted in 579,501 YPLLs.

Editorial Note: In 2001, excessive alcohol use was responsible for approximately 75,000 preventable deaths and 2.3 million YPLLs in the United States. The majority of these deaths involved males (72%) and the majority of the deaths among males involved those 35 years and older (75%). Approximately half of the total deaths and two-thirds of the total YPLLs resulted from acute conditions. Moreover, the BAC level used in this analysis for defining an alcohol-attributable injury death (0.10 g/dL or over) is higher than the BAC level used by the National Institute for Alcohol Abuse and Alcoholism[8] to define binge drinking (0.08 g/dL and over); as a result, all of the injury deaths were attributable to binge alcohol use (more than five drinks per occasion for men; more than four drinks per occasion for women).

The findings described in this report are similar to recent estimates of AADs attributable to excessive drinking in the United States.[1] In contrast, earlier estimates of alcohol-related deaths[9] were higher than the estimates in this analysis and other recent estimates[1] because they were calculated by using a different methodology and were based on mortality from all levels of alcohol consumption, not just excessive drinking.

The 2.3 million YPLLs for excessive drinking is approximately half of the total YPLLs that were caused by smoking in 1999, the most recent year for which this estimate is available,[10] even though mortality attributable to tobacco use is nearly six times higher than that attributable to excessive drinking. This difference exists because many AADs, particularly those caused by injuries, primarily affect youth and young adults, and deaths attributable to tobacco use are uncommon in this population.

The findings in this report are subject to at least six limitations.

1. Data on alcohol use, which are used to calculate indirect estimates of AAFs, are based on self-reports and might underestimate the true prevalence of excessive alcohol use because of underreporting of alcohol use by survey respondents and sampling non-coverage.

2. The risk estimates used in ARDI were calculated by using average daily alcohol consumption levels that begin at levels greater than those typically used to define excessive drinking in the United States.

3. Deaths among former drinkers, who might have discontinued their drinking because of alcohol-related health problems, are not included in the calculation of AAFs, even though some of these deaths might have been alcohol-attributable.

Table 69.1. Number of deaths attributable to the harmful effects of excessive alcohol used by cause and sex–United States, 2001.

Cause	Deaths		
	Male	**Female**	**Total**
Chronic conditions			
Acute pancreatitis	370	364	734
Alcohol abuse	1,804	517	2,321
Alcohol cardiomyopathy	443	56	499
Alcohol dependence syndrome	2,770	750	3,520
Alcohol polyneuropathy	3	0	3
Alcohol-induced chronic pancreatitis	224	71	295
Alcoholic gastritis	6	2	8
Alcoholic liver disease	8,927	3,274	12,201
Alcoholic myopathy	2	0	2
Alcoholic psychosis	564	178	742
Breast cancer	*	352	352
Cholelithiasis	0	0	0
Chronic hepatitis	3	3	6
Chronic pancreatitis	126	106	232
Degeneration of nervous system attributable to alcohol	93	21	114
Epilepsy	96	81	177
Esophageal cancer	394	53	447
Esophageal varices	50	21	71
Fetal alcohol syndrome	3	2	5
Fetus and newborn affected by maternal use of alcohol	0	1	1
Gastroesophageal hemorrhage	19	9	28
Hypertension	632	552	1,184
Ischemic heart disease	635	273	908
Laryngeal cancer	203	30	233
Liver cancer	518	172	690
Liver cirrhosis, unspecified	3,917	2,802	6,719
Low birthweight, prematurity, and intrauterine growth retardation	96	50	146
Oropharyngeal cancer	303	57	360
Portal hypertension	23	14	37
Prostate cancer	233	*	233
Psoriasis	0	0	0

Table 69.1. Number of deaths attributable to the harmful effects of excessive alcohol used by cause and sex–United States, 2001.

Cause	Male	Female	Total
Chronic conditions, continued			
Spontaneous abortion	*	0	0
Stroke, hemorrhagic	1,399	290	1,690
Stroke, ischemic	520	191	711
Supraventricular cardiac dysrhythmia	73	92	165
Total[t]	24,448	10,385	34,833
Acute conditions			
Air-space transport	122	37	159
Alcohol poisoning	253	78	331
Aspiration	97	99	196
Child maltreatment	100	71	171
Drowning	671	141	812
Excessive blood alcohol concentration	1	1	2
Fall injuries	2,560	2,206	4,766
Fire injuries	702	465	1,167
Firearm injuries	113	18	131
Homicide	5,963	1,692	7,655
Hypothermia	164	83	247
Motor-vehicle-non-traffic injuries	171	33	204
Motor-vehicle-traffic injuries	10,674	3,000	13,674
Occupational and machine injuries	121	6	127
Injuries from other road vehicle crashes	170	653	231
Poisoning (not alcohol)	2,782	1,182	3,964
Suicide	5,617	1,352	6,969
Suicide by and exposure to alcohol	21	5	26
Water transport	90	10	100
Total	30,399	10,534	40,933
Total	54,847	20,918	75,766

*Not applicable.

[t]Because of rounding, numbers might not sum to totals.

4. ARDI does not include estimates of AADs for several conditions (tuberculosis, pneumonia, and hepatitis C) for which alcohol is believed to be an important risk factor but for which suitable pooled risk estimates were not available.

5. ARDI exclusively uses the underlying cause of death from vital statistics to identify alcohol-related conditions and does not consider contributing causes of death that might be alcohol-related.

6. Age-specific estimates of AAFs were only available for motor-vehicle traffic deaths, even though alcohol involvement varies by age, particularly for acute conditions.

This analysis illustrates the magnitude of the health consequences of excessive alcohol use in the United States. In addition to estimating the national health effects of alcohol use, ARDI software also can produce state estimates of AADs and YPLLs. Such state-specific analyses are needed because the prevalence of excessive alcohol use, particularly binge drinking, is known to vary substantially by location. State-specific results also can focus discussions of effective public health strategies (for example, increasing alcohol excise taxes and screening for alcohol misuse in clinical settings) to prevent excessive alcohol use and its adverse health and social consequences.

References

1. Mokdad A, Marks J, Stroup D, Gerberding J. Actual causes of death in the United States, 2000. *JAMA* 2004; 291:1238–45.

2. English DR, Holman CDJ, Milne E, et al. *The quantification of drug caused morbidity and mortality in Australia, 1995 edition.* Canberra, Australia: Commonwealth Department of Human Services and Health, 1995.

3. Corrao G, Bagnardi V, Zambon A, Arico S. Exploring the dose-response relationship between alcohol consumption and the risk of several alcohol-related conditions: a meta-analysis. *Addiction* 1999; 94:1551–73.

4. Smith G, Branas C, Miller T. Fatal nontraffic injuries involving alcohol: a meta-analysis. *Ann Emerg* 1999; 33:659–68.

5. Parrish K, Dufour M, Stinson F, Harford T. Average daily alcohol consumption during adult life among decedents with and

without cirrhosis: the 1986 National Mortality Followback Survey. *J Stud Alc* 1993; 54:450–6.

6. National Highway Traffic Safety Administration. *Traffic safety facts 2001*. Washington, DC: National Center for Statistics and Analysis, 2002.

7. World Health Organization. *International guide for monitoring alcohol consumption and related harm*. Geneva, Switzerland: World Health Organization, 2000.

8. U.S. Department of Health and Human Services, National Institutes of Health, National Institute on Alcohol Abuse and Alcoholism. *Newsletter No. 3*. Winter, 2004. Available at http://www.niaaa.nih.gov/publications/Newsletter/winter2004/Newsletter_Number3.pdf.

9. McGinnis JM, Foege WH. Actual causes of death in the United States. *JAMA* 1993; 291:2207–12.

10. U.S. Department of Health and Human Services. The impact of smoking on disease and the benefits of smoking reduction. In: *The health consequences of smoking: a report of the Surgeon General*. Atlanta, Georgia: U.S. Department of Health and Human Services, CDC, National Center for Chronic Disease Prevention and Health Promotion, Office on Smoking and Health, 2004:853–93.

Additional Information

Centers for Disease Control and Prevention (CDC)
1600 Clifton Rd.
Atlanta, GA 30333
Toll-Free: 800-311-3435
Phone: 404-639-3534
Website: http://www.cdc.gov

Chapter 70

Disparities in Deaths from Stroke

Despite declines in deaths from stroke, stroke remained the third leading cause of death in the United States in 2002, and age-adjusted death rates for stroke remained higher among blacks than whites.[1] In 1997, excess deaths from stroke occurred among persons under 65 years in most racial/ethnic minority groups, compared with whites.[2] A younger age distribution among Hispanics and other racial/ethnic groups compared with whites might partly explain the disproportionate burden in deaths at younger ages. To examine disparities in stroke mortality among persons under 75 years, Centers for Disease Control and Prevention (CDC) assessed several characteristics of mortality at younger ages by using death certificate data for 2002. This chapter summarizes the results of that assessment. Overall, 11.9% of all stroke deaths in 2002 occurred among persons under 65 years; the proportion of stroke decedents who were under 65 years was higher among blacks, American Indians/Alaska Natives, and Asians/Pacific Islanders, compared with whites. In addition, the mean ages of stroke decedents were statistically significantly lower in these racial groups than among whites. Blacks had more than twice the age-specific death rates from stroke than whites under 75 years of age. Approximately 3,400 excess stroke deaths would not have occurred among blacks in 2002 if blacks had had the same death rates for stroke as whites under 65 years of age. Moreover, age-adjusted estimates of years of potential

"Disparities in Deaths from Stroke among Persons Aged Less Than 75 Years—United States, 2002," *Morbidity and Mortality Weekly (MMWR)*, May 20, 2005; 54(19); 477–481, Centers for Disease Control and Prevention (CDC).

life lost (YPLL) before age 75 from stroke were more than twice as high for blacks than for all other racial groups. Reducing premature death from stroke in these groups will require early prevention, detection, treatment, and control of risk factors for stroke in young and middle-aged adults.

National and state mortality statistics used in this assessment were based on information from death certificates from all 50 states and the District of Columbia (DC). Demographic data (race/ethnicity, sex, and age) on death certificates were provided by funeral directors or family members. Stroke-related deaths were defined as those for which the underlying causes reported on the death certificate by a physician, medical examiner, or coroner were classified according to International Classification of Diseases, Tenth Revision (ICD–10) codes I60–I69. Age-specific excess deaths for racial groups were calculated by subtracting the expected number of deaths (the population number in a racial group multiplied by the death rate of whites) from the observed number of deaths within each age-specific group.[2] YPLL before age 75 was calculated as the sum of the differences between 75 years and the midpoint of each of eight age groups less than 75 years.[3] Age-adjusted estimates for YPLL before age 75 (per 100,000 persons under 75 years of age) in 2002 were calculated by using the 2000 U.S. standard population.[3] The mean age at death for all stroke decedents was also calculated. Age-adjusted death rates (per 100,000 population) and 95% confidence intervals (CIs) were calculated by using the 2000 U.S. standard population.[1]

Among U.S. residents, 162,672 stroke deaths occurred in 2002, with an age-adjusted death rate of 56.2 per 100,000 (Table 70.1). Age-adjusted rates were higher among blacks (76.3) than whites (54.2). The overall mean age of a stroke decedent was 79.6 years; however, males had a younger mean age at stroke death than females. Blacks, American Indians/Alaska Natives, and Asians/Pacific Islanders had younger mean ages than whites, and the mean age at stroke death was also younger among Hispanics than among non-Hispanics. Of all stroke deaths in 2002, a total of 19,376 (11.9%) occurred among persons under age 65. The proportion of stroke decedents under 65 was higher among men than women, higher in other racial groups than among whites, and higher among Hispanics than among non-Hispanics. Overall, 568,575 YPLL occurred before age 75 from stroke in 2002; this number resulted in an age-adjusted estimate of 208.5 per 100,000 population under 75 years of age. Higher age-adjusted estimates of YPLL were observed in males (227.9) compared with females (190.7) and were more than doubled in blacks (475.3) compared with whites (173.7).

Compared with whites, age-specific death rates for blacks were 2.5 times, 3.5 times, 2.8 times, and 1.9 times higher at ages 0–44, 45–54, 55–64, and 65–74 years, respectively. This resulted in 3,453.9 excess stroke deaths among blacks under 65 years of age (606.5 at age 0–44 years, 1,352.5 at age 45–54 years, and 1,494.9 at age 55–64 years). Age-specific death rates among American Indians/Alaskan Natives and Asians/Pacific Islanders were slightly higher than among whites for age 55–64 years only. Compared with non-Hispanics, Hispanics had lower or similar age-specific death rates for stroke (CDC, unpublished data, 2005).

Age-adjusted death rates, mean age at stroke death, and the proportion of stroke deaths that occurred under 65 years of age varied among states and DC. In 2002, the age-adjusted death rate for stroke ranged from 37.4 per 100,000 in New York to 74.3 in Arkansas. The mean age of stroke decedents ranged from 75.5 years in Alaska to 83.4 years in North Dakota. The proportion of stroke deaths occurring under 65 years of age ranged from 6.3% in Iowa to 18.2% in Louisiana and 18.3% in DC. Age-adjusted estimates of YPLL from stroke before age 75 (per 100,000 population under 75 years) ranged from 132.7 in Vermont to 361.0 in Mississippi in 2002.

Findings of This Report

The findings in this report demonstrate racial and ethnic disparities in stroke mortality under 75 years of age. In 2002, the mean age of stroke decedents was 79.6 years, and only 11.9% of all stroke deaths occurred among persons under 65 years. However, considerable differences by race/ethnicity and by area of residence occurred in the proportion of deaths under 65 years and by race/ethnicity in age-specific mortality rates, excess deaths, and YPLL before age 75 years. Whereas a younger age distribution among Hispanics and other racial groups compared with whites might explain some of the higher proportions of deaths under 65 years of age, stroke decedents in these groups die at a younger age than non-Hispanics and whites. Stroke death at younger ages contributes to 8% of the lower life expectancy in blacks compared with whites after accounting for heart disease (27.4%), cancer (19.4%), and homicide (9.7%).[4] Racial and ethnic disparities might also be explained by differences in stroke risk factors among population subgroups and younger adults. For example, among adults aged 45–54 years, during 1998–2002, a statistically higher prevalence of self-reported diabetes was observed for Hispanics than non-Hispanic whites in several states with the highest proportions of Hispanics.[5] Hispanics and non-Hispanic blacks also have a higher prevalence of overweight, obesity, and physical inactivity than non-Hispanics whites, [3, 6] whereas self-reported high blood pressure is higher in blacks than whites.[3, 6] In certain communities, the prevalence of hypertension, diabetes, and obesity among American Indians and blacks is considerably higher than in the general population.[7] Cigarette smoking tends to be more common in American Indian communities than in other racial or ethnic communities.[7] To eliminate these disparities in stroke mortality among persons under 75 years of age, public health strategies should focus on detecting and reducing stroke risk factors and improving access to health-care and preventive-care services among young and middle-aged adults in racial and ethnic subgroups at high risk.

Variations among states might reflect differences in lifestyle and stroke risk factors.[6] States with the highest proportion of stroke deaths occurring at ages under 65 years are in the southern region of the United States, which includes a higher percentage of adults with stroke risk factors, such as hypertension, smoking, obesity, and physical inactivity.[6] The disproportionate number of stroke deaths among persons under 65 years in Alaska, Nevada, and New Mexico might reflect the demographics of those states, which have greater proportions of American Indian/Alaska Native communities and a high prevalence of stroke risk factors.

The findings in this report are subject to at least two limitations. First, death certificate data are subject to error in the certification of underlying causes of death.[1] Second, underreporting of American Indian/Alaska Native, Asian/Pacific Islander, and Hispanic origin on death certificates might lead to underestimates of the proportion of stroke deaths among persons under 65 years of age among these populations.[1, 8]

Premature death is only part of the health impact of strokes in young and middle-aged adults. An estimated 942,000 hospitalizations for stroke occurred in 2002; of these, 28% occurred among patients under 65 years of age.[9] Approximately 2.3% of whites and 2.7% of blacks living in U.S. households in 2000–2001 reported a history of stroke; approximately half of black stroke survivors and one-third of white stroke survivors were under age 65.[10] Black stroke survivors experienced more limitations of activities than white survivors.[10] The elimination of stroke risk is crucial for reducing not only death but also stroke disability, thereby improving both the quality of life and life expectancy. Campaigns that increase awareness of stroke warning signs and symptoms should be continued, particularly among

Table 70.1. Total number of stroke deaths, age-adjusted death rate,* mean age at death, percentage of stroke decedents under 65 years of age, and years of potential life lost (YPLL) before age 75 years, by selected characteristics: United States 2002.

Characteristic	Total	Rate	Mean age (yrs.)	Aged less than 65 years (%)	YPLL from stroke before age 75 years
Sex					
Men	62,622	56.5	76.3	16.7	300,442
Women	100,050	55.2	81.6	8.9	268,133
Race					
White	139,719	54.2	80.7	9.5	397,680
Black	18,856	76.3	72.6	27.8	145,543
American Indian/Alaska Native	567	37.5	71.4	29.6	4,835
Asian/Pacific Islander	3,530	29.4	75.4	20.5	20,518
Hispanic origin[1]					
Hispanic	6,451	41.3	72.6	26.3	50,516
Non-Hispanic	155,852	56.8	79.9	11.3	516,540
Total	162,672	56.2	79.6	11.9	568,575

*Per 100,000 population; adjusted to the standard 2000 U.S. population.

[1]Hispanics and non-Hispanics include members of any race. Decedents with missing information about Hispanic origin were excluded from this category.

575

young adults who might perceive stroke as a health condition limited to the aging population.

References

1. Kochanek KD, Murphy SL, Anderson RN, Scott C. Deaths: final data for 2002. *Natl Vital Stat Rep 2004*; 53.

2. CDC. Age-specific excess deaths associated with stroke among racial/ethnic minority populations: United States, 1997. *MMWR 2000*; 49:94–7.

3. National Center for Health Statistics. *Health, United States, 2004* with chartbook on trends in the health of Americans. Hyattsville, MD: US Department of Health and Human Services, CDC, National Center for Health Statistics; 2004.

4. CDC. Influence of homicide on racial disparity in life expectancy: United States, 1998. *MMWR 2001*; 50:780–3.

5. CDC. Prevalence of diabetes among Hispanics–selected areas, 1998–2002. *MMWR 2004*; 53:941–3.

6. CDC. State-specific prevalence of selected chronic disease-related characteristics–Behavioral Risk Factor Surveillance System, 2001. In: Surveillance Summaries, August 22, 2003. *MMWR 2003*; 52(No. SS-8).

7. CDC. REACH 2010 surveillance for health status in minority communities: United States, 2001–2002. In: Surveillance Summaries, August 27, 2004. *MMWR 2004*; 53(No. SS-6).

8. Rosenberg HM, Maurer JD, Sorlie PD, et al. Quality of death rates and Hispanic origin: a summary of current research, 1999. *Vital Health Stat 1999*; 2(128).

9. DeFrances CJ, Hall MJ. *2002 National Hospital Discharge Survey. Advance data from vital and health statistics; no. 342.* Hyattsville, MD: US Department of Health and Human Services, CDC, National Center for Health Statistics; 2004.

10. CDC. Differences in disability among black and white stroke survivors: United States, 2000–2001. *MMWR 2005*; 54:3–6.

Chapter 71

Use of Health Care Resources at the End of Life

Summary: This project aimed to understand how resources, including hospitalizations, hospice, home care services, are utilized at the end of life and the relationship with site of death and costs.

Background: Over the last two decades, there has been much controversy about spending at the end of life. The concern has focused on several key perceptions: costs of care at the end of life are very, very high—about 27% of all Medicare expenditures; deaths are too high-tech and de-personalized; and comfort measures, such as hospice, are under-utilized. Unfortunately, there are woefully few data on costs and resource utilization at the end of life. The last analysis of costs at the end of life reported on Medicare costs was from 1988. The last analysis of the use of hospice at the end of life and its effects on costs report on data from 1992 and only reported on Medicare cancer decedents. These data have major deficiencies in that they predate the substantial efforts to reduce hospitalization rates and length of stay; the growth of managed care; and the focus of national attention on improving care at the end of life and use of hospice. Furthermore, almost all available data come from Medicare and therefore focus on the resource utilization of decedents over 65 years of age. Fully one-third of all decedents in the United States are under 65 years of age.

Excerpted from "End-of-Life Resource Use," National Institutes of Health Clinical Center, 2003.

Methodology: Initially both Harvard Pilgrim Health Care (a managed care organization with both a staff model component and an independent practice association [IPA] component) and Massachusetts Blue Cross and Blue Shield thought they could provide expenditure data on all their decedents. Both those covered in managed care programs and those under 65 years of age. Unfortunately, after working with both organizations for over a year, it became clear that they either did not have the expenditure data or did not collect the expenditure data linked to mortality in a format that could be analyzed. Instead, 1996 Medicare data from Massachusetts and California was used, merging Medicare's denominator files with each state's 1996 death certificate files. Only beneficiaries continuously enrolled in both Parts A and B Medicare insurance over the entire last 12 months of life were retained. In Massachusetts, 42,452 Medicare decedents met the criteria. In California 20% of decedents were used comprising 33,684 people. Decedents were divided by their insurance status into three groups:

- those continuously enrolled in a fee-for-service (FFS) plan for the last 12 months of life;

- those continuously enrolled in a managed care organization plan (MCO) for the last 12 months of life; and

- those that changed between FFS and MCO during the last 12 months of life.

Total expenditures were calculated as the sum of HCFA payments and payments from other sources of insurance for Medicare covered services. The study examined expenditures and services provided including hospice and chemotherapy use for decedents for 30-day periods from the date of death back 12 months.

Results: Some of the most salient results can be summarized as follows:

- Expenditures over the last year of life are on average $28,588 for Massachusetts decedents and $27,814 for California decedents (1996 dollars).

- Patients dying of chronic obstructive pulmonary disease (COPD) have the highest expenditures—$35,145 in Massachusetts and $33,269 in California—and patients dying of cancer having the second highest expenditures.

- Expenditures rise exponentially as death approaches, with the last month of life accounting for approximately 32% of the entire last year of expenditures in Massachusetts and 38% in California.

- Overall hospice is still predominantly used by cancer patients. In Massachusetts 70% of all hospice patients have cancer, in California 00%. Indeed, in Massachusetts 33% of all cancer patients receive hospice and just under 50% do so in California.

- Managed care patients are much more likely to receive hospice care at the end of life than patients who have fee for service insurance.

- There is a substantial reduction in expenditures and resource utilization with increasing age. This age-based rationing is not accounted for by co-morbidities.

- There is a reverse racial disparity in expenditures at the end of life: African Americans receive approximately 50% more resources in the last year of life compared to whites. In Massachusetts, expenditures in the last year of life for whites was $28,200 and for African Americans $42,200, in California for whites it was $26,300 and for African Americans $40,700.

- A substantial proportion of patients who die of cancer receive chemotherapy at the end of life. In Massachusetts 33% receive chemotherapy in the last six months, 23% in the last three months and 9% in the last month of life. Similarly in California, 26%, 20% and 9% respectively.

- Chemotherapy use is similar for cancers that tend to be chemotherapy responsive and those that tend to be chemotherapy unresponsive. However the duration of chemotherapy use is lower for unresponsive cancers.

Future Directions: These data are limited in two main ways: generalizability and age of the data. Furthermore, one of the most intriguing results, the disparities in the use of resources at the end of life according to race, was based on very small numbers.

The data from Massachusetts and California suggest important trends in the location of death. In 1996, in these states, approximately 40% of deaths were in hospital. This appears to be a dramatic shift out of the hospital at end of life.

Part Ten

Additional Help
and Information

Chapter 72

Glossary of End-of-Life Terms

Advance Medical Directives: Advance directives are used to give other people, including health care providers, information about your wishes for medical care. Advance directives are important in case there is ever a time when you are not physically or mentally able to speak for yourself and make your wishes known. The most common types of advance directives are the living will and the durable power of attorney for health care.

Allodynia: When pain is caused by something that does not normally cause pain (such as clothing touching the skin).

Analgesic Medications: Medications used to prevent or treat pain.

Antidepressant: Medications used to treat depression, and also used to treat chronic pain. Antidepressants can also be helpful for pain-related symptoms, like sleep problems and muscle spasms.

Anxiolytic: Medications used to treat anxiety, and also used to treat chronic pain. Anxiolytics reduce pain-related anxiety, help relax muscles, and can help a person cope with pain.

Unmarked definitions in this chapter are from StopPain.org, Beth Israel Medical Center, New York, NY. © 2000–2005 Continuum Health Partners, Inc. Reprinted with permission. Terms marked [1] are from "Cognitive Disorders and Delirium PDQ®: Supportive Care–Patient," PDQ® Cancer Information Summary, National Cancer Institute, Bethesda, MD, updated November 2005, available at http://cancer.gov. Accessed March 1, 2006.

Assessment: In health care, a process used to learn about a patient's condition. This may include a complete medical history, medical tests, a physical exam, a test of learning skills, tests to find out if the patient is able to carry out the tasks of daily living, a mental health evaluation, and a review of social support and community resources available to the patient. [1]

Bereavement: The act of grieving someone's death.

Caregiver: Any person who provides care for the physical and emotional needs of a family member or friend.

Causalgia (Complex Regional Pain Syndrome II): Pain, usually burning, that is associated with autonomic changes—change in color of the skin, change in temperature, change in sweating, swelling. Causalgia occurs after a nerve injury.

Central Nervous System: The brain and the spinal cord.

Clinical Trials: Carefully planned and monitored experiments to test a new drug or treatment.

Complementary Medicine: Approaches to medical treatment that are outside of mainstream medical training. Complementary medicine treatments used for pain include: acupuncture, low-level laser therapy, meditation, aroma therapy, Chinese medicine, dance therapy, music therapy, massage, herbalism, therapeutic touch, yoga, osteopathy, chiropractic treatments, naturopathy, and homeopathy.

Computed Tomography (CT/CAT) Scanning: A painless technique used to produce a picture of a cross-section, or slice, of a part of the body. X-rays are used to produce this picture.

Constipation: Difficulty having a bowel movement.

Dehydration: A condition caused by the loss of too much water from the body. Severe diarrhea or vomiting can cause dehydration. [1]

Delirium: A disturbance of the brain function that causes confusion and changes in alertness, attention, thinking and reasoning, memory, emotions, sleeping patterns, and coordination. These symptoms may start suddenly, are due to some type of medical problem, and they may get worse or better multiple times.

Depression: A mental condition marked by ongoing feelings of sadness, despair, loss of energy, and difficulty dealing with normal daily life. Other symptoms of depression include feelings of worthlessness and hopelessness, loss of pleasure in activities, changes in eating or sleeping habits, and thoughts of death or suicide. Depression can affect anyone, and can be successfully treated. Depression affects 15–25% of cancer patients. [1]

Diagnosis: The process of identifying a disease by the signs and symptoms. [1]

Disorder: In medicine, a disturbance of normal functioning of the mind or body. Disorders may be caused by genetic factors, disease, or trauma. [1]

Do-Not-Resuscitate (DNR) Orders: Instructions written by a doctor telling other health care providers not to try to restart a patient's heart, using cardiopulmonary resuscitation (CPR) or other related treatments, if his/her heart stops beating. Usually, DNR orders are written after a discussion between a doctor and the patient and/or family members. DNR orders are written for people who are very unlikely to have a successful result from CPR—those who are terminally ill or those who are elderly and frail.

Durable Power of Attorney for Health Care: A legal document that specifies one or more individuals (called a health care proxy) you would like to make medical decisions for you if you are unable to do so yourself.

Dyspnea: Difficulty in breathing.

End-of-Life Care: Doctors and caregivers provide care to patients approaching the end of life that is focused on comfort, respect for decisions, support for the family, and treatments to help psychological and spiritual concerns.

Entitlement: A federal program (such as Social Security or unemployment benefits) that guarantees a certain level of benefits to those who meet requirements set by law.

EPEC (Education for Physicians on End-of-Life Care): A project designed to educate physicians across the United States about providing good end-of-life care for patients. EPEC includes a curriculum used to train doctors in clinical knowledge and skills they need to care for dying patients.

Ethics: A system of moral principles and rules that are used as standards for professional conduct. Many hospitals and other health care facilities have ethics committees that can help doctors, other health care providers, patients, and their family members in making difficult decisions regarding medical care.

Fatigue: A feeling of becoming tired easily, being unable to complete usual activity, feeling weak, and difficulty concentrating.

Fibromyalgia: A pain disorder in which a person feels widespread pain and stiffness in the muscles, fatigue, and other symptoms.

Hospice: A special way of caring for people with terminal illnesses and their families by meeting the patient's physical, emotional, social, and spiritual needs, as well as the needs of the family. The goals of hospice are to keep the patient as comfortable as possible by relieving pain and other symptoms; to prepare for a death that follows the wishes and needs of the patient; and to reassure both the patient and family members by helping them to understand and manage what is happening.

Hospice Home Care: Most hospice patients receive care while living in their homes. Home hospice patients have family members or friends who provide most of their care, with help and support from the trained hospice team. The hospice team visits at the house to provide medical and nursing care, emotional support, counseling, information, instruction, and practical help. A home care aide may also be available to help with daily care, if needed.

Hyperalgesia: Extreme sensitivity to pain.

Hyperpathia: An exaggerated response to something that causes pain, with continued pain after the cause of the pain is no longer present.

Incontinence: Inability to control the flow of urine from the bladder (urinary incontinence) or the escape of stool from the rectum (fecal incontinence). [1]

Informed Consent: The process of making decisions about medical care that are based on open, honest communication between the health care provider and the patient and/or the patient's family members.

Living Will: A legal document which outlines the kinds of medical care a patient wants and does not want. The living will is used only if the patient becomes unable to make decisions for him/herself.

Magnetic Resonance Imaging (MRI): A painless technique that uses magnetic fields and radio waves (without radiation) to create clear cross-sectional pictures of the body.

Multidisciplinary: In medicine, a term used to describe a treatment planning approach or team that includes a number of doctors and other health care professionals who are experts in different specialties (disciplines). [1]

Myofascial Pain: Muscle pain and tenderness.

Nerve Blocks: Injections of anesthetic (or numbing) substances into nerves in order to reduce pain.

Nutrition/Hydration: Intravenous (IV) fluid and nutritional supplements given to patients who are unable to eat or drink by mouth, or those who are dehydrated or malnourished.

Opioid: A type of medication related to opium. Opioids are strong analgesics. Opioids include morphine, codeine, and a large number of synthetic (man-made) drugs like methadone and fentanyl.

Pain: An unpleasant feeling that may or may not be related to an injury, illness, or other bodily trauma. Pain is complex and differs from person to person.

Pain, Acute: Pain that has a known cause and occurs for a limited time. Acute pain usually responds to treatment with analgesic medications and treatment of the cause of the pain.

Pain, Chronic: Pain that occurs for more than one month after healing of an injury, that occurs repeatedly over months, or is due to a lesion that is not expected to heal.

Pain Due to Nerve Injury: Pain caused by an injury or other problem in the nervous system.

Palliative Care: The total care of patients with progressive, incurable illness. In palliative care, the focus of care is on quality of life. Control of pain and other physical symptoms, and psychological, social, and spiritual problems is considered most important.

Patient-Controlled Analgesia (PCA): Pain medication given through an IV or epidural catheter. Patients control the dose of medication they take, depending on how much is needed to control the pain.

PCA is usually used for patients recovering from intra-abdominal, major orthopedic, or thoracic surgery, and for chronic pain states such as those due to cancer.

Peripheral Nervous System: The nerves throughout the body that send messages to the central nervous system.

Peripheral Neuropathy: Pain caused by an injury or other problem with the peripheral nervous system.

Phantom Pain: Pain that develops after an amputation. To the patient, the pain feels like it is coming from the missing body part.

Pharmacotherapy: The treatment of diseases and symptoms with medications.

Physician-Assisted Suicide: Actions by a doctor that help a patient commit suicide. Though the doctor may provide medication, a prescription, or take other steps, the patient takes his/her own life (for instance, by swallowing the pills that are expected to bring about death).

Postherpetic Neuralgia (PHN): Painful condition following shingles (herpes zoster).

Psychological Approaches: Techniques used to help patients cope with their pain and deal with emotional factors that can increase pain. Such strategies include biofeedback, imagery, hypnosis, relaxation training, stress management, cognitive-behavioral therapy, and family counseling.

Reflex Sympathetic Dystrophy (Complex Regional Pain Syndrome I): Pain, usually burning, that is associated with autonomic changes—change in color of the skin, change in temperature, change in sweating, swelling. Reflex sympathetic dystrophy is caused by injury to bone, joint, or soft tissues.

Rehabilitation: Treatment for an injury, illness, or pain with the goal of restoring function.

Side Effect: A problem that occurs when treatment affects healthy tissues or organs. Some common side effects of cancer treatment are fatigue, pain, nausea, vomiting, decreased blood cell counts, hair loss, and mouth sores. [1]

Standard Therapy: In medicine, treatment that experts agree is appropriate, accepted, and widely used. Health care providers are obligated to provide patients with standard therapy. Also called standard of care or best practice. [1]

Symptom: An indication that a person has a condition or disease. Some examples of symptoms are headache, fever, fatigue, nausea, vomiting, and pain. [1]

Terminal Disease: Disease that cannot be cured and will cause death. [1]

Treatment Withdrawal: A syndrome that might occur when a medication that has been used regularly to treat pain is no longer used, or when the dose is decreased. Showing symptoms of withdrawal does not mean that a patient is addicted to his/her pain medication.

Trigeminal Neuralgia: A disorder of the trigeminal nerve that causes brief attacks of severe pain in the lips, cheeks, gums, or chin on one side of the face.

Chapter 73

Support Groups for End-of-Life Issues

American Association of Suicidology
5221 Wisconsin Ave., N.W.
Washington, DC 20016
Phone: 202-237-2280
Website: http://www.suicidology.org
E-mail: info@suicidology.org

AAS provides an online listing by state of suicide survivors support groups.

American Cancer Society
1599 Clifton Rd., N.E.
Atlanta, GA 30329-4251
Toll-Free: 800-227-2345
Phone: 404-320-3333
Website: http://www.cancer.org

ACS has information about types of support groups and how to find online and local support.

Compassionate Friends
P.O. Box 3696
Oak Brook, IL 60522-3696

Resources in this chapter were compiled from several sources deemed reliable. All contact information was verified and updated in March 2006.

Toll-Free: 877-969-0010
Fax: 630-990-0246
Website: http://www.compassionatefriends.org
E-mail: nationaloffice@compassionatefriends.org

Compassionate Friends offers support groups and resources for parents who have had a child die and children who have had a sibling die.

First Candle/SIDS Alliance
1314 Bedford Ave.
Suite 210
Baltimore, MD 21208
Toll-Free: 800-221-7437
Phone: 410-653-8226
Website: http://www.sidsalliance.org
E-mail: info@firstcandle.org

First Candle has an online state-by-state list of grief support groups available for families affected by infant death.

GriefShare
P.O. Box 1739
Wake Forest, NC 27588
Toll-Free: 800-395-5755
Website: http://griefshare.org
E-mail: info@griefshare.org

GriefShare offers resources and an online directory of support groups in the U.S. and Canada that feature biblical teaching on grief and recovery topics.

Leukemia & Lymphoma Society
1311 Mamaroneck Ave.
White Plains, NY 10605
Toll-Free: 800-955-4572
Phone: 914-949-5213
Fax: 914-949-6691
Website: http://www.leukemia-lymphoma.org

Leukemia & Lymphoma Society has an online listing of family support groups for anyone affected by blood cancer.

National Hospice and Palliative Care Organization
1700 Diagonal Rd., Suite 625
Alexandria, VA 22314
Toll-Free: 800-658-8898
Phone: 703-837-1500; Fax: 703-837-1233
Website: http://www.nhpco.org
E-mail: nhpco_info@nhpco.org

NHPCO offers an online discussion forum of end-of-life issues.

National SHARE Office
St. Joseph Health Center
300 First Capitol Dr.
St. Charles, MO 63301-2893
Toll-Free: 800-821-6819
Phone: 636-947-6164; Fax: 636-947-7486
Website: http://www.nationalshareoffice.com
E-mail: share@nationalshareoffice.com

National SHARE has an online directory of support groups for families who have experienced the death of a baby.

Suicide Prevention Resource Center
55 Chapel Street
Newton, MA 02458-1060
Toll-Free: 877-GET-SPRC (438-7772)
TTY: 617-964-5448
Website: http://www.sprc.org
E-mail: info@sprc.org

Suicide Prevention Resource Center has Internet links to suicide survivor support groups and resources for survivors of suicide.

TAPS (Tragedy Assistance Program for Survivors, Inc.)
1621 Connecticut, N.W., Suite 300
Washington, DC 20009
Toll-Free: 800-959-TAPS (8277)
Phone: 202-588-8277; Fax: 202-638-5312
Website: http://www.taps.org

TAPS serves the families and friends of those who have died while serving in the Armed Forces. Services include a military survivor peer support network, grief counseling referral, caseworker assistance, and crisis information.

Well Spouse Foundation
63 W. Main St., Suite H
Freehold, NJ 07728
Toll-Free: 800-838-0873
Website: http://www.wellspouse.org

Well Spouse Foundation offers monthly group meetings to support wives, husbands, and partners of the chronically ill.

Yellow Ribbon
P.O. Box 644
Westminster, CO 80036-0644
Phone: 303-429-3530
Fax: 303-426-4496
Website: http://www.yellowribbon.org
E-mail: ask4help@yellowribbon.org

Yellow Ribbon has an online directory of suicide survivors support group information available at http://www.yellowribbon.org/Survivor SupportGroups.html.

Editor's Note: Local hospitals, libraries, mental health organizations, and churches may also be able to direct you to support groups available in your home area.

Chapter 74

Resources for Information about Death and Dying

Administration on Aging
330 Independence Ave., S.W.
Washington, DC 20201
Phone: 202-619-0724
Fax: 202-357-3560
Website: http://www.aoa.gov
E-mail: aoainfo@aoa.gov

AGS Foundation for Health in Aging
350 Fifth Ave.
Suite 801
New York, NY 10118
Toll-Free: 800-563-4916
Phone: 212-755-6810
Fax: 212-832-8646
Website: http://www.healthinaging.org
E-mail: staff@healthinaging.org

AIDS Info
P.O. Box 6303
Rockville MD 20849-6303
Toll-Free: 800-HIV-0440 (800-448-0440)
Toll-Free TTY: 888-480-3739
Phone: 301-519-0459
Fax: 301-519-6616
Website: http://aidsinfo.nih.gov
E-mail: contactus@aidsinfo.nih.gov

ALS Association
27001 Agoura Rd.
Suite 150
Calabasas Hills, CA 91301
Phone: 818-880-9007
Website: http://www.alsa.org
E-mail: alsinfo@alsa-national.org

Resources in this chapter were compiled from several sources deemed reliable. All contact information was verified and updated in March 2006.

Alzheimer's Association
225 N. Michigan Ave., Suite 1700
Chicago, IL 60601
Toll-Free: 800-272-3900
Fax: 312-335-1110
Website: http://www.alz.org
E-mail: info@alz.org

Alzheimer's Disease Education and Referral Center (ADEAR)
P.O. Box 8250
Silver Spring, MD 20907-8250
Toll-Free: 800-438-4380
Website: http://
www.alzheimers.org

American Academy of Hospice and Palliative Medicine
4700 W. Lake Ave.
Glenview IL 60025
Phone: 847-375-4712
Fax: 877-734-8671
Website: http://www.aahpm.org
E-mail: info@aahpm.org

American Association of Homes and Services for the Aging
2519 Connecticut Ave., N.W.
Washington, DC 20008
Phone: 202-783-2242
Website: http://www.aahsa.org

American Association of Retired People (AARP)
601 E Street, N.W.
Washington, DC 20049
Toll-Free: 888-687-2277
Website: http://www.aarp.org

American Association of Suicidology
5221 Wisconsin Ave., N.W.
Washington, DC 20016
Phone: 202-237-2280
Website: http://
www.suicidology.org
E-mail: info@suicidology.org

American Chronic Pain Association (ACPA)
P.O. Box 850
Rocklin, CA 95677
Toll-Free: 800-533-3231
Fax: 916-632-3208
Website: http://www.theacpa.org
E-mail: ACPA@pacbell.net

American Hospice Foundation
2120 L Street, N.W.
Suite 200
Washington, DC 20037
Phone: 202-223-0204
Fax: 202-223-0208
Website: http://
www.americanhospice.org
E-mail:
ahf@americanhospice.org

American Pain Foundation
201 N. Charles St.
Suite 710
Baltimore, MD 21201-4111
Toll-Free: 888-615-PAIN (7246)
Fax: 410-385-1832
Website: http://
www.painfoundation.org
E-mail: info@painfoundation.org

American Pain Society
4700 W. Lake Ave.
Glenview IL 60025
Phone: 847-375-4715
Fax: 877-734-8758
Website: http://
www.ampainsoc.org
E-mail: info@ampainsoc.org

Americans for Better Care of the Dying
1700 Diagonal Rd.
Suite 635
Alexandria, VA 22314
Phone: 703-647-8505
Fax: 703-837-1233
Website: http://www.abcd-caring.org
E-mail: info@abcd-caring.org

Association for Death Education and Counseling (ADEC)
60 Revere Dr., Suite 500
Northbrook, IL 60062
Phone: 847-509-0403
Fax: 847-480-9282
Website: http://www.adec.org
E-mail: adec@adec.org

Association of Professional Chaplains
1701 E. Woodfield Rd., Suite 760
Schaumburg, IL 60173
Phone: 847-240-1014
Fax: 847-240-1015
Website: http://
www.professionalchaplains.org
E-mail:
info@professionalchaplains.org

Bereaved Parents of the USA
National Office
P.O. Box 95
Park Forest, IL 60466
Phone: 708-748-7866
Website: http://
www.bereavedparentsusa.org

Cancer Care, Inc.
275 Seventh Ave.
New York, NY 10001
Toll-Free: 800-813-HOPE (4673)
Website: http://
www.cancercare.org
E-mail: info@cancercare.org

Centers for Disease Control and Prevention (CDC)
1600 Clifton Rd.
Atlanta, GA 30333
Toll-Free: 800-311-3435
Phone: 404-639-3534
Website: http://www.cdc.gov

Centers for Medicare and Medicaid Services
Toll-Free: 800-MEDICARE (800-633-4227)
Toll-Free TTY: 877-486-2048
Websites: http://
www.medicare.gov or http://
www.cms.hhs.gov

Children's Hospice International
901 N. Pitt St., Suite 230
Alexandria, VA 22314
Toll-Free: 800-242-4453
http://www.chionline.org

Commission on Accreditation of Rehabilitation Facilities
4891 E. Grant Rd.
Tucson, AZ 85712
Toll-Free Voice/TTY: 888-281-6531
Phone: 520-325-1044
Fax: 520-318-1129
Website: http://www.carf.org

Compassion & Choices
P.O. Box 101810
Denver, CO 80250-1810
Toll-Free: 800-247-7421
Fax: 303-639-1224
Website: http://www.compassionindying.org

Compassionate Friends
P.O. Box 3696
Oak Brook, IL 60522-3696
Toll-Free: 877-969-0010
Fax: 630-990-0246
Website: http://www.compassionatefriends.org
E-mail: nationaloffice@compassionatefriends.org

Dougy Center for Grieving Children and Families
P.O. Box 86852
Portland, OR 97286
Toll-Free: 866-775-5683
Phone: 503-775-5683
Fax: 503-777-3097
Website: http://www.dougy.org
E-mail: help@dougy.org

Eldercare Locator
Administration on Aging
330 Independence Ave., S.W.
Washington, DC 20201
Toll-Free: 800-677-1116
Phone: 202-619-7501
Website: http://www.eldercare.gov
E-mail: eldercarelocator@spherix.com

Family Caregiver Alliance
180 Montgomery St., Suite 1100
San Francisco, CA 94104
Toll-Free: 800-445-8106
Phone: 415-434-3388
Website: http://caregiver.org
E-mail: info@caregiver.org

Federal Trade Commission
Consumer Response Center
600 Pennsylvania Ave., N.W.
Washington, DC 20580
Toll-Free: 877-FTC-HELP (382-4357)
Toll-Free TDD: 866-653-4261
Website: http://www.ftc.gov

First Candle/SIDS Alliance
1314 Bedford Ave., Suite 210
Baltimore, MD 21208
Toll-Free: 800-221-7437
Phone: 410-653-8226
Website: http://www.sidsalliance.org
E-mail: info@firstcandle.org

Funeral Consumers Alliance
33 Patchen Road
South Burlington, VT 05403
Toll-Free: 800-765-0107
Website: http://www.funerals.org

George Washington Institute for Spirituality and Health (GWish)
2131 K Street, N.W.
Suite #510
Washington, DC 20037-1898
Phone: 202-496-6409
Fax: 202-496-6413
Website: http://www.gwish.org

Hospice Education Institute
3 Unity Square
P.O. Box 98
Machiasport, ME 04655-0098
Toll-Free: 800-331-1620
Phone: 207-255-8800
Fax: 207-255-8008
Website: http://www.hospiceworld.org
E-mail: info@hospiceworld.org

Hospice Foundation of America
1621 Connecticut Ave., N.W.,
Suite 300
Washington, DC 20009
Toll-Free: 800-854-3402
Fax: 202-638-5312
Website: http://www.hospicefoundation.org
E-mail: info@hospicefoundation.org

International Cemetery and Funeral Association
107 Carpenter Dr., Suite 100
Sterling, VA 20164
Toll-Free: 800-645-7700
Phone: 703-391-8400
Fax: 703-391-8416
Website: http://www.icfa.org

Joint Commission on Accreditation of Healthcare Organizations
One Renaissance Blvd.
Oakbrook Terrace, IL 60181
Phone: 630-792-5800
Website: http://www.jcaho.org
Quality Check® Website: http://www.qualitycheck.org
E-mail: customerservice@jcaho.org

National Association for Home Care
228 7th St., S.E.
Washington, DC 20003
Phone: 202-547-7424
Fax: 202-547-3540
Website: http://www.nahc.org

National Association of Area Agencies on Aging
1730 Rhode Island Ave., N.W.,
Suite 1200
Washington, DC 20036
Phone: 202-872-0888
Fax: 202-872-0057
Website: http://www.n4a.org

National Association of Catholic Chaplains
3501 S. Lake Dr.
P.O. Box 070473
Milwaukee, WI 53207-0473
Phone: 414-483-4898
Fax: 414-483-6712
Website: http://www.nacc.org
E-mail: info@nacc.org

National Association of State Units on Aging
1201 15th St., N.W., Suite 350
Washington, DC 20005
Phone: 202-898-2578
Fax: 202-898-2583
Website: http://www.nasua.org
E-mail: info@nasua.org

National Cancer Institute
6116 Executive Blvd.
Suite 3036A, MSC 8322
Bethesda, MD 20892-8322
Toll-Free: 800-4-CANCER (800-422-6237)
Toll-Free TTY: 800-332-8615
Website: http://www.cancer.gov
E-mail:
cancergovstaff@mail.nih.gov

National Family Caregivers Association
10400 Connecticut Ave., Suite 500
Kensington, MD 20895-3944
Toll-Free: 800-896-3650
Phone: 301-942-6430
Fax: 301-942-2302
Website: http://www.nfcacares.org
E-mail:
info@thefamilycaregiver.org

National Funeral Directors Association
Funeral Service Consumer
Assistance Program
13625 Bishop's Dr.
Brookfield, WI 53005-6607
Toll-Free: 800-228-6332
Phone: 262-789-1880
Fax: 262-789-6977
Website: http://www.nfda.org
E-mail: nfda@nfda.org

National Hospice and Palliative Care Organization
1700 Diagonal Rd., Suite 625
Alexandria, VA 22314
Toll-Free: 800-658-8898
Phone: 703-837-1500
Fax: 703-837-1233
Website: http://www.nhpco.org
E-mail: nhpco_info@nhpco.org

National Institute on Aging (NIA)
Bldg. 31, Room 5C27
31 Center Dr., MSC 2292
Bethesda, MD 20892
Toll-Free: 800-222-2225
Phone: 301-496-1752
Fax: 301-496-1072
Toll-Free TTY: 800-222-4225
Website: http://www.nia.nih.gov

National SHARE Office
St. Joseph Health Center
300 First Capitol Dr.
St. Charles, MO 63301-2893
Toll-Free: 800-821-6819
Phone: 636-947-6164
Fax: 636-947-7486
Website: http://
www.nationalshareoffice.com
E-mail: share
@nationalshareoffice.com

Safe Kids USA
1301 Pennsylvania Ave., N.W.,
Suite 1000
Washington, DC 20004
Phone: 202-662-0600
Fax: 202-393-2072
Website: http://
www.usa.safekids.org

Social Security Administration
Office of Public Inquiries
Windsor Park Building
6401 Security Blvd.
Baltimore, MD 21235
Toll-Free: 800-772-1213
Toll-Free TTY: 800-325-0778
Website: http://www.ssa.gov

Society of Critical Care Medicine
701 Lee St., Suite 200
Des Plaines, IL 60016
Phone: 847-827-6888
Fax: 847-827-6886
Website: http://www.sccm.org
E-mail: info@sccm.org

Substance Abuse and Mental Health Services Administration
1 Choke Cherry Rd.
Room 8-1036
Rockville, MD 20857
Toll-Free Suicide Prevention
Hotline: 800-273-8255
Toll-Free TTY: 800-799-4889
Website: http://www.samhsa.gov

Suicide Prevention Resource Center
55 Chapel St.
Newton, MA 02458-1060
Toll-Free: 877-GET-SPRC (438-7772)
TTY: 617-964-5448
Website: http://www.sprc.org
E-mail: info@sprc.org

U.S. Department of Labor
Frances Perkins Building
200 Constitution Ave., N.W.
Washington, DC 20210
Toll-Free: 866-4-USWAGE (487-9243)
Toll-Free TTY: 877-889-5627
Website: http://www.dol.gov

Visiting Nurse Associations of America
99 Summer St., Suite 1700
Boston, MA 02110
Phone: 617-737-3200
Fax: 617-737-1144
Website: http://www.vnaa.org.
E-mail: vnaa@vnaa.org

Yellow Ribbon
P.O. Box 644
Westminster, CO 80036-0644
Phone: 303-429-3530
Fax: 303-426-4496
Website: http://www.yellowribbon.org
E-mail: ask4help@yellowribbon.org

601

Index

Index

Page numbers followed by 'n' indicate a footnote. Page numbers in *italics* indicate a table or illustration.

605

Health Reference Series
COMPLETE CATALOG

List price $87 per volume. **School and library price $78 per volume.**

Adolescent Health Sourcebook

Basic Consumer Health Information about Common Medical, Mental, and Emotional Concerns in Adolescents, Including Facts about Acne, Body Piercing, Mononucleosis, Nutrition, Eating Disorders, Stress, Depression, Behavior Problems, Peer Pressure, Violence, Gangs, Drug Use, Puberty, Sexuality, Pregnancy, Learning Disabilities, and More

Along with a Glossary of Terms and Other Resources for Further Help and Information

Edited by Chad T. Kimball. 658 pages. 2002. 0-7808-0248-9.

"It is written in clear, nontechnical language aimed at general readers. . . . Recommended for public libraries, community colleges, and other agencies serving health care consumers."
— *American Reference Books Annual, 2003*

"Recommended for school and public libraries. Parents and professionals dealing with teens will appreciate the easy-to-follow format and the clearly written text. This could become a 'must have' for every high school teacher." — *E-Streams, Jan '03*

"A good starting point for information related to common medical, mental, and emotional concerns of adolescents." — *School Library Journal, Nov '02*

"This book provides accurate information in an easy to access format. It addresses topics that parents and caregivers might not be aware of and provides practical, useable information."
— *Doody's Health Sciences Book Review Journal, Sep-Oct '02*

"Recommended reference source."
— *Booklist, American Library Association, Sep '02*

AIDS Sourcebook, 3rd Edition

Basic Consumer Health Information about Acquired Immune Deficiency Syndrome (AIDS) and Human Immunodeficiency Virus (HIV) Infection, Including Facts about Transmission, Prevention, Diagnosis, Treatment, Opportunistic Infections, and Other Complications, with a Section for Women and Children, Including Details about Associated Gynecological Concerns, Pregnancy, and Pediatric Care

Along with Updated Statistical Information, Reports on Current Research Initiatives, a Glossary, and Directories of Internet, Hotline, and Other Resources

Edited by Dawn D. Matthews. 664 pages. 2003. 0-7808-0631-X.

The 3rd edition of the AIDS Sourcebook, part of Omnigraphics' *Health Reference Series*, is a welcome update. . . . This resource is highly recommended for academic and public libraries."
— *American Reference Books Annual, 2004*

"Excellent sourcebook. This continues to be a highly recommended book. There is no other book that provides as much information as this book provides."
— *AIDS Book Review Journal, Dec-Jan '00*

"Recommended reference source."
— *Booklist, American Library Association, Dec '99*

Alcoholism Sourcebook

Basic Consumer Health Information about the Physical and Mental Consequences of Alcohol Abuse, Including Liver Disease, Pancreatitis, Wernicke-Korsakoff Syndrome (Alcoholic Dementia), Fetal Alcohol Syndrome, Heart Disease, Kidney Disorders, Gastrointestinal Problems, and Immune System Compromise and Featuring Facts about Addiction, Detoxification, Alcohol Withdrawal, Recovery, and the Maintenance of Sobriety

Along with a Glossary and Directories of Resources for Further Help and Information

Edited by Karen Bellenir. 613 pages. 2000. 0-7808-0325-6.

"This title is one of the few reference works on alcoholism for general readers. For some readers this will be a welcome complement to the many self-help books on the market. Recommended for collections serving general readers and consumer health collections."
— *E-Streams, Mar '01*

"This book is an excellent choice for public and academic libraries."
— *American Reference Books Annual, 2001*

"Recommended reference source."
— *Booklist, American Library Association, Dec '00*

"Presents a wealth of information on alcohol use and abuse and its effects on the body and mind, treatment, and prevention." — *SciTech Book News, Dec '00*

"Important new health guide which packs in the latest consumer information about the problems of alcoholism." — *Reviewer's Bookwatch, Nov '00*

SEE ALSO Drug Abuse Sourcebook, Substance Abuse Sourcebook

Allergies Sourcebook, 2nd Edition

Basic Consumer Health Information about Allergic Disorders, Triggers, Reactions, and Related Symptoms, Including Anaphylaxis, Rhinitis, Sinusitis, Asthma, Dermatitis, Conjunctivitis, and Multiple Chemical Sensitivity

Along with Tips on Diagnosis, Prevention, and Treatment, Statistical Data, a Glossary, and a Directory of Sources for Further Help and Information

Edited by Annemarie S. Muth. 598 pages. 2002. 0-7808-0376-0.

"This book brings a great deal of useful material together. . . . This is an excellent addition to public and consumer health library collections."
— American Reference Books Annual, 2003

"This second edition would be useful to laypersons with little or advanced knowledge of the subject matter. This book would also serve as a resource for nursing and other health care professions students. It would be useful in public, academic, and hospital libraries with consumer health collections." *— E-Streams, Jul '02*

Alternative Medicine Sourcebook

SEE *Complementary & Alternative Medicine Sourcebook, 3rd Edition*

Alzheimer's Disease Sourcebook, 3rd Edition

Basic Consumer Health Information about Alzheimer's Disease, Other Dementias, and Related Disorders, Including Multi-Infarct Dementia, AIDS Dementia Complex, Dementia with Lewy Bodies, Huntington's Disease, Wernicke-Korsakoff Syndrome (Alcohol-Reated Dementia), Delirium, and Confusional States

Along with Information for People Newly Diagnosed with Alzheimer's Disease and Caregivers, Reports Detailing Current Research Efforts in Prevention, Diagnosis, and Treatment, Facts about Long-Term Care Issues, and Listings of Sources for Additional Information

Edited by Karen Bellenir. 645 pages. 2003. 0-7808-0666-2.

"This very informative and valuable tool will be a great addition to any library serving consumers, students and health care workers."
— American Reference Books Annual, 2004

"This is a valuable resource for people affected by dementias such as Alzheimer's. It is easy to navigate and includes important information and resources."
— Doody's Review Service, Feb '04

"Recommended reference source."
— Booklist, American Library Association, Oct '99

SEE ALSO *Brain Disorders Sourcebook*

Arthritis Sourcebook, 2nd Edition

Basic Consumer Health Information about Osteoarthritis, Rheumatoid Arthritis, Other Rheumatic Disorders, Infectious Forms of Arthritis, and Diseases with Symptoms Linked to Arthritis, Featuring Facts about Diagnosis, Pain Management, and Surgical Therapies

Along with Coping Strategies, Research Updates, a Glossary, and Resources for Additional Help and Information

Edited by Amy L. Sutton. 593 pages. 2004. 0-7808-0667-0.

"This easy-to-read volume is recommended for consumer health collections within public or academic libraries." *—E-Streams, May '05*

"As expected, this updated edition continues the excellent reputation of this series in providing sound, usable health information. . . . Highly recommended."
— American Reference Books Annual, 2005

"Excellent reference." *— The Bookwatch, Jan '05*

Asthma Sourcebook, 2nd Edition

Basic Consumer Health Information about the Causes, Symptoms, Diagnosis, and Treatment of Asthma in Infants, Children, Teenagers, and Adults, Including Facts about Different Types of Asthma, Common Co-Occurring Conditions, Asthma Management Plans, Triggers, Medications, and Medication Delivery Devices

Along with Asthma Statistics, Research Updates, a Glossary, a Directory of Asthma-Related Resources, and More

Edited by Karen Bellenir. 609 pages. 2006. 0-7808-0866-5.

"A worthwhile reference acquisition for public libraries and academic medical libraries whose readers desire a quick introduction to the wide range of asthma information." *— Choice, Association of College & Research Libraries, Jun '01*

"Recommended reference source."
— Booklist, American Library Association, Feb '01

"Highly recommended." *— The Bookwatch, Jan '01*

"There is much good information for patients and their families who deal with asthma daily."
— American Medical Writers Association Journal, Winter '01

"This informative text is recommended for consumer health collections in public, secondary school, and community college libraries and the libraries of universities with a large undergraduate population."
— American Reference Books Annual, 2001

Attention Deficit Disorder Sourcebook

Basic Consumer Health Information about Attention Deficit/Hyperactivity Disorder in Children and Adults, Including Facts about Causes, Symptoms, Diagnostic Criteria, and Treatment Options Such as Medications, Behavior Therapy, Coaching, and Homeopathy

Along with Reports on Current Research Initiatives, Legal Issues, and Government Regulations, and Featuring a Glossary of Related Terms, Internet Resources, and a List of Additional Reading Material

Edited by Dawn D. Matthews. 470 pages. 2002. 0-7000-0624-7.

"Recommended reference source."
— Booklist, American Library Association, Jan '03

"This book is recommended for all school libraries and the reference or consumer health sections of public libraries." — American Reference Books Annual, 2003

■

Back & Neck Sourcebook, 2nd Edition

Basic Consumer Health Information about Spinal Pain, Spinal Cord Injuries, and Related Disorders, Such as Degenerative Disk Disease, Osteoarthritis, Scoliosis, Sciatica, Spina Bifida, and Spinal Stenosis, and Featuring Facts about Maintaining Spinal Health, Self-Care, Pain Management, Rehabilitative Care, Chiropractic Care, Spinal Surgeries, and Complementary Therapies

Along with Suggestions for Preventing Back and Neck Pain, a Glossary of Related Terms, and a Directory of Resources

Edited by Amy L. Sutton. 633 pages. 2004. 0-7808-0738-3.

"Recommended . . . an easy to use, comprehensive medical reference book." — E-Streams, Sep '05

"The strength of this work is its basic, easy-to-read format. Recommended." — Reference and User Services Quarterly, American Library Association, Winter '97

■

Blood & Circulatory Disorders Sourcebook, 2nd Edition

Basic Consumer Health Information about the Blood and Circulatory System and Related Disorders, Such as Anemia and Other Hemoglobin Diseases, Cancer of the Blood and Associated Bone Marrow Disorders, Clotting and Bleeding Problems, and Conditions That Affect the Veins, Blood Vessels, and Arteries, Including Facts about the Donation and Transplantation of Bone Marrow, Stem Cells, and Blood and Tips for Keeping the Blood and Circulatory System Healthy

Along with a Glossary of Related Terms and Resources for Additional Help and Information

Edited by Amy L. Sutton. 659 pages. 2005. 0-7808-0746-4.

"Highly recommended pick for basic consumer health reference holdings at all levels."
— The Bookwatch, Aug '05

"Recommended reference source."
— Booklist, American Library Association, Feb '99

"An important reference sourcebook written in simple language for everyday, non-technical users. "
— Reviewer's Bookwatch, Jan '99

Brain Disorders Sourcebook, 2nd Edition

Basic Consumer Health Information about Acquired and Traumatic Brain Injuries, Infections of the Brain, Epilepsy and Seizure Disorders, Cerebral Palsy, and Degenerative Neurological Disorders, Including Amyotrophic Lateral Sclerosis (ALS), Dementias, Multiple Sclerosis, and More

Along with Information on the Brain's Structure and Function, Treatment and Rehabilitation Options, Reports on Current Research Initiatives, a Glossary of Terms Related to Brain Disorders and Injuries, and a Directory of Sources for Further Help and Information

Edited by Sandra J. Judd. 625 pages. 2005. 0-7808-0744-8.

"Highly recommended pick for basic consumer health reference holdings at all levels."
— The Bookwatch, Aug '05

"Belongs on the shelves of any library with a consumer health collection." — E-Streams, Mar '00

"Recommended reference source."
— Booklist, American Library Association, Oct '99

SEE ALSO Alzheimer's Disease Sourcebook

■

Breast Cancer Sourcebook, 2nd Edition

Basic Consumer Health Information about Breast Cancer, Including Facts about Risk Factors, Prevention, Screening and Diagnostic Methods, Treatment Options, Complementary and Alternative Therapies, Post-Treatment Concerns, Clinical Trials, Special Risk Populations, and New Developments in Breast Cancer Research

Along with Breast Cancer Statistics, a Glossary of Related Terms, and a Directory of Resources for Additional Help and Information

Edited by Sandra J. Judd. 595 pages. 2004. 0-7808-0668-9.

"This book will be an excellent addition to public, community college, medical, and academic libraries."
— American Reference Books Annual, 2006

"It would be a useful reference book in a library or on loan to women in a support group."
— Cancer Forum, Mar '03

"Recommended reference source."
— Booklist, American Library Association, Jan '02

"This reference source is highly recommended. It is quite informative, comprehensive and detailed in nature, and yet it offers practical advice in easy-to-read language. It could be thought of as the 'bible' of breast cancer for the consumer." — E-Streams, Jan '02

"From the pros and cons of different screening methods and results to treatment options, Breast Cancer Sourcebook provides the latest information on the subject."
— Library Bookwatch, Dec '01

"This thoroughgoing, very readable reference covers all aspects of breast health and cancer.... Readers will find

629

much to consider here. Recommended for all public and patient health collections."
— *Library Journal, Sep '01*

SEE ALSO *Cancer Sourcebook for Women, Women's Health Concerns Sourcebook*

■

Breastfeeding Sourcebook

Basic Consumer Health Information about the Benefits of Breastmilk, Preparing to Breastfeed, Breastfeeding as a Baby Grows, Nutrition, and More, Including Information on Special Situations and Concerns Such as Mastitis, Illness, Medications, Allergies, Multiple Births, Prematurity, Special Needs, and Adoption

Along with a Glossary and Resources for Additional Help and Information

Edited by Jenni Lynn Colson. 388 pages. 2002. 0-7808-0332-9.

"Particularly useful is the information about professional lactation services and chapters on breastfeeding when returning to work. . . . *Breastfeeding Sourcebook* will be useful for public libraries, consumer health libraries, and technical schools offering nurse assistant training, especially in areas where Internet access is problematic."
— *American Reference Books Annual, 2003*

SEE ALSO *Pregnancy & Birth Sourcebook*

■

Burns Sourcebook

Basic Consumer Health Information about Various Types of Burns and Scalds, Including Flame, Heat, Cold, Electrical, Chemical, and Sun Burns

Along with Information on Short-Term and Long-Term Treatments, Tissue Reconstruction, Plastic Surgery, Prevention Suggestions, and First Aid

Edited by Allan R. Cook. 604 pages. 1999. 0-7808-0204-7.

"This is an exceptional addition to the series and is highly recommended for all consumer health collections, hospital libraries, and academic medical centers."
— *E-Streams, Mar '00*

"This key reference guide is an invaluable addition to all health care and public libraries in confronting this ongoing health issue."
— *American Reference Books Annual, 2000*

"Recommended reference source."
— *Booklist, American Library Association, Dec '99*

SEE ALSO *Dermatological Disorders Sourcebook*

■

Cancer Sourcebook, 4th Edition

Basic Consumer Health Information about Major Forms and Stages of Cancer, Featuring Facts about Head and Neck Cancers, Lung Cancers, Gastrointestinal Cancers, Genitourinary Cancers, Lymphomas, Blood Cell Cancers, Endocrine Cancers, Skin Cancers, Bone Cancers, Sarcomas, and Others, and Including Information about Cancer Treatments and Therapies,

Identifying and Reducing Cancer Risks, and Strategies for Coping with Cancer and the Side Effects of Treatment

Along with a Cancer Glossary, Statistical and Demographic Data, and a Directory of Sources for Additional Help and Information

Edited by Karen Bellenir. 1,119 pages. 2003. 0-7808-0633-6.

"With cancer being the second leading cause of death for Americans, a prodigious work such as this one, which locates centrally so much cancer-related information, is clearly an asset to this nation's citizens and others."
— *Journal of the National Medical Association, 2004*

"This title is recommended for health sciences and public libraries with consumer health collections."
— *E-Streams, Feb '01*

". . . can be effectively used by cancer patients and their families who are looking for answers in a language they can understand. Public and hospital libraries should have it on their shelves."
— *American Reference Books Annual, 2001*

"Recommended reference source."
— *Booklist, American Library Association, Dec '00*

SEE ALSO *Breast Cancer Sourcebook, Cancer Sourcebook for Women, Pediatric Cancer Sourcebook, Prostate Cancer Sourcebook*

■

Cancer Sourcebook for Women, 3rd Edition

Basic Consumer Health Information about Leading Causes of Cancer in Women, Featuring Facts about Gynecologic Cancers and Related Concerns, Such as Breast Cancer, Cervical Cancer, Endometrial Cancer, Uterine Sarcoma, Vaginal Cancer, Vulvar Cancer, and Common Non-Cancerous Gynecologic Conditions, in Addition to Facts about Lung Cancer, Colorectal Cancer, and Thyroid Cancer in Women

Along with Information about Cancer Risk Factors, Screening and Prevention, Treatment Options, and Tips on Coping with Life after Cancer Treatment, a Glossary of Cancer Terms, and a Directory of Resources for Additional Help and Information

Edited by Amy L. Sutton. 715 pages. 2006. 0-7808-0867-3.

"An excellent addition to collections in public, consumer health, and women's health libraries."
— *American Reference Books Annual, 2003*

"Overall, the information is excellent, and complex topics are clearly explained. As a reference book for the consumer it is a valuable resource to assist them to make informed decisions about cancer and its treatments."
— *Cancer Forum, Nov '02*

"Highly recommended for academic and medical reference collections."
— *Library Bookwatch, Sep '02*

"This is a highly recommended book for any public or consumer library, being reader friendly and containing accurate and helpful information."
— *E-Streams, Aug '02*

"Recommended reference source."
—*Booklist, American Library Association, Jul '02*

SEE ALSO *Breast Cancer Sourcebook, Women's Health Concerns Sourcebook*

Cardiovascular Diseases & Disorders Sourcebook, 3rd Edition

Basic Consumer Health Information about Heart and Vascular Diseases and Disorders, Such as Angina, Heart Attacks, Arrhythmias, Cardiomyopathy, Valve Disease, Atherosclerosis, and Aneurysms, with Information about Managing Cardiovascular Risk Factors and Maintaining Heart Health, Medications and Procedures Used to Treat Cardiovascular Disorders, and Concerns of Special Significance to Women

Along with Reports on Current Research Initiatives, a Glossary of Related Medical Terms, and a Directory of Sources for Further Help and Information

Edited by Sandra J. Judd. 713 pages. 2005. 0-7808-0739-1.

"This updated sourcebook is still the best first stop for comprehensive introductory information on cardiovascular diseases."
—*American Reference Books Annual, 2006*

"Recommended for public libraries and libraries supporting health care professionals."
—*E-Streams, Sep '05*

"This should be a standard health library reference."
—*The Bookwatch, Jun '05*

"Recommended reference source."
—*Booklist, American Library Association, Dec '00*

". . . comprehensive format provides an extensive overview on this subject."
—*Choice, Association of College & Research Libraries*

Caregiving Sourcebook

Basic Consumer Health Information for Caregivers, Including a Profile of Caregivers, Caregiving Responsibilities and Concerns, Tips for Specific Conditions, Care Environments, and the Effects of Caregiving

Along with Facts about Legal Issues, Financial Information, and Future Planning, a Glossary, and a Listing of Additional Resources

Edited by Joyce Brennfleck Shannon. 600 pages. 2001. 0-7808-0331-0.

"Essential for most collections."
—*Library Journal, Apr 1, 2002*

"An ideal addition to the reference collection of any public library. Health sciences information professionals may also want to acquire the *Caregiving Sourcebook* for their hospital or academic library for use as a ready reference tool by health care workers interested in aging and caregiving." —*E-Streams, Jan '02*

"Recommended reference source."
—*Booklist, American Library Association, Oct '01*

Child Abuse Sourcebook

Basic Consumer Health Information about the Physical, Sexual, and Emotional Abuse of Children, with Additional Facts about Neglect, Munchausen Syndrome by Proxy (MSBP), Shaken Baby Syndrome, and Controversial Issues Related to Child Abuse, Such as Withholding Medical Care, Corporal Punishment, and Child Maltreatment in Youth Sports, and Featuring Facts about Child Protective Services, Foster Care, Adoption, Parenting Challenges, and Other Abuse Prevention Efforts

Along with a Glossary of Related Terms and Resources for Additional Help and Information

Edited by Dawn D. Matthews. 620 pages. 2004. 0-7808-0705-7.

"A valuable and highly recommended resource for school, academic and public libraries whether used on its own or as a starting point for more in-depth research." —*E-Streams, Apr '05*

"Every week the news brings cases of child abuse or neglect, so it is useful to have a source that supplies so much helpful information. . . . Recommended. Public and academic libraries, and child welfare offices."
—*Choice, Association of College & Research Libraries, Mar '05*

"Packed with insights on all kinds of issues, from foster care and adoption to parenting and abuse prevention."
—*The Bookwatch, Nov '04*

SEE ALSO: *Domestic Violence Sourcebook, 2nd Edition*

Childhood Diseases & Disorders Sourcebook

Basic Consumer Health Information about Medical Problems Often Encountered in Pre-Adolescent Children, Including Respiratory Tract Ailments, Ear Infections, Sore Throats, Disorders of the Skin and Scalp, Digestive and Genitourinary Diseases, Infectious Diseases, Inflammatory Disorders, Chronic Physical and Developmental Disorders, Allergies, and More

Along with Information about Diagnostic Tests, Common Childhood Surgeries, and Frequently Used Medications, with a Glossary of Important Terms and Resource Directory

Edited by Chad T. Kimball. 662 pages. 2003. 0-7808-0458-9.

"This is an excellent book for new parents and should be included in all health care and public libraries."
—*American Reference Books Annual, 2004*

SEE ALSO: *Healthy Children Sourcebook*

Colds, Flu & Other Common Ailments Sourcebook

Basic Consumer Health Information about Common Ailments and Injuries, Including Colds, Coughs, the Flu, Sinus Problems, Headaches, Fever, Nausea and

Vomiting, Menstrual Cramps, Diarrhea, Constipation, Hemorrhoids, Back Pain, Dandruff, Dry and Itchy Skin, Cuts, Scrapes, Sprains, Bruises, and More

Along with Information about Prevention, Self-Care, Choosing a Doctor, Over the Counter Medications, Folk Remedies, and Alternative Therapies, and Including a Glossary of Important Terms and a Directory of Resources for Further Help and Information

Edited by Chad T. Kimball. 638 pages. 2001. 0-7808-0435-X.

"A good starting point for research on common illnesses. It will be a useful addition to public and consumer health library collections."
— American Reference Books Annual, 2002

"Will prove valuable to any library seeking to maintain a current, comprehensive reference collection of health resources. . . . Excellent reference."
— The Bookwatch, Aug '01

"Recommended reference source."
— Booklist, American Library Association, Jul '01

■

Communication Disorders Sourcebook

Basic Information about Deafness and Hearing Loss, Speech and Language Disorders, Voice Disorders, Balance and Vestibular Disorders, and Disorders of Smell, Taste, and Touch

Edited by Linda M. Ross. 533 pages. 1996. 0-7808-0077-X.

"This is skillfully edited and is a welcome resource for the layperson. It should be found in every public and medical library."   — Booklist Health Sciences Supplement, American Library Association, Oct '97

■

Complementary & Alternative Medicine Sourcebook, 3rd Edition

Basic Consumer Health Information about Complementary and Alternative Medical Therapies, Including Acupuncture, Ayurveda, Traditional Chinese Medicine, Herbal Medicine, Homeopathy, Naturopathy, Biofeedback, Hypnotherapy, Yoga, Art Therapy, Aromatherapy, Clinical Nutrition, Vitamin and Mineral Supplements, Chiropractic, Massage, Reflexology, Crystal Therapy, Therapeutic Touch, and More

Along with Facts about Alternative and Complementary Treatments for Specific Conditions Such as Cancer, Diabetes, Osteoarthritis, Chronic Pain, Menopause, Gastrointestinal Disorders, Headaches, and Mental Illness, a Glossary, and a Resource List for Additional Help and Information

Edited by Sandra J. Judd. 657 pages. 2006. 0-7808-0864-9.

"Recommended for public, high school, and academic libraries that have consumer health collections. Hospital libraries that also serve the public will find this to be a useful resource."   — E-Streams, Feb '03

"Recommended reference source."
— Booklist, American Library Association, Jan '03

"An important alternate health reference."
— MBR Bookwatch, Oct '02

"A great addition to the reference collection of every type of library." — American Reference Books Annual, 2000

■

Congenital Disorders Sourcebook

Basic Information about Disorders Acquired during Gestation, Including Spina Bifida, Hydrocephalus, Cerebral Palsy, Heart Defects, Craniofacial Abnormalities, Fetal Alcohol Syndrome, and More

Along with Current Treatment Options and Statistical Data

Edited by Karen Bellenir. 607 pages. 1997. 0-7808-0205-5.

"Recommended reference source."
— Booklist, American Library Association, Oct '97

SEE ALSO Pregnancy & Birth Sourcebook

■

Consumer Issues in Health Care Sourcebook

Basic Information about Health Care Fundamentals and Related Consumer Issues, Including Exams and Screening Tests, Physician Specialties, Choosing a Doctor, Using Prescription and Over-the-Counter Medications Safely, Avoiding Health Scams, Managing Common Health Risks in the Home, Care Options for Chronically or Terminally Ill Patients, and a List of Resources for Obtaining Help and Further Information

Edited by Karen Bellenir. 618 pages. 1998. 0-7808-0221-7.

"Both public and academic libraries will want to have a copy in their collection for readers who are interested in self-education on health issues."
— American Reference Books Annual, 2000

"The editor has researched the literature from government agencies and others, saving readers the time and effort of having to do the research themselves. Recommended for public libraries."
— Reference and User Services Quarterly, American Library Association, Spring '99

"Recommended reference source."
— Booklist, American Library Association, Dec '98

■

Contagious Diseases Sourcebook

Basic Consumer Health Information about Infectious Diseases Spread by Person-to-Person Contact through Direct Touch, Airborne Transmission, Sexual Contact, or Contact with Blood or Other Body Fluids, Including Hepatitis, Herpes, Influenza, Lice, Measles, Mumps, Pinworm, Ringworm, Severe Acute Respiratory Syndrome (SARS), Streptococcal Infections, Tuberculosis, and Others

Along with Facts about Disease Transmission, Antimicrobial Resistance, and Vaccines, with a Glossary and Directories of Resources for More Information

Edited by Karen Bellenir. 643 pages. 2004. 0-7808-0736-7.

"This easy-to-read volume is recommended for consumer health collections within public or academic libraries." —*E-Streams, May '05*

"This informative book is highly recommended for public libraries, consumer health collections, and secondary schools and undergraduate libraries." —*American Reference Books Annual, 2005*

"Excellent reference." —*The Bookwatch, Jan '05*

Contagious & Non-Contagious Infectious Diseases Sourcebook

Basic Information about Contagious Diseases like Measles, Polio, Hepatitis B, and Infectious Mononucleosis, and Non-Contagious Infectious Diseases like Tetanus and Toxic Shock Syndrome, and Diseases Occurring as Secondary Infections Such as Shingles and Reye Syndrome

Along with Vaccination, Prevention, and Treatment Information, and a Section Describing Emerging Infectious Disease Threats

Edited by Karen Bellenir and Peter D. Dresser. 566 pages. 1996. 0-7808-0075-3.

SEE ALSO Infectious Diseases Sourcebook

Death & Dying Sourcebook, 2nd Edition

Basic Consumer Health Information about End-of-Life Care and Related Perspectives and Ethical Issues, Including End-of-Life Symptoms and Treatments, Pain Management, Quality-of-Life Concerns, the Use of Life Support, Patients' Rights and Privacy Issues, Advance Directives, Physician-Assisted Suicide, Caregiving, Organ and Tissue Donation, Autopsies, Funeral Arrangements, and Grief

Along with Statistical Data, Information about the Leading Causes of Death, a Glossary, and Directories of Support Groups and Other Resources

Edited by Joyce Brennfleck Shannon. 653 pages. 2006. 0-7808-0871-1.

"Public libraries, medical libraries, and academic libraries will all find this sourcebook a useful addition to their collections." —*American Reference Books Annual, 2001*

"An extremely useful resource for those concerned with death and dying in the United States." —*Respiratory Care, Nov '00*

"Recommended reference source." —*Booklist, American Library Association, Aug '00*

"This book is a definite must for all those involved in end-of-life care." —*Doody's Review Service, 2000*

Dental Care & Oral Health Sourcebook, 2nd Edition

Basic Consumer Health Information about Dental Care, Including Oral Hygiene, Dental Visits, Pain Management, Cavities, Crowns, Bridges, Dental Implants, and Fillings, and Other Oral Health Concerns, Such as Gum Disease, Bad Breath, Dry Mouth, Genetic and Developmental Abnormalities, Oral Cancers, Orthodontics, and Temporomandibular Disorders

Along with Updates on Current Research in Oral Health, a Glossary, a Directory of Dental and Oral Health Organizations, and Resources for People with Dental and Oral Health Disorders

Edited by Amy L. Sutton. 609 pages. 2003. 0-7808-0634-4.

"This book could serve as a turning point in the battle to educate consumers in issues concerning oral health." —*American Reference Books Annual, 2004*

"Unique source which will fill a gap in dental sources for patients and the lay public. A valuable reference tool even in a library with thousands of books on dentistry. Comprehensive, clear, inexpensive, and easy to read and use. It fills an enormous gap in the health care literature." —*Reference & User Services Quarterly, American Library Association, Summer '98*

"Recommended reference source." —*Booklist, American Library Association, Dec '97*

Depression Sourcebook

Basic Consumer Health Information about Unipolar Depression, Bipolar Disorder, Postpartum Depression, Seasonal Affective Disorder, and Other Types of Depression in Children, Adolescents, Women, Men, the Elderly, and Other Selected Populations

Along with Facts about Causes, Risk Factors, Diagnostic Criteria, Treatment Options, Coping Strategies, Suicide Prevention, a Glossary, and a Directory of Sources for Additional Help and Information

Edited by Karen Belleni. 602 pages. 2002. 0-7808-0611-5.

"*Depression Sourcebook* is of a very high standard. Its purpose, which is to serve as a reference source to the lay reader, is very well served." —*Journal of the National Medical Association, 2004*

"Invaluable reference for public and school library collections alike." —*Library Bookwatch, Apr '03*

"Recommended for purchase." —*American Reference Books Annual, 2003*

Dermatological Disorders Sourcebook, 2nd Edition

Basic Consumer Health Information about Conditions and Disorders Affecting the Skin, Hair, and Nails, Such as Acne, Rosacea, Rashes, Dermatitis, Pigmentation Disorders, Birthmarks, Skin Cancer, Skin Injuries, Psoriasis, Scleroderma, and Hair Loss, Including Facts about Medications and Treatments for Dermatological

Disorders and Tips for Maintaining Healthy Skin, Hair, and Nails

Along with Information about How Aging Affects the Skin, a Glossary of Related Terms, and a Directory of Resources for Additional Help and Information

Edited by Amy L. Sutton. 645 pages. 2005. 0-7808-0795-2.

"... comprehensive, easily read reference book."
—*Doody's Health Sciences Book Reviews, Oct '97*

SEE ALSO *Burns Sourcebook*

■

Diabetes Sourcebook, 3rd Edition

Basic Consumer Health Information about Type 1 Diabetes (Insulin-Dependent or Juvenile-Onset Diabetes), Type 2 Diabetes (Noninsulin-Dependent or Adult-Onset Diabetes), Gestational Diabetes, Impaired Glucose Tolerance (IGT), and Related Complications, Such as Amputation, Eye Disease, Gum Disease, Nerve Damage, and End-Stage Renal Disease, Including Facts about Insulin, Oral Diabetes Medications, Blood Sugar Testing, and the Role of Exercise and Nutrition in the Control of Diabetes

Along with a Glossary and Resources for Further Help and Information

Edited by Dawn D. Matthews. 622 pages. 2003. 0-7808-0629-8.

"This edition is even more helpful than earlier versions. . . . It is a truly valuable tool for anyone seeking readable and authoritative information on diabetes."
— *American Reference Books Annual, 2004*

"An invaluable reference." — *Library Journal, May '00*

Selected as one of the 250 "Best Health Sciences Books of 1999." — *Doody's Rating Service, Mar-Apr '00*

"Provides useful information for the general public."
— *Healthlines, University of Michigan Health Management Research Center, Sep/Oct '99*

". . . provides reliable mainstream medical information . . . belongs on the shelves of any library with a consumer health collection." — *E-Streams, Sep '99*

"Recommended reference source."
— *Booklist, American Library Association, Feb '99*

■

Diet & Nutrition Sourcebook, 3rd Edition

Basic Consumer Health Information about Dietary Guidelines and the Food Guidance System, Recommended Daily Nutrient Intakes, Serving Proportions, Weight Control, Vitamins and Supplements, Nutrition Issues for Different Life Stages and Lifestyles, and the Needs of People with Specific Medical Concerns, Including Cancer, Celiac Disease, Diabetes, Eating Disorders, Food Allergies, and Cardiovascular Disease

Along with Facts about Federal Nutrition Support Programs, a Glossary of Nutrition and Dietary Terms, and Directories of Additional Resources for More Information about Nutrition

Edited by Joyce Brennfleck Shannon. 633 pages. 2006. 0-7808-0800-2.

"This book is an excellent source of basic diet and nutrition information." — *Booklist Health Sciences Supplement, American Library Association, Dec '00*

"This reference document should be in any public library, but it would be a very good guide for beginning students in the health sciences. If the other books in this publisher's series are as good as this, they should all be in the health sciences collections."
— *American Reference Books Annual, 2000*

"This book is an excellent general nutrition reference for consumers who desire to take an active role in their health care for prevention. Consumers of all ages who select this book can feel confident they are receiving current and accurate information." — *Journal of Nutrition for the Elderly, Vol. 19, No. 4, 2000*

SEE ALSO *Digestive Diseases & Disorders Sourcebook, Eating Disorders Sourcebook, Gastrointestinal Diseases & Disorders Sourcebook, Vegetarian Sourcebook*

■

Digestive Diseases & Disorders Sourcebook

Basic Consumer Health Information about Diseases and Disorders that Impact the Upper and Lower Digestive System, Including Celiac Disease, Constipation, Crohn's Disease, Cyclic Vomiting Syndrome, Diarrhea, Diverticulosis and Diverticulitis, Gallstones, Heartburn, Hemorrhoids, Hernias, Indigestion (Dyspepsia), Irritable Bowel Syndrome, Lactose Intolerance, Ulcers, and More

Along with Information about Medications and Other Treatments, Tips for Maintaining a Healthy Digestive Tract, a Glossary, and Directory of Digestive Diseases Organizations

Edited by Karen Bellenir. 335 pages. 2000. 0-7808-0327-2.

"This title would be an excellent addition to all public or patient-research libraries."
— *American Reference Books Annual, 2001*

"This title is recommended for public, hospital, and health sciences libraries with consumer health collections." — *E-Streams, Jul-Aug '00*

"Recommended reference source."
— *Booklist, American Library Association, May '00*

SEE ALSO *Eating Disorders Sourcebook, Gastrointestinal Diseases & Disorders Sourcebook*

■

Disabilities Sourcebook

Basic Consumer Health Information about Physical and Psychiatric Disabilities, Including Descriptions of Major Causes of Disability, Assistive and Adaptive Aids, Workplace Issues, and Accessibility Concerns

Along with Information about the Americans with Disabilities Act, a Glossary, and Resources for Additional Help and Information

Edited by Dawn D. Matthews. 616 pages. 2000. 0-7808-0389-2.

"It is a must for libraries with a consumer health section." —*American Reference Books Annual, 2002*

"A much needed addition to the Omnigraphics Health Reference Series. A current reference work to provide people with disabilities, their families, caregivers or those who work with them, a broad range of information in one volume, has not been available until now. . . . It is recommended for all public and academic library reference collections." —*E-Streams, May '01*

"An excellent source book in easy-to-read format covering many current topics; highly recommended for all libraries." —*Choice, Association of College & Research Libraries, Jan '01*

"Recommended reference source."
—*Booklist, American Library Association, Jul '00*

<hr>

Domestic Violence Sourcebook, 2nd Edition

Basic Consumer Health Information about the Causes and Consequences of Abusive Relationships, Including Physical Violence, Sexual Assault, Battery, Stalking, and Emotional Abuse, and Facts about the Effects of Violence on Women, Men, Young Adults, and the Elderly, with Reports about Domestic Violence in Selected Populations, and Featuring Facts about Medical Care, Victim Assistance and Protection, Prevention Strategies, Mental Health Services, and Legal Issues

Along with a Glossary of Related Terms and Resources for Additional Help and Information

Edited by Dawn D. Matthews. 628 pages. 2004. 0-7808-0669-7.

"Educators, clergy, medical professionals, police, and victims and their families will benefit from this realistic and easy-to-understand resource." —*American Reference Books Annual, 2005*

"Recommended for all collections supporting consumer health information. It should also be considered for any collection needing general, readable information on domestic violence." —*E-Streams, Jan '05*

"This sourcebook complements other books in its field, providing a one-stop resource . . . Recommended." —*Choice, Association of College & Research Libraries, Jan '05*

"Interested lay persons should find the book extremely beneficial. . . . A copy of *Domestic Violence and Child Abuse Sourcebook* should be in every public library in the United States." —*Social Science & Medicine, No. 56, 2003*

"This is important information. The Web has many resources but this sourcebook fills an important societal need. I am not aware of any other resources of this type." —*Doody's Review Service, Sep '01*

"Recommended reference source."
—*Booklist, American Library Association, Apr '01*

"Important pick for college-level health reference libraries." —*The Bookwatch, Mar '01*

"Because this problem is so widespread and because this book includes a lot of issues within one volume, this work is recommended for all public libraries." —*American Reference Books Annual, 2001*

SEE ALSO *Child Abuse Sourcebook*

<hr>

Drug Abuse Sourcebook, 2nd Edition

Basic Consumer Health Information about Illicit Substances of Abuse and the Misuse of Prescription and Over-the-Counter Medications, Including Depressants, Hallucinogens, Inhalants, Marijuana, Stimulants, and Anabolic Steroids

Along with Facts about Related Health Risks, Treatment Programs, Prevention Programs, a Glossary of Abuse and Addiction Terms, a Glossary of Drug-Related Street Terms, and a Directory of Resources for More Information

Edited by Catherine Ginther. 607 pages. 2004. 0-7808-0740-5.

"Commendable for organizing useful, normally scattered government and association-produced data into a logical sequence." —*American Reference Books Annual, 2006*

"This easy-to-read volume is recommended for consumer health collections within public or academic libraries." —*E-Streams, Sep '05*

"An excellent library reference."
—*The Bookwatch, May '05*

"Containing a wealth of information, this book will be useful to the college student just beginning to explore the topic of substance abuse. This resource belongs in libraries that serve a lower-division undergraduate or community college clientele as well as the general public." —*Choice, Association of College & Research Libraries, Jun '01*

"Recommended reference source."
—*Booklist, American Library Association, Feb '01*

SEE ALSO *Alcoholism Sourcebook, Substance Abuse Sourcebook*

<hr>

Ear, Nose & Throat Disorders Sourcebook, 2nd Edition

Basic Consumer Health Information about Disorders of the Ears, Hearing Loss, Vestibular Disorders, Nasal and Sinus Problems, Throat and Vocal Cord Disorders, and Otolaryngologic Cancers, Including Facts about Ear Infections and Injuries, Genetic and Congenital Deafness, Sensorineural Hearing Disorders, Tinnitus, Vertigo, Ménière Disease, Rhinitis, Sinusitis, Snoring, Sore Throats, Hoarseness, and More

Along with Reports on Current Research Initiatives, a Glossary of Related Medical Terms, and a Directory of Sources for Further Help and Information

Edited by Sandra J. Judd. 625 pages. 2006. 0-7808-0872-X.

"Overall, this sourcebook is helpful for the consumer seeking information on ENT issues. It is recommended for public libraries."
—American Reference Books Annual, 1999

"Recommended reference source."
—Booklist, American Library Association, Dec '98

■

Eating Disorders Sourcebook

Basic Consumer Health Information about Eating Disorders, Including Information about Anorexia Nervosa, Bulimia Nervosa, Binge Eating, Body Dysmorphic Disorder, Pica, Laxative Abuse, and Night Eating Syndrome

Along with Information about Causes, Adverse Effects, and Treatment and Prevention Issues, and Featuring a Section on Concerns Specific to Children and Adolescents, a Glossary, and Resources for Further Help and Information

Edited by Dawn D. Matthews. 322 pages. 2001. 0-7808-0335-3.

"Recommended for health science libraries that are open to the public, as well as hospital libraries. This book is a good resource for the consumer who is concerned about eating disorders." *— E-Streams, Mar '02*

"This volume is another convenient collection of excerpted articles. Recommended for school and public library patrons; lower-division undergraduates; and two-year technical program students."
—Choice, Association of College & Research Libraries, Jan '02

"Recommended reference source."
— Booklist, American Library Association, Oct '01

SEE ALSO *Diet & Nutrition Sourcebook, Digestive Diseases & Disorders Sourcebook, Gastrointestinal Diseases & Disorders Sourcebook*

■

Emergency Medical Services Sourcebook

Basic Consumer Health Information about Preventing, Preparing for, and Managing Emergency Situations, When and Who to Call for Help, What to Expect in the Emergency Room, the Emergency Medical Team, Patient Issues, and Current Topics in Emergency Medicine

Along with Statistical Data, a Glossary, and Sources of Additional Help and Information

Edited by Jenni Lynn Colson. 494 pages. 2002. 0-7808-0420-1.

"Handy and convenient for home, public, school, and college libraries. Recommended."
— Choice, Association of College & Research Libraries, Apr '03

"This reference can provide the consumer with answers to most questions about emergency care in the United States, or it will direct them to a resource where the answer can be found."
—American Reference Books Annual, 2003

"Recommended reference source."
— Booklist, American Library Association, Feb '03

■

Endocrine & Metabolic Disorders Sourcebook

Basic Information for the Layperson about Pancreatic and Insulin-Related Disorders Such as Pancreatitis, Diabetes, and Hypoglycemia; Adrenal Gland Disorders Such as Cushing's Syndrome, Addison's Disease, and Congenital Adrenal Hyperplasia; Pituitary Gland Disorders Such as Growth Hormone Deficiency, Acromegaly, and Pituitary Tumors; Thyroid Disorders Such as Hypothyroidism, Graves' Disease, Hashimoto's Disease, and Goiter; Hyperparathyroidism; and Other Diseases and Syndromes of Hormone Imbalance or Metabolic Dysfunction

Along with Reports on Current Research Initiatives

Edited by Linda M. Shin. 574 pages. 1998. 0-7808-0207-1.

"Omnigraphics has produced another needed resource for health information consumers."
—American Reference Books Annual, 2000

"Recommended reference source."
— Booklist, American Library Association, Dec '98

■

Environmental Health Sourcebook, 2nd Edition

Basic Consumer Health Information about the Environment and Its Effect on Human Health, Including the Effects of Air Pollution, Water Pollution, Hazardous Chemicals, Food Hazards, Radiation Hazards, Biological Agents, Household Hazards, Such as Radon, Asbestos, Carbon Monoxide, and Mold, and Information about Associated Diseases and Disorders, Including Cancer, Allergies, Respiratory Problems, and Skin Disorders

Along with Information about Environmental Concerns for Specific Populations, a Glossary of Related Terms, and Resources for Further Help and Information

Edited by Dawn D. Matthews. 673 pages. 2003. 0-7808-0632-8.

"This recently updated edition continues the level of quality and the reputation of the numerous other volumes in Omnigraphics' Health Reference Series."
—American Reference Books Annual, 2004

"An excellent updated edition."
— The Bookwatch, Oct '03

"Recommended reference source."
— Booklist, American Library Association, Sep '98

"This book will be a useful addition to anyone's library." *—Choice Health Sciences Supplement, Association of College & Research Libraries, May '98*

"... a good survey of numerous environmentally induced physical disorders ... a useful addition to anyone's library."
— *Doody's Health Sciences Book Reviews, Jan '98*

■

Environmentally Induced Disorders Sourcebook

SEE Environmental Health Sourcebook, 2nd Edition

■

Ethnic Diseases Sourcebook

Basic Consumer Health Information for Ethnic and Racial Minority Groups in the United States, Including General Health Indicators and Behaviors, Ethnic Diseases, Genetic Testing, the Impact of Chronic Diseases, Women's Health, Mental Health Issues, and Preventive Health Care Services

Along with a Glossary and a Listing of Additional Resources

Edited by Joyce Brennfleck Shannon. 664 pages. 2001. 0-7808-0336-1.

"Recommended for health sciences libraries where public health programs are a priority."
— *E-Streams, Jan '02*

"Not many books have been written on this topic to date, and the *Ethnic Diseases Sourcebook* is a strong addition to the list. It will be an important introductory resource for health consumers, students, health care personnel, and social scientists. It is recommended for public, academic, and large hospital libraries."
— *American Reference Books Annual, 2002*

"Recommended reference source."
— *Booklist, American Library Association, Oct '01*

"Will prove valuable to any library seeking to maintain a current, comprehensive reference collection of health resources.... An excellent source of health information about genetic disorders which affect particular ethnic and racial minorities in the U.S."
— *The Bookwatch, Aug '01*

■

Eye Care Sourcebook, 2nd Edition

Basic Consumer Health Information about Eye Care and Eye Disorders, Including Facts about the Diagnosis, Prevention, and Treatment of Common Refractive Problems Such as Myopia, Hyperopia, Astigmatism, and Presbyopia, and Eye Diseases, Including Glaucoma, Cataract, Age-Related Macular Degeneration, and Diabetic Retinopathy

Along with a Section on Vision Correction and Refractive Surgeries, Including LASIK and LASEK, a Glossary, and Directories of Resources for Additional Help and Information

Edited by Amy L. Sutton. 543 pages. 2003. 0-7808-0635-2.

"... a solid reference tool for eye care and a valuable addition to a collection."
— *American Reference Books Annual, 2004*

■

Family Planning Sourcebook

Basic Consumer Health Information about Planning for Pregnancy and Contraception, Including Traditional Methods, Barrier Methods, Hormonal Methods, Permanent Methods, Future Methods, Emergency Contraception, and Birth Control Choices for Women at Each Stage of Life

Along with Statistics, a Glossary, and Sources of Additional Information

Edited by Amy Marcaccio Keyzer. 520 pages. 2001. 0-7808-0379-5.

"Recommended for public, health, and undergraduate libraries as part of the circulating collection."
— *E-Streams, Mar '02*

"Information is presented in an unbiased, readable manner, and the sourcebook will certainly be a necessary addition to those public and high school libraries where Internet access is restricted or otherwise problematic." — *American Reference Books Annual, 2002*

"Recommended reference source."
— *Booklist, American Library Association, Oct '01*

"Will prove valuable to any library seeking to maintain a current, comprehensive reference collection of health resources. . . . Excellent reference."
— *The Bookwatch, Aug '01*

SEE ALSO *Pregnancy & Birth Sourcebook*

■

Fitness & Exercise Sourcebook, 2nd Edition

Basic Consumer Health Information about the Fundamentals of Fitness and Exercise, Including How to Begin and Maintain a Fitness Program, Fitness as a Lifestyle, the Link between Fitness and Diet, Advice for Specific Groups of People, Exercise as It Relates to Specific Medical Conditions, and Recent Research in Fitness and Exercise

Along with a Glossary of Important Terms and Resources for Additional Help and Information

Edited by Kristen M. Gledhill. 646 pages. 2001. 0-7808-0334-5.

"This work is recommended for all general reference collections."
— *American Reference Books Annual, 2002*

"Highly recommended for public, consumer, and school grades fourth through college." — *E-Streams, Nov '01*

"Recommended reference source."
— *Booklist, American Library Association, Oct '01*

"The information appears quite comprehensive and is considered reliable. . . . This second edition is a welcomed addition to the series."
— *Doody's Review Service, Sep '01*

Food & Animal Borne Diseases Sourcebook

Basic Information about Diseases That Can Be Spread to Humans through the Ingestion of Contaminated Food or Water or by Contact with Infected Animals and Insects, Such as Botulism, E. Coli, Hepatitis A, Trichinosis, Lyme Disease, and Rabies

Along with Information Regarding Prevention and Treatment Methods, and Including a Special Section for International Travelers Describing Diseases Such as Cholera, Malaria, Travelers' Diarrhea, and Yellow Fever, and Offering Recommendations for Avoiding Illness

Edited by Karen Bellenir and Peter D. Dresser. 535 pages. 1995. 0-7808-0033-8.

"Targeting general readers and providing them with a single, comprehensive source of information on selected topics, this book continues, with the excellent caliber of its predecessors, to catalog topical information on health matters of general interest. Readable and thorough, this valuable resource is highly recommended for all libraries."
— Academic Library Book Review, Summer '96

"A comprehensive collection of authoritative information."
— Emergency Medical Services, Oct '95

Food Safety Sourcebook

Basic Consumer Health Information about the Safe Handling of Meat, Poultry, Seafood, Eggs, Fruit Juices, and Other Food Items, and Facts about Pesticides, Drinking Water, Food Safety Overseas, and the Onset, Duration, and Symptoms of Foodborne Illnesses, Including Types of Pathogenic Bacteria, Parasitic Protozoa, Worms, Viruses, and Natural Toxins

Along with the Role of the Consumer, the Food Handler, and the Government in Food Safety; a Glossary, and Resources for Additional Help and Information

Edited by Dawn D. Matthews. 339 pages. 1999. 0-7808-0326-4.

"This book is recommended for public libraries and universities with home economic and food science programs."
— E-Streams, Nov '00

"Recommended reference source."
— Booklist, American Library Association, May '00

"This book takes the complex issues of food safety and foodborne pathogens and presents them in an easily understood manner. [It does] an excellent job of covering a large and often confusing topic."
— American Reference Books Annual, 2000

Forensic Medicine Sourcebook

Basic Consumer Information for the Layperson about Forensic Medicine, Including Crime Scene Investigation, Evidence Collection and Analysis, Expert Testimony, Computer-Aided Criminal Identification, Digital Imaging in the Courtroom, DNA Profiling, Accident Reconstruction, Autopsies, Ballistics, Drugs and

Explosives Detection, Latent Fingerprints, Product Tampering, and Questioned Document Examination

Along with Statistical Data, a Glossary of Forensics Terminology, and Listings of Sources for Further Help and Information

Edited by Annemarie S. Muth. 574 pages. 1999. 0-7808-0232-2.

"Given the expected widespread interest in its content and its easy to read style, this book is recommended for most public and all college and university libraries."
— E-Streams, Feb '01

"Recommended for public libraries."
— Reference & User Services Quarterly, American Library Association, Spring 2000

"Recommended reference source."
— Booklist, American Library Association, Feb '00

"A wealth of information, useful statistics, references are up-to-date and extremely complete. This wonderful collection of data will help students who are interested in a career in any type of forensic field. It is a great resource for attorneys who need information about types of expert witnesses needed in a particular case. It also offers useful information for fiction and nonfiction writers whose work involves a crime. A fascinating compilation. All levels."
— Choice, Association of College & Research Libraries, Jan '00

"There are several items that make this book attractive to consumers who are seeking certain forensic data. . . . This is a useful current source for those seeking general forensic medical answers."
— American Reference Books Annual, 2000

Gastrointestinal Diseases & Disorders Sourcebook, 2nd Edition

Basic Consumer Health Information about the Upper and Lower Gastrointestinal (GI) Tract, Including the Esophagus, Stomach, Intestines, Rectum, Liver, and Pancreas, with Facts about Gastroesophageal Reflux Disease, Gastritis, Hernias, Ulcers, Celiac Disease, Diverticulitis, Irritable Bowel Syndrome, Hemorrhoids, Gastrointestinal Cancers, and Other Diseases and Disorders Related to the Digestive Process

Along with Information about Commonly Used Diagnostic and Surgical Procedures, Statistics, Reports on Current Research Initiatives and Clinical Trials, a Glossary, and Resources for Additional Help and Information

Edited by Sandra J. Judd. 681 pages. 2006. 0-7808-0798-7.

". . . very readable form. The successful editorial work that brought this material together into a useful and understandable reference makes accessible to all readers information that can help them more effectively understand and obtain help for digestive tract problems."
— Choice, Association of College & Research Libraries, Feb '97

SEE ALSO *Diet & Nutrition Sourcebook, Digestive Diseases & Disorders, Eating Disorders Sourcebook*

Genetic Disorders Sourcebook, 3rd Edition

Basic Consumer Health Information about Hereditary Diseases and Disorders, Including Facts about the Human Genome, Genetic Inheritance Patterns, Disorders Associated with Specific Genes, Such as Sickle Cell Disease, Hemophilia, and Cystic Fibrosis, Chromosome Disorders, Such as Down Syndrome, Fragile X Syndrome, and Turner Syndrome, and Complex Diseases and Disorders Resulting from the Interaction of Environmental and Genetic Factors, Such as Allergies, Cancer, and Obesity

Along with Facts about Genetic Testing, Suggestions for Parents of Children with Special Needs, Reports on Current Research Initiatives, a Glossary of Genetic Terminology, and Resources for Additional Help and Information

Edited by Karen Bellenir. 777 pages. 2004. 0-7808-0742-1.

"This text is recommended for any library with an interest in providing consumer health resources."
— *E-Streams, Aug '05*

"This is a valuable resource for anyone wishing to have an understandable description of any of the topics or disorders included. The editor succeeds in making complex genetic issues understandable."
— *Doody's Book Review Service, May '05*

"A good acquisition for public libraries."
— *American Reference Books Annual, 2005*

"Excellent reference." — *The Bookwatch, Jan '05*

"Recommended reference source."
— *Booklist, American Library Association, Apr '01*

"Important pick for college-level health reference libraries." — *The Bookwatch, Mar '01*

Head Trauma Sourcebook

Basic Information for the Layperson about Open-Head and Closed-Head Injuries, Treatment Advances, Recovery, and Rehabilitation

Along with Reports on Current Research Initiatives

Edited by Karen Bellenir. 414 pages. 1997. 0-7808-0208-X.

Headache Sourcebook

Basic Consumer Health Information about Migraine, Tension, Cluster, Rebound and Other Types of Headaches, with Facts about the Cause and Prevention of Headaches, the Effects of Stress and the Environment, Headaches during Pregnancy and Menopause, and Childhood Headaches

Along with a Glossary and Other Resources for Additional Help and Information

Edited by Dawn D. Matthews. 362 pages. 2002. 0-7808-0337-X.

"Highly recommended for academic and medical reference collections." — *Library Bookwatch, Sep '02*

Health Insurance Sourcebook

Basic Information about Managed Care Organizations, Traditional Fee-for-Service Insurance, Insurance Portability and Pre-Existing Conditions Clauses, Medicare, Medicaid, Social Security, and Military Health Care

Along with Information about Insurance Fraud

Edited by Wendy Wilcox. 530 pages. 1997. 0-7808-0222-5.

"Particularly useful because it brings much of this information together in one volume. This book will be a handy reference source in the health sciences library, hospital library, college and university library, and medium to large public library."
— *Medical Reference Services Quarterly, Fall '98*

Awarded "Books of the Year Award"
— *American Journal of Nursing, 1997*

"The layout of the book is particularly helpful as it provides easy access to reference material. A most useful addition to the vast amount of information about health insurance. The use of data from U.S. government agencies is most commendable. Useful in a library or learning center for healthcare professional students."
— *Doody's Health Sciences Book Reviews, Nov '97*

Healthy Aging Sourcebook

Basic Consumer Health Information about Maintaining Health through the Aging Process, Including Advice on Nutrition, Exercise, and Sleep, Help in Making Decisions about Midlife Issues and Retirement, and Guidance Concerning Practical and Informed Choices in Health Consumerism

Along with Data Concerning the Theories of Aging, Different Experiences in Aging by Minority Groups, and Facts about Aging Now and Aging in the Future; and Featuring a Glossary, a Guide to Consumer Help, Additional Suggested Reading, and Practical Resource Directory

Edited by Jenifer Swanson. 536 pages. 1999. 0-7808-0390-6.

"Recommended reference source."
— *Booklist, American Library Association, Feb '00*

SEE ALSO *Physical & Mental Issues in Aging Sourcebook*

Healthy Children Sourcebook

Basic Consumer Health Information about the Physical and Mental Development of Children between the Ages of 3 and 12, Including Routine Health Care, Preventative Health Services, Safety and First Aid, Healthy Sleep, Dental Care, Nutrition, and Fitness, and Featuring Parenting Tips on Such Topics as Bed-

wetting, Choosing Day Care, Monitoring TV and Other Media, and Establishing a Foundation for Substance Abuse Prevention

Along with a Glossary of Commonly Used Pediatric Terms and Resources for Additional Help and Information.

Edited by Chad T. Kimball. 647 pages. 2003. 0-7808-0247-0.

"It is hard to imagine that any other single resource exists that would provide such a comprehensive guide of timely information on health promotion and disease prevention for children aged 3 to 12."
—*American Reference Books Annual, 2004*

"The strengths of this book are many. It is clearly written, presented and structured."
—*Journal of the National Medical Association, 2004*

SEE ALSO Childhood Diseases & Disorders Sourcebook

Healthy Heart Sourcebook for Women

Basic Consumer Health Information about Cardiac Issues Specific to Women, Including Facts about Major Risk Factors and Prevention, Treatment and Control Strategies, and Important Dietary Issues

Along with a Special Section Regarding the Pros and Cons of Hormone Replacement Therapy and Its Impact on Heart Health, and Additional Help, Including Recipes, a Glossary, and a Directory of Resources

Edited by Dawn D. Matthews. 336 pages. 2000. 0-7808-0329-9.

"A good reference source and recommended for all public, academic, medical, and hospital libraries."
—*Medical Reference Services Quarterly, Summer '01*

"Because of the lack of information specific to women on this topic, this book is recommended for public libraries and consumer libraries."
—*American Reference Books Annual, 2001*

"Contains very important information about coronary artery disease that all women should know. The information is current and presented in an easy-to-read format. The book will make a good addition to any library."
—*American Medical Writers Association Journal, Summer '00*

"Important, basic reference."
—*Reviewer's Bookwatch, Jul '00*

SEE ALSO Cardiovascular Diseases & Disorders Sourcebook, Women's Health Concerns Sourcebook

Heart Diseases & Disorders Sourcebook

SEE Cardiovascular Diseases & Disorders Sourcebook, 3rd Edition

Hepatitis Sourcebook

Basic Consumer Health Information about Hepatitis A, Hepatitis B, Hepatitis C, and Other Forms of Hepatitis, Including Autoimmune Hepatitis, Alcoholic Hepatitis, Nonalcoholic Steatohepatitis, and Toxic Hepatitis, with Facts about Risk Factors, Screening Methods, Diagnostic Tests, and Treatment Options

Along with Information on Liver Health, Tips for People Living with Chronic Hepatitis, Reports on Current Research Initiatives, a Glossary of Terms Related to Hepatitis, and a Directory of Sources for Further Help and Information

Edited by Sandra J. Judd. 597 pages. 2005. 0-7808-0749-9.

"Highly recommended."
—*American Reference Books Annual, 2006*

Household Safety Sourcebook

Basic Consumer Health Information about Household Safety, Including Information about Poisons, Chemicals, Fire, and Water Hazards in the Home

Along with Advice about the Safe Use of Home Maintenance Equipment, Choosing Toys and Nursery Furniture, Holiday and Recreation Safety, a Glossary, and Resources for Further Help and Information

Edited by Dawn D. Matthews. 606 pages. 2002. 0-7808-0338-8.

"This work will be useful in public libraries with large consumer health and wellness departments."
—*American Reference Books Annual, 2003*

"As a sourcebook on household safety this book meets its mark. It is encyclopedic in scope and covers a wide range of safety issues that are commonly seen in the home."
—*E-Streams, Jul '02*

Hypertension Sourcebook

Basic Consumer Health Information about the Causes, Diagnosis, and Treatment of High Blood Pressure, with Facts about Consequences, Complications, and Co-Occurring Disorders, Such as Coronary Heart Disease, Diabetes, Stroke, Kidney Disease, and Hypertensive Retinopathy, and Issues in Blood Pressure Control, Including Dietary Choices, Stress Management, and Medications

Along with Reports on Current Research Initiatives and Clinical Trials, a Glossary, and Resources for Additional Help and Information

Edited by Dawn D. Matthews and Karen Bellenir. 613 pages. 2004. 0-7808-0674-3.

"Academic, public, and medical libraries will want to add the *Hypertension Sourcebook* to their collections."
—*E-Streams, Aug '05*

"The strength of this source is the wide range of information given about hypertension."
—*American Reference Books Annual, 2005*

Immune System Disorders Sourcebook, 2nd Edition

Basic Consumer Health Information about Disorders of the Immune System, Including Immune System Function and Response, Diagnosis of Immune Disorders, Information about Inherited Immune Disease, Acquired Immune Disease, and Autoimmune Diseases, Including Primary Immune Deficiency, Acquired Immunodeficiency Syndrome (AIDS), Lupus, Multiple Sclerosis, Type 1 Diabetes, Rheumatoid Arthritis, and Graves' Disease

Along with Treatments, Tips for Coping with Immune Disorders, a Glossary, and a Directory of Additional Resources.

Edited by Joyce Brennfleck Shannon. 671 pages. 2005. 0-7808-0748-0

"Highly recommended for academic and public libraries." — *American Reference Books Annual, 2006*

"The updated second edition is a 'must' for any consumer health library seeking a solid resource covering the treatments, symptoms, and options for immune disorder sufferers. . . . An excellent guide."
— *MBR Bookwatch, Jan '06*

■

Infant & Toddler Health Sourcebook

Basic Consumer Health Information about the Physical and Mental Development of Newborns, Infants, and Toddlers, Including Neonatal Concerns, Nutrition Recommendations, Immunization Schedules, Common Pediatric Disorders, Assessments and Milestones, Safety Tips, and Advice for Parents and Other Caregivers

Along with a Glossary of Terms and Resource Listings for Additional Help

Edited by Jenifer Swanson. 585 pages. 2000. 0-7808-0246-2.

"As a reference for the general public, this would be useful in any library." — *E-Streams, May '01*

"Recommended reference source."
— *Booklist, American Library Association, Feb '01*

"This is a good source for general use."
— *American Reference Books Annual, 2001*

■

Infectious Diseases Sourcebook

Basic Consumer Health Information about Non-Contagious Bacterial, Viral, Prion, Fungal, and Parasitic Diseases Spread by Food and Water, Insects and Animals, or Environmental Contact, Including Botulism, E. Coli, Encephalitis, Legionnaires' Disease, Lyme Disease, Malaria, Plague, Rabies, Salmonella, Tetanus, and Others, and Facts about Newly Emerging Diseases, Such as Hantavirus, Mad Cow Disease, Monkeypox, and West Nile Virus

Along with Information about Preventing Disease Transmission, the Threat of Bioterrorism, and Current

Research Initiatives, with a Glossary and Directory of Resources for More Information

Edited by Karen Bellenir. 634 pages. 2004. 0-7808-0675-1.

"This reference continues the excellent tradition of the *Health Reference Series* in consolidating a wealth of information on a selected topic into a format that is easy to use and accessible to the general public."
— *American Reference Books Annual, 2005*

"Recommended for public and academic libraries."
— *E-Streams, Jan '05*

■

Injury & Trauma Sourcebook

Basic Consumer Health Information about the Impact of Injury, the Diagnosis and Treatment of Common and Traumatic Injuries, Emergency Care, and Specific Injuries Related to Home, Community, Workplace, Transportation, and Recreation

Along with Guidelines for Injury Prevention, a Glossary, and a Directory of Additional Resources

Edited by Joyce Brennfleck Shannon. 696 pages. 2002. 0-7808-0421-X.

"This publication is the most comprehensive work of its kind about injury and trauma."
— *American Reference Books Annual, 2003*

"This sourcebook provides concise, easily readable, basic health information about injuries. . . . This book is well organized and an easy to use reference resource suitable for hospital, health sciences and public libraries with consumer health collections."
— *E-Streams, Nov '02*

"Practitioners should be aware of guides such as this in order to facilitate their use by patients and their families." — *Doody's Health Sciences Book Review Journal, Sep-Oct '02*

"Recommended reference source."
— *Booklist, American Library Association, Sep '02*

"Highly recommended for academic and medical reference collections." — *Library Bookwatch, Sep '02*

■

Kidney & Urinary Tract Diseases & Disorders Sourcebook

SEE *Urinary Tract & Kidney Diseases & Disorders Sourcebook, 2nd Edition*

■

Learning Disabilities Sourcebook, 2nd Edition

Basic Consumer Health Information about Learning Disabilities, Including Dyslexia, Developmental Speech and Language Disabilities, Non-Verbal Learning Disorders, Developmental Arithmetic Disorder, Developmental Writing Disorder, and Other Conditions That Impede Learning Such as Attention Deficit/ Hyperactivity Disorder, Brain Injury, Hearing Impairment, Kline-felter Syndrome, Dyspraxia, and Tourette's Syndrome

Along with Facts about Educational Issues and Assistive Technology, Coping Strategies, a Glossary of Related Terms, and Resources for Further Help and Information

Edited by Dawn D. Matthews. 621 pages. 2003. 0-7808-0626-3.

"The second edition of Learning Disabilities Sourcebook far surpasses the earlier edition in that it is more focused on information that will be useful as a consumer health resource."
— American Reference Books Annual, 2004

"Teachers as well as consumers will find this an essential guide to understanding various syndromes and their latest treatments. [An] invaluable reference for public and school library collections alike."
— Library Bookwatch, Apr '03

Named "Outstanding Reference Book of 1999."
— New York Public Library, Feb 2000

"An excellent candidate for inclusion in a public library reference section. It's a great source of information. Teachers will also find the book useful. Definitely worth reading."
— Journal of Adolescent & Adult Literacy, Feb 2000

"Readable . . . provides a solid base of information regarding successful techniques used with individuals who have learning disabilities, as well as practical suggestions for educators and family members. Clear language, concise descriptions, and pertinent information for contacting multiple resources add to the strength of this book as a useful tool." — Choice, Association of College & Research Libraries, Feb '99

"Recommended reference source."
— Booklist, American Library Association, Sep '98

"A useful resource for libraries and for those who don't have the time to identify and locate the individual publications." — Disability Resources Monthly, Sep '98

Leukemia Sourcebook

Basic Consumer Health Information about Adult and Childhood Leukemias, Including Acute Lymphocytic Leukemia (ALL), Chronic Lymphocytic Leukemia (CLL), Acute Myelogenous Leukemia (AML), Chronic Myelogenous Leukemia (CML), and Hairy Cell Leukemia, and Treatments Such as Chemotherapy, Radiation Therapy, Peripheral Blood Stem Cell and Marrow Transplantation, and Immunotherapy

Along with Tips for Life During and After Treatment, a Glossary, and Directories of Additional Resources

Edited by Joyce Brennfleck Shannon. 587 pages. 2003. 0-7808-0627-1.

"Unlike other medical books for the layperson, . . . the language does not talk down to the reader. . . . This volume is highly recommended for all libraries."
— American Reference Books Annual, 2004

"... a fine title which ranges from diagnosis to alternative treatments, staging, and tips for life during and after diagnosis." — The Bookwatch, Dec '03

Liver Disorders Sourcebook

Basic Consumer Health Information about the Liver and How It Works; Liver Diseases, Including Cancer, Cirrhosis, Hepatitis, and Toxic and Drug Related Diseases; Tips for Maintaining a Healthy Liver; Laboratory Tests, Radiology Tests, and Facts about Liver Transplantation

Along with a Section on Support Groups, a Glossary, and Resource Listings

Edited by Joyce Brennfleck Shannon. 591 pages. 2000. 0-7808-0383-3.

"A valuable resource."
— American Reference Books Annual, 2001

"This title is recommended for health sciences and public libraries with consumer health collections."
— E-Streams, Oct '00

"Recommended reference source."
— Booklist, American Library Association, Jun '00

Lung Disorders Sourcebook

Basic Consumer Health Information about Emphysema, Pneumonia, Tuberculosis, Asthma, Cystic Fibrosis, and Other Lung Disorders, Including Facts about Diagnostic Procedures, Treatment Strategies, Disease Prevention Efforts, and Such Risk Factors as Smoking, Air Pollution, and Exposure to Asbestos, Radon, and Other Agents

Along with a Glossary and Resources for Additional Help and Information

Edited by Dawn D. Matthews. 678 pages. 2002. 0-7808-0339-6.

"This title is a great addition for public and school libraries because it provides concise health information on the lungs."
— American Reference Books Annual, 2003

"Highly recommended for academic and medical reference collections." — Library Bookwatch, Sep '02

SEE ALSO Respiratory Diseases & Disorders Sourcebook

Medical Tests Sourcebook, 2nd Edition

Basic Consumer Health Information about Medical Tests, Including Age-Specific Health Tests, Important Health Screenings and Exams, Home-Use Tests, Blood and Specimen Tests, Electrical Tests, Scope Tests, Genetic Testing, and Imaging Tests, Such as X-Rays, Ultrasound, Computed Tomography, Magnetic Resonance Imaging, Angiography, and Nuclear Medicine

Along with a Glossary and Directory of Additional Resources

Edited by Joyce Brennfleck Shannon. 654 pages. 2004. 0-7808-0670-0.

"Recommended for hospital and health sciences libraries with consumer health collections."
— *E-Streams, Mar '00*

"This is an overall excellent reference with a wealth of general knowledge that may aid those who are reluctant to get vital tests performed."
— *Today's Librarian, Jan '00*

"A valuable reference guide."
— *American Reference Books Annual, 2000*

■

Men's Health Concerns Sourcebook, 2nd Edition

Basic Consumer Health Information about the Medical and Mental Concerns of Men, Including Theories about the Shorter Male Lifespan, the Leading Causes of Death and Disability, Physical Concerns of Special Significance to Men, Reproductive and Sexual Concerns, Sexually Transmitted Diseases, Men's Mental and Emotional Health, and Lifestyle Choices That Affect Wellness, Such as Nutrition, Fitness, and Substance Use

Along with a Glossary of Related Terms and a Directory of Organizational Resources in Men's Health

Edited by Robert Aquinas McNally. 644 pages. 2004. 0-7808-0671-9.

"A very accessible reference for non-specialist general readers and consumers." — *The Bookwatch, Jun '04*

"This comprehensive resource and the series are highly recommended."
— *American Reference Books Annual, 2000*

"Recommended reference source."
— *Booklist, American Library Association, Dec '98*

■

Mental Health Disorders Sourcebook, 3rd Edition

Basic Consumer Health Information about Mental and Emotional Health and Mental Illness, Including Facts about Depression, Bipolar Disorder, and Other Mood Disorders, Phobias, Post-Traumatic Stress Disorder (PTSD), Obsessive-Compulsive Disorder, and Other Anxiety Disorders, Impulse Control Disorders, Eating Disorders, Personality Disorders, and Psychotic Disorders, Including Schizophrenia and Dissociative Disorders

Along with Statistical Information, a Special Section Concerning Mental Health Issues in Children and Adolescents, a Glossary, and Directories of Resources for Additional Help and Information

Edited by Karen Bellenir. 661 pages. 2005. 0-7808-0747-2.

"Recommended for public libraries and academic libraries with an undergraduate program in psychology."
— *American Reference Books Annual, 2006*

"Recommended reference source."
— *Booklist, American Library Association, Jun '00*

■

Mental Retardation Sourcebook

Basic Consumer Health Information about Mental Retardation and Its Causes, Including Down Syndrome, Fetal Alcohol Syndrome, Fragile X Syndrome, Genetic Conditions, Injury, and Environmental Sources

Along with Preventive Strategies, Parenting Issues, Educational Implications, Health Care Needs, Employment and Economic Matters, Legal Issues, a Glossary, and a Resource Listing for Additional Help and Information

Edited by Joyce Brennfleck Shannon. 642 pages. 2000. 0-7808-0377-9.

"Public libraries will find the book useful for reference and as a beginning research point for students, parents, and caregivers."
— *American Reference Books Annual, 2001*

"The strength of this work is that it compiles many basic fact sheets and addresses for further information in one volume. It is intended and suitable for the general public. This sourcebook is relevant to any collection providing health information to the general public."
— *E-Streams, Nov '00*

"From preventing retardation to parenting and family challenges, this covers health, social and legal issues and will prove an invaluable overview."
— *Reviewer's Bookwatch, Jul '00*

■

Movement Disorders Sourcebook

Basic Consumer Health Information about Neurological Movement Disorders, Including Essential Tremor, Parkinson's Disease, Dystonia, Cerebral Palsy, Huntington's Disease, Myasthenia Gravis, Multiple Sclerosis, and Other Early-Onset and Adult-Onset Movement Disorders, Their Symptoms and Causes, Diagnostic Tests, and Treatments

Along with Mobility and Assistive Technology Information, a Glossary, and a Directory of Additional Resources

Edited by Joyce Brennfleck Shannon. 655 pages. 2003. 0-7808-0628-X.

". . . a good resource for consumers and recommended for public, community college and undergraduate libraries." — *American Reference Books Annual, 2004*

■

Muscular Dystrophy Sourcebook

Basic Consumer Health Information about Congenital, Childhood-Onset, and Adult-Onset Forms of Muscular Dystrophy, Such as Duchenne, Becker, Emery-Dreifuss, Distal, Limb-Girdle, Facioscapulohumeral (FSHD), Myotonic, and Ophthalmoplegic Muscular Dystro-

phies, Including Facts about Diagnostic Tests, Medical and Physical Therapies, Management of Co-Occurring Conditions, and Parenting Guidelines

Along with Practical Tips for Home Care, a Glossary, and Directories of Additional Resources

Edited by Joyce Brennfleck Shannon. 577 pages. 2004. 0-7808-0676-X.

"This book is highly recommended for public and academic libraries as well as health care offices that support the information needs of patients and their families."
— E-Streams, Apr '05

"Excellent reference." — The Bookwatch, Jan '05

Obesity Sourcebook

Basic Consumer Health Information about Diseases and Other Problems Associated with Obesity, and Including Facts about Risk Factors, Prevention Issues, and Management Approaches

Along with Statistical and Demographic Data, Information about Special Populations, Research Updates, a Glossary, and Source Listings for Further Help and Information

Edited by Wilma Caldwell and Chad T. Kimball. 376 pages. 2001. 0-7808-0333-7.

"The book synthesizes the reliable medical literature on obesity into one easy-to-read and useful resource for the general public."
— American Reference Books Annual, 2002

"This is a very useful resource book for the lay public."
— Doody's Review Service, Nov '01

"Well suited for the health reference collection of a public library or an academic health science library that serves the general population." — E-Streams, Sep '01

"Recommended reference source."
— Booklist, American Library Association, Apr '01

"Recommended pick both for specialty health library collections and any general consumer health reference collection." — The Bookwatch, Apr '01

Ophthalmic Disorders Sourcebook

SEE Eye Care Sourcebook, 2nd Edition

Oral Health Sourcebook

SEE Dental Care & Oral Health Sourcebook, 2nd Edition

Osteoporosis Sourcebook

Basic Consumer Health Information about Primary and Secondary Osteoporosis and Juvenile Osteoporosis and Related Conditions, Including Fibrous Dysplasia,

Gaucher Disease, Hyperthyroidism, Hypophosphatasia, Myeloma, Osteopetrosis, Osteogenesis Imperfecta, and Paget's Disease

Along with Information about Risk Factors, Treatments, Traditional and Non-Traditional Pain Management, a Glossary of Related Terms, and a Directory of Resources

Edited by Allan R. Cook. 584 pages. 2001. 0-7808-0239-X.

"This would be a book to be kept in a staff or patient library. The targeted audience is the layperson, but the therapist who needs a quick bit of information on a particular topic will also find the book useful."
— Physical Therapy, Jan '02

"This resource is recommended as a great reference source for public, health, and academic libraries, and is another triumph for the editors of Omnigraphics."
— American Reference Books Annual, 2002

"Recommended for all public libraries and general health collections, especially those supporting patient education or consumer health programs."
— E-Streams, Nov '01

"Will prove valuable to any library seeking to maintain a current, comprehensive reference collection of health resources. . . . From prevention to treatment and associated conditions, this provides an excellent survey."
— The Bookwatch, Aug '01

"Recommended reference source."
— Booklist, American Library Association, Jul '01

SEE ALSO Healthy Aging Sourcebook, Physical & Mental Issues in Aging Sourcebook, Women's Health Concerns Sourcebook

---

Pain Sourcebook, 2nd Edition

Basic Consumer Health Information about Specific Forms of Acute and Chronic Pain, Including Muscle and Skeletal Pain, Nerve Pain, Cancer Pain, and Disorders Characterized by Pain, Such as Fibromyalgia, Shingles, Angina, Arthritis, and Headaches

Along with Information about Pain Medications and Management Techniques, Complementary and Alternative Pain Relief Options, Tips for People Living with Chronic Pain, a Glossary, and a Directory of Sources for Further Information

Edited by Karen Bellenir. 670 pages. 2002. 0-7808-0612-3.

"A source of valuable information. . . . This book offers help to nonmedical people who need information about pain and pain management. It is also an excellent reference for those who participate in patient education."
— Doody's Review Service, Sep '02

"Highly recommended for academic and medical reference collections." — Library Bookwatch, Sep '02

"The text is readable, easily understood, and well indexed. This excellent volume belongs in all patient education libraries, consumer health sections of public libraries, and many personal collections."
— American Reference Books Annual, 1999

"The information is basic in terms of scholarship and is appropriate for general readers. Written in journalistic style . . . intended for non-professionals. Quite thorough in its coverage of different pain conditions and summarizes the latest clinical information regarding pain treatment." — *Choice, Association of College and Research Libraries, Jun '98*

"Recommended reference source."
— *Booklist, American Library Association, Mar '98*

■

Pediatric Cancer Sourcebook

Basic Consumer Health Information about Leukemias, Brain Tumors, Sarcomas, Lymphomas, and Other Cancers in Infants, Children, and Adolescents, Including Descriptions of Cancers, Treatments, and Coping Strategies

Along with Suggestions for Parents, Caregivers, and Concerned Relatives, a Glossary of Cancer Terms, and Resource Listings

Edited by Edward J. Prucha. 587 pages. 1999. 0-7808-0245-4.

"An excellent source of information. Recommended for public, hospital, and health science libraries with consumer health collections." — *E-Streams, Jun '00*

"Recommended reference source."
— *Booklist, American Library Association, Feb '00*

"A valuable addition to all libraries specializing in health services and many public libraries."
— *American Reference Books Annual, 2000*

SEE ALSO Childhood Diseases & Disorders Sourcebook, Healthy Children Sourcebook

■

Physical & Mental Issues in Aging Sourcebook

Basic Consumer Health Information on Physical and Mental Disorders Associated with the Aging Process, Including Concerns about Cardiovascular Disease, Pulmonary Disease, Oral Health, Digestive Disorders, Musculoskeletal and Skin Disorders, Metabolic Changes, Sexual and Reproductive Issues, and Changes in Vision, Hearing, and Other Senses

Along with Data about Longevity and Causes of Death, Information on Acute and Chronic Pain, Descriptions of Mental Concerns, a Glossary of Terms, and Resource Listings for Additional Help

Edited by Jenifer Swanson. 660 pages. 1999. 0-7808-0233-0.

"This is a treasure of health information for the layperson." — *Choice Health Sciences Supplement, Association of College & Research Libraries, May '00*

"Recommended for public libraries."
— *American Reference Books Annual, 2000*

"Recommended reference source."
— *Booklist, American Library Association, Oct '99*

SEE ALSO Healthy Aging Sourcebook

Podiatry Sourcebook

Basic Consumer Health Information about Foot Conditions, Diseases, and Injuries, Including Bunions, Corns, Calluses, Athlete's Foot, Plantar Warts, Hammertoes and Clawtoes, Clubfoot, Heel Pain, Gout, and More

Along with Facts about Foot Care, Disease Prevention, Foot Safety, Choosing a Foot Care Specialist, a Glossary of Terms, and Resource Listings for Additional Information

Edited by M. Lisa Weatherford. 380 pages. 2001. 0-7808-0215-2.

"Recommended reference source."
— *Booklist, American Library Association, Feb '02*

"There is a lot of information presented here on a topic that is usually only covered sparingly in most larger comprehensive medical encyclopedias."
— *American Reference Books Annual, 2002*

■

Pregnancy & Birth Sourcebook, 2nd Edition

Basic Consumer Health Information about Conception and Pregnancy, Including Facts about Fertility, Infertility, Pregnancy Symptoms and Complications, Fetal Growth and Development, Labor, Delivery, and the Postpartum Period, as Well as Information about Maintaining Health and Wellness during Pregnancy and Caring for a Newborn

Along with Information about Public Health Assistance for Low-Income Pregnant Women, a Glossary, and Directories of Agencies and Organizations Providing Help and Support

Edited by Amy L. Sutton. 626 pages. 2004. 0-7808-0672-7.

"Will appeal to public and school reference collections strong in medicine and women's health. . . . Deserves a spot on any medical reference shelf."
— *The Bookwatch, Jul '04*

"A well-organized handbook. Recommended."
— *Choice, Association of College & Research Libraries, Apr '98*

"Recommended reference source."
— *Booklist, American Library Association, Mar '98*

"Recommended for public libraries."
— *American Reference Books Annual, 1998*

SEE ALSO Breastfeeding Sourcebook, Congenital Disorders Sourcebook, Family Planning Sourcebook

■

Prostate Cancer Sourcebook

Basic Consumer Health Information about Prostate Cancer, Including Information about the Associated Risk Factors, Detection, Diagnosis, and Treatment of Prostate Cancer

Along with Information on Non-Malignant Prostate Conditions, and Featuring a Section Listing Support and Treatment Centers and a Glossary of Related Terms

Edited by Dawn D. Matthews. 358 pages. 2001. 0-7808-0324-8.

"Recommended reference source."
— *Booklist, American Library Association, Jan '02*

"A valuable resource for health care consumers seeking information on the subject. . . . All text is written in a clear, easy-to-understand language that avoids technical jargon. Any library that collects consumer health resources would strengthen their collection with the addition of the Prostate Cancer Sourcebook."
— *American Reference Books Annual, 2002*

SEE ALSO *Men's Health Concerns Sourcebook*

■

Prostate & Urological Disorders Sourcebook

Basic Consumer Health Information about Urogenital and Sexual Disorders in Men, Including Prostate and Other Andrological Cancers, Prostatitis, Benign Prostatic Hyperplasia, Testicular and Penile Trauma, Cryptorchidism, Peyronie Disease, Erectile Dysfunction, and Male Factor Infertility, and Facts about Commonly Used Tests and Procedures, Such as Prostatectomy, Vasectomy, Vasectomy Reversal, Penile Implants, and Semen Analysis

Along with a Glossary of Andrological Terms and a Directory of Resources for Additional Information

Edited by Karen Bellenir. 631 pages. 2005. 0-7808-0797-9.

■

Public Health Sourcebook

Basic Information about Government Health Agencies, Including National Health Statistics and Trends, Healthy People 2000 Program Goals and Objectives, the Centers for Disease Control and Prevention, the Food and Drug Administration, and the National Institutes of Health

Along with Full Contact Information for Each Agency

Edited by Wendy Wilcox. 698 pages. 1998. 0-7808-0220-9.

"Recommended reference source."
— *Booklist, American Library Association, Sep '98*

"This consumer guide provides welcome assistance in navigating the maze of federal health agencies and their data on public health concerns."
— *SciTech Book News, Sep '98*

■

Reconstructive & Cosmetic Surgery Sourcebook

Basic Consumer Health Information on Cosmetic and Reconstructive Plastic Surgery, Including Statistical Information about Different Surgical Procedures, Things to Consider Prior to Surgery, Plastic Surgery Techniques and Tools, Emotional and Psychological Considerations, and Procedure-Specific Information

Along with a Glossary of Terms and a Listing of Resources for Additional Help and Information

Edited by M. Lisa Weatherford. 374 pages. 2001. 0-7808-0214-4.

"An excellent reference that addresses cosmetic and medically necessary reconstructive surgeries. . . . The style of the prose is calm and reassuring, discussing the many positive outcomes now available due to advances in surgical techniques."
— *American Reference Books Annual, 2002*

"Recommended for health science libraries that are open to the public, as well as hospital libraries that are open to the patients. This book is a good resource for the consumer interested in plastic surgery."
— *E-Streams, Dec '01*

"Recommended reference source."
— *Booklist, American Library Association, Jul '01*

■

Rehabilitation Sourcebook

Basic Consumer Health Information about Rehabilitation for People Recovering from Heart Surgery, Spinal Cord Injury, Stroke, Orthopedic Impairments, Amputation, Pulmonary Impairments, Traumatic Injury, and More, Including Physical Therapy, Occupational Therapy, Speech/Language Therapy, Massage Therapy, Dance Therapy, Art Therapy, and Recreational Therapy

Along with Information on Assistive and Adaptive Devices, a Glossary, and Resources for Additional Help and Information

Edited by Dawn D. Matthews. 531 pages. 1999. 0-7808-0236-5.

"This is an excellent resource for public library reference and health collections."
— *American Reference Books Annual, 2001*

"Recommended reference source."
— *Booklist, American Library Association, May '00*

■

Respiratory Diseases & Disorders Sourcebook

Basic Information about Respiratory Diseases and Disorders, Including Asthma, Cystic Fibrosis, Pneumonia, the Common Cold, Influenza, and Others, Featuring Facts about the Respiratory System, Statistical and Demographic Data, Treatments, Self-Help Management Suggestions, and Current Research Initiatives

Edited by Allan R. Cook and Peter D. Dresser. 771 pages. 1995. 0-7808-0037-0.

"Designed for the layperson and for patients and their families coping with respiratory illness. . . . an extensive array of information on diagnosis, treatment, management, and prevention of respiratory illnesses for the general reader." — *Choice, Association of College & Research Libraries, Jun '96*

"A highly recommended text for all collections. It is a comforting reminder of the power of knowledge that good books carry between their covers."
— *Academic Library Book Review, Spring '96*

"A comprehensive collection of authoritative information presented in a nontechnical, humanitarian style for patients, families, and caregivers."
— Association of Operating Room Nurses, Sep/Oct '95

SEE ALSO Lung Disorders Sourcebook

■

Sexually Transmitted Diseases Sourcebook, 3rd Edition

Basic Consumer Health Information about Chlamydial Infections, Gonorrhea, Hepatitis, Herpes, HIV/AIDS, Human Papillomavirus, Pubic Lice, Scabies, Syphilis, Trichomoniasis, Vaginal Infections, and Other Sexually Transmitted Diseases, Including Facts about Risk Factors, Symptoms, Diagnosis, Treatment, and the Prevention of Sexually Transmitted Infections

Along with Updates on Current Research Initiatives, a Glossary of Related Terms, and Resources for Additional Help and Information

Edited by Amy L. Sutton. 629 pages. 2006. 0-7808-0824-X.

"Recommended for consumer health collections in public libraries, and secondary school and community college libraries."
— American Reference Books Annual, 2002

"Every school and public library should have a copy of this comprehensive and user-friendly reference book."
— Choice, Association of College & Research Libraries, Sep '01

"This is a highly recommended book. This is an especially important book for all school and public libraries."
— AIDS Book Review Journal, Jul-Aug '01

"Recommended reference source."
— Booklist, American Library Association, Apr '01

■

Skin Disorders Sourcebook

SEE Dermatological Disorders Sourcebook, 2nd Edition

■

Sleep Disorders Sourcebook, 2nd Edition

Basic Consumer Health Information about Sleep and Sleep Disorders, Including Insomnia, Sleep Apnea, Restless Legs Syndrome, Narcolepsy, Parasomnias, and Other Health Problems That Affect Sleep, Plus Facts about Diagnostic Procedures, Treatment Strategies, Sleep Medications, and Tips for Improving Sleep Quality

Along with a Glossary of Related Terms and Resources for Additional Help and Information

Edited by Amy L. Sutton. 567 pages. 2005. 0-7808-0743-X.

"This book will be useful for just about everybody, especially the 40 million Americans with sleep disorders."
— American Reference Books Annual, 2006

"Recommended for public libraries and libraries supporting health care professionals." — E-Streams, Sep '05

". . . key medical library acquisition."
— The Bookwatch, Jun '05

■

Smoking Concerns Sourcebook

Basic Consumer Health Information about Nicotine Addiction and Smoking Cessation, Featuring Facts about the Health Effects of Tobacco Use, Including Lung and Other Cancers, Heart Disease, Stroke, and Respiratory Disorders, Such as Emphysema and Chronic Bronchitis

Along with Information about Smoking Prevention Programs, Suggestions for Achieving and Maintaining a Smoke-Free Lifestyle, Statistics about Tobacco Use, Reports on Current Research Initiatives, a Glossary of Related Terms, and Directories of Resources for Additional Help and Information

Edited by Karen Bellenir. 621 pages. 2004. 0-7808-0323-X.

"Provides everything needed for the student or general reader seeking practical details on the effects of tobacco use." — The Bookwatch, Mar '05

"Public libraries and consumer health care libraries will find this work useful."
— American Reference Books Annual, 2005

■

Sports Injuries Sourcebook, 2nd Edition

Basic Consumer Health Information about the Diagnosis, Treatment, and Rehabilitation of Common Sports-Related Injuries in Children and Adults

Along with Suggestions for Conditioning and Training, Information and Prevention Tips for Injuries Frequently Associated with Specific Sports and Special Populations, a Glossary, and a Directory of Additional Resources

Edited by Joyce Brennfleck Shannon. 614 pages. 2002. 0-7808-0604-2.

"This is an excellent reference for consumers and it is recommended for public, community college, and undergraduate libraries."
— American Reference Books Annual, 2003

"Recommended reference source."
— Booklist, American Library Association, Feb '03

■

Stress-Related Disorders Sourcebook

Basic Consumer Health Information about Stress and Stress-Related Disorders, Including Stress Origins and Signals, Environmental Stress at Work and Home, Mental and Emotional Stress Associated with Depression, Post-Traumatic Stress Disorder, Panic Disorder, Suicide, and the Physical Effects of Stress on the Cardiovascular, Immune, and Nervous Systems

Along with Stress Management Techniques, a Glossary, and a Listing of Additional Resources

Edited by Joyce Brennfleck Shannon. 610 pages. 2002. 0-7808-0560-7.

"Well written for a general readership, the *Stress-Related Disorders Sourcebook* is a useful addition to the health reference literature."
— *American Reference Books Annual, 2003*

"I am impressed by the amount of information. It offers a thorough overview of the causes and consequences of stress for the layperson. . . . A well-done and thorough reference guide for professionals and nonprofessionals alike." — *Doody's Review Service, Dec '02*

Stroke Sourcebook

Basic Consumer Health Information about Stroke, Including Ischemic, Hemorrhagic, Transient Ischemic Attack (TIA), and Pediatric Stroke, Stroke Triggers and Risks, Diagnostic Tests, Treatments, and Rehabilitation Information

Along with Stroke Prevention Guidelines, Legal and Financial Information, a Glossary, and a Directory of Additional Resources

Edited by Joyce Brennfleck Shannon. 606 pages. 2003. 0-7808-0630-1.

"This volume is highly recommended and should be in every medical, hospital, and public library."
— *American Reference Books Annual, 2004*

"Highly recommended for the amount and variety of topics and information covered." — *Choice, Nov '03*

Substance Abuse Sourcebook

Basic Health-Related Information about the Abuse of Legal and Illegal Substances Such as Alcohol, Tobacco, Prescription Drugs, Marijuana, Cocaine, and Heroin; and Including Facts about Substance Abuse Prevention Strategies, Intervention Methods, Treatment and Recovery Programs, and a Section Addressing the Special Problems Related to Substance Abuse during Pregnancy

Edited by Karen Bellenir. 573 pages. 1996. 0-7808-0038-9.

"A valuable addition to any health reference section. Highly recommended."
— *The Book Report, Mar/Apr '97*

". . . a comprehensive collection of substance abuse information that's both highly readable and compact. Families and caregivers of substance abusers will find the information enlightening and helpful, while teachers, social workers and journalists should benefit from the concise format. Recommended."
— *Drug Abuse Update, Winter '96/'97*

SEE ALSO *Alcoholism Sourcebook, Drug Abuse Sourcebook*

Surgery Sourcebook

Basic Consumer Health Information about Inpatient and Outpatient Surgeries, Including Cardiac, Vascular, Orthopedic, Ocular, Reconstructive, Cosmetic, Gynecologic, and Ear, Nose, and Throat Procedures and More

Along with Information about Operating Room Policies and Instruments, Laser Surgery Techniques, Hospital Errors, Statistical Data, a Glossary, and Listings of Sources for Further Help and Information

Edited by Annemarie S. Muth and Karen Bellenir. 596 pages. 2002. 0-7808-0380-9.

"Large public libraries and medical libraries would benefit from this material in their reference collections."
— *American Reference Books Annual, 2004*

"Invaluable reference for public and school library collections alike." — *Library Bookwatch, Apr '03*

Thyroid Disorders Sourcebook

Basic Consumer Health Information about Disorders of the Thyroid and Parathyroid Glands, Including Hypothyroidism, Hyperthyroidism, Graves Disease, Hashimoto Thyroiditis, Thyroid Cancer, and Parathyroid Disorders, Featuring Facts about Symptoms, Risk Factors, Tests, and Treatments

Along with Information about the Effects of Thyroid Imbalance on Other Body Systems, Environmental Factors That Affect the Thyroid Gland, a Glossary, and a Directory of Additional Resources

Edited by Joyce Brennfleck Shannon. 599 pages. 2005. 0-7808-0745-6.

"Recommended for consumer health collections."
— *American Reference Books Annual, 2006*

"Highly recommended pick for basic consumer health reference holdings at all levels."
— *The Bookwatch, Aug '05*

Transplantation Sourcebook

Basic Consumer Health Information about Organ and Tissue Transplantation, Including Physical and Financial Preparations, Procedures and Issues Relating to Specific Solid Organ and Tissue Transplants, Rehabilitation, Pediatric Transplant Information, the Future of Transplantation, and Organ and Tissue Donation

Along with a Glossary and Listings of Additional Resources

Edited by Joyce Brennfleck Shannon. 628 pages. 2002. 0-7808-0322-1.

"Along with these advances [in transplantation technology] have come a number of daunting questions for potential transplant patients, their families, and their health care providers. This reference text is the best single tool to address many of these questions. . . . It will be a much-needed addition to the reference collections in health care, academic, and large public libraries."
— *American Reference Books Annual, 2003*

"Recommended for libraries with an interest in offering consumer health information." — *E-Streams, Jul '02*

"This is a unique and valuable resource for patients facing transplantation and their families."
— *Doody's Review Service, Jun '02*

Traveler's Health Sourcebook

Basic Consumer Health Information for Travelers, Including Physical and Medical Preparations, Transportation Health and Safety, Essential Information about Food and Water, Sun Exposure, Insect and Snake Bites, Camping and Wilderness Medicine, and Travel with Physical or Medical Disabilities

Along with International Travel Tips, Vaccination Recommendations, Geographical Health Issues, Disease Risks, a Glossary, and a Listing of Additional Resources

Edited by Joyce Brennfleck Shannon. 613 pages. 2000. 0-7808-0384-1.

"Recommended reference source."
— *Booklist, American Library Association, Feb '01*

"This book is recommended for any public library, any travel collection, and especially any collection for the physically disabled."
— *American Reference Books Annual, 2001*

SEE ALSO Worldwide Health Sourcebook

Urinary Tract & Kidney Diseases & Disorders Sourcebook, 2nd Edition

Basic Consumer Health Information about the Urinary System, Including the Bladder, Urethra, Ureters, and Kidneys, with Facts about Urinary Tract Infections, Incontinence, Congenital Disorders, Kidney Stones, Cancers of the Urinary Tract and Kidneys, Kidney Failure, Dialysis, and Kidney Transplantation

Along with Statistical and Demographic Information, Reports on Current Research in Kidney and Urologic Health, a Summary of Commonly Used Diagnostic Tests, a Glossary of Related Terms, and a Directory of Resources for Additional Help and Information

Edited by Ivy L. Alexander. 649 pages. 2005. 0-7808-0750-2.

"A good choice for a consumer health information library or for a medical library needing information to refer to their patients."
— *American Reference Books Annual, 2006*

Vegetarian Sourcebook

Basic Consumer Health Information about Vegetarian Diets, Lifestyle, and Philosophy, Including Definitions of Vegetarianism and Veganism, Tips about Adopting Vegetarianism, Creating a Vegetarian Pantry, and Meeting Nutritional Needs of Vegetarians, with Facts Regarding Vegetarianism's Effect on Pregnant and Lactating Women, Children, Athletes, and Senior Citizens

Along with a Glossary of Commonly Used Vegetarian Terms and Resources for Additional Help and Information

Edited by Chad T. Kimball. 360 pages. 2002. 0-7808-0439-2.

"Organizes into one concise volume the answers to the most common questions concerning vegetarian diets and lifestyles. This title is recommended for public and secondary school libraries." — *E-Streams, Apr '03*

"Invaluable reference for public and school library collections alike." — *Library Bookwatch, Apr '03*

"The articles in this volume are easy to read and come from authoritative sources. The book does not necessarily support the vegetarian diet but instead provides the pros and cons of this important decision. The Vegetarian Sourcebook is recommended for public libraries and consumer health libraries."
— *American Reference Books Annual, 2003*

SEE ALSO Diet & Nutrition Sourcebook

Women's Health Concerns Sourcebook, 2nd Edition

Basic Consumer Health Information about the Medical and Mental Concerns of Women, Including Maintaining Health and Wellness, Gynecological Concerns, Breast Health, Sexuality and Reproductive Issues, Menopause, Cancer in Women, Leading Causes of Death and Disability among Women, Physical Concerns of Special Significance to Women, and Women's Mental and Emotional Health

Along with a Glossary of Related Terms and Directories of Resources for Additional Help and Information

Edited by Amy L. Sutton. 746 pages. 2004. 0-7808-0673-5.

"This is a useful reference book, which makes the reader knowledgeable about several issues that concern women's health. It is recommended for public libraries and home library collections." — *E-Streams, May '05*

"A useful addition to public and consumer health library collections."
— *American Reference Books Annual, 2005*

"A highly recommended title."
— *The Bookwatch, May '04*

"Handy compilation. There is an impressive range of diseases, devices, disorders, procedures, and other physical and emotional issues covered . . . well organized, illustrated, and indexed." — *Choice, Association of College & Research Libraries, Jan '98*

SEE ALSO Breast Cancer Sourcebook, Cancer Sourcebook for Women, Healthy Heart Sourcebook for Women, Osteoporosis Sourcebook

Workplace Health & Safety Sourcebook

Basic Consumer Health Information about Workplace Health and Safety, Including the Effect of Workplace Hazards on the Lungs, Skin, Heart, Ears, Eyes, Brain, Reproductive Organs, Musculoskeletal System, and Other Organs and Body Parts

Along with Information about Occupational Cancer, Personal Protective Equipment, Toxic and Hazardous Chemicals, Child Labor, Stress, and Workplace Violence

Edited by Chad T. Kimball. 626 pages. 2000. 0-7808-0231-4.

"As a reference for the general public, this would be useful in any library." — *E-Streams, Jun '01*

"Provides helpful information for primary care physicians and other caregivers interested in occupational medicine. . . . General readers; professionals."
— *Choice, Association of College & Research Libraries, May '01*

"Recommended reference source."
— *Booklist, American Library Association, Feb '01*

"Highly recommended." — *The Bookwatch, Jan '01*

■

Worldwide Health Sourcebook

Basic Information about Global Health Issues, Including Malnutrition, Reproductive Health, Disease Dispersion and Prevention, Emerging Diseases, Risky Health Behaviors, and the Leading Causes of Death

Along with Global Health Concerns for Children, Women, and the Elderly, Mental Health Issues, Research and Technology Advancements, and Economic, Environmental, and Political Health Implications, a Glossary, and a Resource Listing for Additional Help and Information

Edited by Joyce Brennfleck Shannon. 614 pages. 2001. 0-7808-0330-2.

"Named an Outstanding Academic Title."
— *Choice, Association of College & Research Libraries, Jan '02*

"Yet another handy but also unique compilation in the extensive Health Reference Series, this is a useful work because many of the international publications reprinted or excerpted are not readily available. Highly recommended." — *Choice, Association of College & Research Libraries, Nov '01*

"Recommended reference source."
— *Booklist, American Library Association, Oct '01*

SEE ALSO Traveler's Health Sourcebook

650

Teen Health Series
Helping Young Adults Understand, Manage, and Avoid Serious Illness

List price $65 per volume. **School and library price $58 per volume.**

Alcohol Information for Teens
Health Tips about Alcohol and Alcoholism
Including Facts about Underage Drinking, Preventing Teen Alcohol Use, Alcohol's Effects on the Brain and the Body, Alcohol Abuse Treatment, Help for Children of Alcoholics, and More

Edited by Joyce Brennfleck Shannon. 370 pages. 2005. 0-7808-0741-3.

"Boxed facts and tips add visual interest to the well-researched and clearly written text."
— *Curriculum Connection, Apr '06*

Allergy Information for Teens
Health Tips about Allergic Reactions Such as Anaphylaxis, Respiratory Problems, and Rashes
Including Facts about Identifying and Managing Allergies to Food, Pollen, Mold, Animals, Chemicals, Drugs, and Other Substances

Edited by Karen Bellenir. 410 pages. 2006. 0-7808-0799-5.

Asthma Information for Teens
Health Tips about Managing Asthma and Related Concerns
Including Facts about Asthma Causes, Triggers, Symptoms, Diagnosis, and Treatment

Edited by Karen Bellenir. 386 pages. 2005. 0-7808-0770-7.

"Highly recommended for medical libraries, public school libraries, and public libraries."
— *American Reference Books Annual, 2006*

"It is so clearly written and well organized that even hesitant readers will be able to find the facts they need, whether for reports or personal information. . . . A succinct but complete resource."
— *School Library Journal, Sep '05*

Cancer Information for Teens
Health Tips about Cancer Awareness, Prevention, Diagnosis, and Treatment
Including Facts about Frequently Occurring Cancers, Cancer Risk Factors, and Coping Strategies for Teens Fighting Cancer or Dealing with Cancer in Friends or Family Members

Edited by Wilma R. Caldwell. 428 pages. 2004. 0-7808-0678-6.

"Recommended for school libraries, or consumer libraries that see a lot of use by teens."
— *E-Streams, May 2005*

"A valuable educational tool."
— *American Reference Books Annual, 2005*

"Young adults and their parents alike will find this new addition to the *Teen Health Series* an important reference to cancer in teens."
— *Children's Bookwatch, Feb '05*

Diabetes Information for Teens
Health Tips about Managing Diabetes and Preventing Related Complications
Including Information about Insulin, Glucose Control, Healthy Eating, Physical Activity, and Learning to Live with Diabetes

Edited by Sandra Augustyn Lawton. 410 pages. 2006. 0-7808-0811-8.

Diet Information for Teens, 2nd Edition
Health Tips about Diet and Nutrition
Including Facts about Dietary Guidelines, Food Groups, Nutrients, Healthy Meals, Snacks, Weight Control, Medical Concerns Related to Diet, and More

Edited by Karen Bellenir. 432 pages. 2006. 0-7808-0820-7.

"Full of helpful insights and facts throughout the book. . . . An excellent resource to be placed in public libraries or even in personal collections."
— *American Reference Books Annual, 2002*

"Recommended for middle and high school libraries and media centers as well as academic libraries that educate future teachers of teenagers. It is also a suitable addition to health science libraries that serve patrons who are interested in teen health promotion and education."
— *E-Streams, Oct '01*

"This comprehensive book would be beneficial to collections that need information about nutrition, dietary guidelines, meal planning, and weight control. . . . This reference is so easy to use that its purchase is recommended."
— *The Book Report, Sep-Oct '01*

651

"This book is written in an easy to understand format describing issues that many teens face every day, and then provides thoughtful explanations so that teens can make informed decisions. This is an interesting book that provides important facts and information for today's teens." — *Doody's Health Sciences Book Review Journal, Jul-Aug '01*

"A comprehensive compendium of diet and nutrition. The information is presented in a straightforward, plain-spoken manner. This title will be useful to those working on reports on a variety of topics, as well as to general readers concerned about their dietary health." — *School Library Journal, Jun '01*

■

Drug Information for Teens, 2nd Edition

Health Tips about the Physical and Mental Effects of Substance Abuse

Including Information about Marijuana, Inhalants, Club Drugs, Stimulants, Hallucinogens, Opiates, Prescription and Over-the-Counter Drugs, Herbal Products, Tobacco, Alcohol, and More

Edited by Sandra Augustyn Lawton. 468 pages. 2006. 0-7808-0862-2.

"A clearly written resource for general readers and researchers alike." — *School Library Journal*

"This book is well-balanced. . . . a must for public and school libraries." — *VOYA: Voice of Youth Advocates, Dec '03*

"The chapters are quick to make a connection to their teenage reading audience. The prose is straightforward and the book lends itself to spot reading. It should be useful both for practical information and for research, and it is suitable for public and school libraries." — *American Reference Books Annual, 2003*

"Recommended reference source." — *Booklist, American Library Association, Feb '03*

"This is an excellent resource for teens and their parents. Education about drugs and substances is key to discouraging teen drug abuse and this book provides this much needed information in a way that is interesting and factual." — *Doody's Review Service, Dec '02*

■

Eating Disorders Information for Teens

Health Tips about Anorexia, Bulimia, Binge Eating, and Other Eating Disorders

Including Information on the Causes, Prevention, and Treatment of Eating Disorders, and Such Other Issues as Maintaining Healthy Eating and Exercise Habits

Edited by Sandra Augustyn Lawton. 337 pages. 2005. 0-7808-0783-9.

"An excellent resource for teens and those who work with them." — *VOYA: Voice of Youth Advocates, Apr '06*

"A welcome addition to high school and undergraduate libraries." — *American Reference Books Annual, 2006*

"This book covers the topic in a lucid manner but delves deeper into every aspect of an eating disorder. A solid addition for any nonfiction or reference collection." — *School Library Journal, Dec '05*

■

Fitness Information for Teens

Health Tips about Exercise, Physical Well-Being, and Health Maintenance

Including Facts about Aerobic and Anaerobic Conditioning, Stretching, Body Shape and Body Image, Sports Training, Nutrition, and Activities for Non-Athletes

Edited by Karen Bellenir. 425 pages. 2004. 0-7808-0679-4.

"Another excellent offering from Omnigraphics in their *Teen Health Series*. . . . This book will be a great addition to any public, junior high, senior high, or secondary school library." — *American Reference Books Annual, 2005*

■

Learning Disabilities Information for Teens

Health Tips about Academic Skills Disorders and Other Disabilities That Affect Learning

Including Information about Common Signs of Learning Disabilities, School Issues, Learning to Live with a Learning Disability, and Other Related Issues

Edited by Sandra Augustyn Lawton. 337 pages. 2005. 0-7808-0796-0.

"This book provides a wealth of information for any reader interested in the signs, causes, and consequences of learning disabilities, as well as related legal rights and educational interventions. . . . Public and academic libraries should want this title for both students and general readers." — *American Reference Books Annual, 2006*

■

Mental Health Information for Teens, 2nd Edition

Health Tips about Mental Wellness and Mental Illness

Including Facts about Mental and Emotional Health, Depression and Other Mood Disorders, Anxiety Disorders, Behavior Disorders, Self-Injury, Psychosis, Schizophrenia, and More

Edited by Karen Bellenir. 400 pages. 2006. 0-7808-0863-0.

"In both language and approach, this user-friendly entry in the *Teen Health Series* is on target for teens needing information on mental health concerns." — *Booklist, American Library Association, Jan '02*

"Readers will find the material accessible and informative, with the shaded notes, facts, and embedded glossary insets adding appropriately to the already interesting and succinct presentation."

— School Library Journal, Jan '02

"This title is highly recommended for any library that serves adolescents and parents/caregivers of adolescents." — E-Streams, Jan '02

"Recommended for high school libraries and young adult collections in public libraries. Both health professionals and teenagers will find this book useful." — American Reference Books Annual, 2002

"This is a nice book written to enlighten the society, primarily teenagers, about common teen mental health issues. It is highly recommended to teachers and parents as well as adolescents." — Doody's Review Service, Dec '01

Sexual Health Information for Teens

Health Tips about Sexual Development, Human Reproduction, and Sexually Transmitted Diseases

Including Facts about Puberty, Reproductive Health, Chlamydia, Human Papillomavirus, Pelvic Inflammatory Disease, Herpes, AIDS, Contraception, Pregnancy, and More

Edited by Deborah A. Stanley. 391 pages. 2003. 0-7808-0445-7.

"This work should be included in all high school libraries and many larger public libraries. . . . highly recommended." — American Reference Books Annual, 2004

"Sexual Health approaches its subject with appropriate seriousness and offers easily accessible advice and information." — School Library Journal, Feb '04

Skin Health Information for Teens

Health Tips about Dermatological Concerns and Skin Cancer Risks

Including Facts about Acne, Warts, Hives, and Other Conditions and Lifestyle Choices, Such as Tanning, Tattooing, and Piercing, That Affect the Skin, Nails, Scalp, and Hair

Edited by Robert Aquinas McNally. 429 pages. 2003. 0-7808-0446-5.

"This volume, as with others in the series, will be a useful addition to school and public library collections." — American Reference Books Annual, 2004

"There is no doubt that this reference tool is valuable." — VOYA: Voice of Youth Advocates, Feb '04

"This volume serves as a one-stop source and should be a necessity for any health collection." — Library Media Connection

Sports Injuries Information for Teens

Health Tips about Sports Injuries and Injury Protection

Including Facts about Specific Injuries, Emergency Treatment, Rehabilitation, Sports Safety, Competition Stress, Fitness, Sports Nutrition, Steroid Risks, and More

Edited by Joyce Brennfleck Shannon. 405 pages. 2003. 0-7808-0447-3.

"This work will be useful in the young adult collections of public libraries as well as high school libraries." — American Reference Books Annual, 2004

Suicide Information for Teens

Health Tips about Suicide Causes and Prevention

Including Facts about Depression, Risk Factors, Getting Help, Survivor Support, and More

Edited by Joyce Brennfleck Shannon. 368 pages. 2005. 0-7808-0737-5.